MW01108998

Nursing
TimeSavers

Respiratory
Disorders

Nursing
TimeSavers

Respiratory Disorders

Springhouse Corporation
Springhouse, Pennsylvania

Staff

Executive Director, Editorial
Stanley Loeb

Senior Publisher
Matthew Cahill

Art Director
John Hubbard

Clinical Manager
Cindy Tryniszewski, RN, MSN

Senior Editor
Michael Shaw

Clinical Editor
Mary Chapman Gyetvan, RN, MSN

Editors
J. Allen Canale, Peter Dechnik, Traci A.
Ginnona, Judd L. Howard, Ann Lenkiewicz,
Carol H. Munson, Art Ofner, Pat Wittig

Copy Editors
Cynthia C. Breuninger (supervisor), Pris-
cilla DeWitt, Nancy Papsin, Jennifer
George Mintzer, Doris Weinstock

Designers
Stephanie Peters (associate art director),
Matie Patterson (senior designer), Kaa-
ren Mitchel, Amy Smith

Illustrators
Kevin Curry, Jacalyn Facciolo, Dan
Fione, Robert Neumann, Judy Newhouse

Manufacturing
Deborah Meiris (director), Pat Dorshaw
(manager), Anna Brindisi, Kate Davis,
T.A. Landis

Production Coordination
Patricia McCloskey

Editorial Assistants
Maree DeRosa, Beverly Lane, Mary Madden

Indexer
Barbara Hodgson

Library of Congress Cataloging-in-Publication Data
Respiratory disorders.
    p. cm. — (Nursing timesavers)
    Includes bibliographical references and
index.
    1. Respiratory system — Diseases —
Nursing   I. Springhouse Corporation. II. Series.
    [DNLM: 1. Nursing Care — methods.
    2. Respiratory Tract Diseases — nursing.
    3. Nursing Process. WY 163 C886r 1993]
RC735.5.C73   1993
610.73'692 — dc20
DNLM/DLC   93-34657
ISBN: 0-87434-657-6   CIP

Contents

Contributors and consultants

Contributors

Kathy Craig, RN, BA
Nurse Consultant
Collegeville, Pa.

Sandra M. Nettina, RN,C, MSN, CRNP
Adult Nurse Practitioner
Mercy Primary Care Group
Baltimore

Consultants

David J. Blanchard, RPh, BS
Pharmacist Specialist
Mary Imogene Basset Hospital
Cooperstown, N.Y.

Janice M. Boutotte, RN, MS, CS
Director of Epidemiology, Case Management and Prevention Services
Division of Tuberculosis Control
Massachusetts Department of Public Health
Jamaica Plain, Mass.

Vicki Buchda, RN, MS
Director, Special Care Unit
Maryvale Samaritan Medical Center
Phoenix, Ariz.

Joan T. Granberry, RN, BS, CCRN
Clinical Nurse III
St. Francis Medical Center
Trenton, N.J.

Nancy L. Kranzley, RN, MS
Pulmonary Clinical Nurse Specialist
The Christ Hospital
Cincinnati

Karen Landis, RN, MS, CCRN
Pulmonary Clinical Nurse Specialist
Lehigh Valley Hospital
Allentown, Pa.

Virginia R. Martin, RN, MSN, OCN
Clinical Manager, Ambulatory Care
Fox Chase Cancer Center
Philadelphia

Steven B. Meisel, PharmD
Assistant Director of Pharmacy
Fairview Southdale Hospital
Minneapolis

Marcella Majors Moreno, RN, MSN
Cardiopulmonary Rehabilitation Nurse Specialist
St. Francis–St. George Hospital
Cincinnati

Ann Smith, RN, MSN, CCRN
Clinical Nurse Specialist, Surgical ICU
Thomas Jefferson University Hospital
Philadelphia

Donald St. Onge, RN, MSN
Pulmonary Clinical Nurse Specialist
Allegheny General Hospital
Pittsburgh

Barbara J. Taptich, RN, MA
Director, Heart Institute
St. Francis Medical Center
Trenton, N.J.

Kathy M. Witta, RN, MSN, CS
Pulmonary Clinical Nurse Specialist and Practitioner
Pulmonary Associates
Newark, Del.
Staff Nurse, Intermediate Medical Care Unit
Hospital of the University of Pennsylvania
Philadelphia

Foreword

Today, no matter where you work, respiratory care requires a wide range of clinical skills. Consider, for a moment, just a fraction of your responsibility:

• recognizing early signs of adult respiratory distress syndrome (ARDS) and providing emergency care

• teaching the patient with chronic obstructive pulmonary disease (COPD) how to improve his quality of life

• monitoring the postoperative patient for such respiratory complications as pneumonia, atelectasis, and pulmonary embolism

• recognizing the patient at risk for tuberculosis, a lung infection reemerging at an alarming rate, with many drug-resistant strains

• interpreting arterial blood gas (ABG) studies to detect crucial changes in respiratory status.

Obviously, the roster of your responsibilities could continue from here. But underlying all of them is a requirement for accuracy, efficiency, and speed brought on by increased patient acuity and shortened hospital stays.

To help you meet this requirement, you need a reliable, up-to-date reference that doesn't waste words or your time. Fortunately, *Respiratory Disorders,* the latest book in the Nursing TimeSavers series, addresses your needs. Concise and easy-to-use, this handbook was developed by nursing professionals — all with years of bedside know-how — who understand the professional demands and time constraints you deal with every day.

Chapter 1 explains how to use the nursing process to provide expert respiratory care. You'll learn how the nursing process can help you identify patient problems, develop a plan of care, set outcomes for the patient, determine the necessary interventions, and evaluate whether outcomes have been achieved. You'll also find concise coverage of key nursing diagnoses encountered in respiratory care.

Chapter 2 provides guidelines for assessing your patient's chief complaint. For instance, if your patient says, "I feel like I can't breathe" or "I coughed up lots of blood this morning," turn to this chapter for a list of questions to ask and assessment techniques to perform. This chapter also covers the four primary signs and symptoms of respiratory dysfunction — dyspnea, cough, chest pain, and hemoptysis — as well as other key chief complaints.

In Chapter 3, you'll find detailed instructions for monitoring your patient's condition and response to interventions. This chapter gives you guidelines for interpreting ABG studies and for performing and interpreting mixed venous oxygen saturation monitoring, pulse oximetry, bedside pulmonary function testing, and apnea monitoring.

Chapters 4 through 10 cover the most frequently encountered respiratory disorders: ARDS, pneumonia, COPD, lung cancer, and many others. To save you time, you'll find that each disorder is organized according to the nursing process with five easy-to-spot headings:

• *Assessment.* This section tells you what health history data, physical examination findings, and diagnostic test results to expect.

• *Nursing diagnosis.* In this section, you'll find the most common nursing diagnoses and related etiologies for each disorder.

- *Planning.* This section identifies patient outcomes for each nursing diagnosis. This feature will ensure that your documentation includes accurate outcome statements.
- *Implementation.* In this section, you'll find complete, step-by-step nursing interventions as well as guidelines for patient teaching.
- *Evaluation.* This section gives the criteria for judging the effectiveness of your nursing care and your patient's progress toward meeting documented outcomes.

Throughout the book, you'll see special graphic devices called logos that direct you to important information and timesaving ideas. The *FactFinder* logo, for instance, highlights key points about a disorder, covering such topics as risk factors, demographics, and prognosis. The *Timesaving tip* logo alerts you to ways to save time as you proceed with your nursing care. The *Assessment TimeSaver* logo helps you organize and expedite the initial step of the nursing process. The *Treatments* logo summarizes the latest medical therapies for each disorder. The *Teaching TimeSaver* logo provides suggestions and guidelines for teaching patients. And the *Discharge TimeSaver* logo signals a checklist of teaching topics, referrals, and follow-up appointments to promote your patient's well-being after hospitalization.

Additionally, *Respiratory Disorders* includes helpful appendices on common respiratory treatments and drugs. The first appendix, on respiratory treatments, covers current procedures for managing respiratory disorders, complete with concise descriptions, indications, and complications. The second appendix, on common respiratory drugs, includes generic and trade names, indications and adult dosages, and adverse reactions. Common and life-threatening adverse reactions are clearly marked.

By providing up-to-date clinical information in a focused, quick-reference format, *Respiratory Disorders* can save you time and help you provide better care for your respiratory patients. Become familiar with this tool and use it at home or at work. A better understanding of respiratory care enhances your confidence — and thereby increases your chances for success — no matter where you practice nursing.

Karen Landis, RN, MS, CCRN
Pulmonary Clinical Nurse Specialist
Lehigh Valley Hospital
Allentown, Pa.

CHAPTER

1

Applying the nursing process to respiratory care

Because of the prevalence of and high mortality from severe acute and chronic respiratory disorders, such as asthma, chronic obstructive pulmonary disease (COPD), cystic fibrosis, and acute airway obstruction, nurses in almost any setting must be able to assess respiratory status, formulate nursing diagnoses, create a plan of care, and intervene effectively. (See *Key points about respiratory disorders.*) In addition, you must educate the patient and members of the family about the disorder and its management. This is especially important if long-term home care is needed. To accomplish all these tasks during the short course of the patient's hospitalization, your care must be efficient and well-organized. By using the nursing process, you can provide expert respiratory care while saving time. You'll use the nursing process to:

• identify patient problems you can treat

• identify patient problems you can help to prevent

• select goals for the patient and determine whether they've been achieved

• develop a plan of care that addresses the patient's actual and potential problems

• determine what kind of assistance the patient needs and who can best provide it

• accurately document your contribution to achieving patient outcomes.

The five steps of the nursing process — assessment, nursing diagnosis, planning, implementation, and evaluation — help you address specific patient needs in an orderly and timely way. Keep in mind, however, that these steps are dynamic and flexible and often overlap.

Assessment

The first step in the nursing process, assessment, is crucial. The quality of data gathered during assessment will affect all subsequent steps in the nursing process. Assessment usually includes taking a health history, performing a physical examination, and reviewing the results of diagnostic tests.

Any patient can develop respiratory complications, regardless of his primary problem. His respiratory status may be compromised by changes in any body system that influence:

• *ventilation*—movement of air in and out of the lungs

• *diffusion*—passive movement of oxygen and carbon dioxide across the alveolocapillary membrane between the lungs and the bloodstream

• *perfusion*—circulation to the lungs and transport of oxygen and carbon dioxide in the blood

• *breathing regulation*—neuromuscular and chemical regulation of air movement.

You can evaluate both subtle and obvious respiratory changes by performing a thorough respiratory assessment.

Timesaving tip: Although a comprehensive assessment is ideal, you may need to assess your patient quickly. When performing a rapid assessment, try to identify the most important clues to your patient's respiratory problem. Let the patient's condition be your guide. For example, if your patient is admitted with pneumonia and has rapid, shallow respirations, central cyanosis, and copious amounts of sputum, provide oxygen and perform a brief, focused assessment. Ask only pertinent questions and phrase them so the patient can nod or give one-word answers. Limit the physical examination to vital signs, general appearance, and an assessment of cardio-pulmonary status. You can perform a more extensive assessment when the patient's condition improves.

For patients experiencing breathing difficulties, anxiety is a common emotion. To calm the patient, ensure privacy and assume a gentle, confident manner. Identify yourself by name as well as professional title. Speak in a conversational tone to put the patient at ease and to encourage him to share information. However, if the patient is acutely ill, be prepared to provide emergency interventions. (See *Quick assessment in a respiratory emergency,* page 4.)

Health history

The health history allows you to explore the patient's chief complaint and its relationship to other symptoms, assess the impact of the illness on the patient and his family, and begin to develop and implement a plan of care. Health history information also helps guide medical diagnosis and subsequent treatment.

When taking the health history, use a systematic approach to avoid overlooking important clues. Be sensitive to the patient's concerns and feelings, and encourage him to formulate his own responses. Be alert for nonverbal signs that seem to contradict verbal responses. For example, the patient may say that he is not short of breath and yet exhibit signs of breathing difficulties, such as nasal flaring and frequent pauses for breath. Explore these apparent contradictions.

Chief complaint

Begin the health history interview by asking about the patient's chief complaint. Chest pain and dyspnea are the two most commonly reported chief complaints for the patient with a respiratory disorder. Other signs and symptoms include cough (either productive

FactFinder
Key points about respiratory disorders

In North America, more than 17 million people have some form of chronic respiratory disease.

Disorders
• Chronic obstructive pulmonary disease, which represents the fifth leading cause of death in the North America, affects about 10 million Americans, with highest morbidity among older men. At least 80%•of these cases result from smoking.
• Asthma, the most common chronic disease of childhood, affects about 7 million Americans. In the last 10 years, the number of patients under age 18 with asthma has increased over 60%.
• Cystic fibrosis, a hereditary disorder, is the most common cause of chronic lung disease in children and young adults.

Causes
• Smoking represents the most common cause of lung cancer and chronic respiratory disorders.
• Industrial pollutants, which can result in occupational lung disease, are also a leading cause of lung disorders. Major occupational lung disorders include silicosis, coal worker's pneumoconiosis, and asbestosis.

or nonproductive), cyanosis, hemoptysis, chills, fever, wheezing, and increased mucus production. If the patient has trouble identifying a single complaint ask, "What made you seek medical care today?" Then let the patient describe his problem in his own words. Record his response verbatim whenever possible. Ask him to describe the onset, location, frequency, and duration of the chief complaint.

Quick assessment in a respiratory emergency

Acute respiratory distress poses an imminent risk of organ damage or death. In a respiratory emergency, you'll need to quickly assess the patient and adapt your skills to meet the demands of the developing emergency. Use the following list as a guide.

Assessing airway, breathing, and circulation (ABCs)
• Is the patient's airway open?
• Is he breathing?
• Does the patient have a pulse?
If these signs are absent, call for help and initiate cardiopulmonary resuscitation.

Observing for danger signs
Look for the following indications of respiratory emergency:
• breathing difficulties, such as tachypnea, labored breathing, or audible breathing (wheezing, stridor, gurgling)
• use of accessory muscles to assist breathing (chest excursion of less than 3″ to 6″ [7.5 to 15 cm], shoulder elevation, intercostal muscle retraction, use of scalene and sternocleidomastoid muscles)
• diminished level of consciousness
• confusion, anxiety, or agitation
• frequent position changes to make breathing easier

• pale, diaphoretic, dusky, or cyanotic skin.

Maximizing your effectiveness
• Adapt your assessment to the patient's condition, available resources, and your level of knowledge and skill.
• Assess ABCs first, and then progress to less vital criteria.
• Focus on gathering data that help define the immediate problem. Trust your clinical impression.
• Don't assume. Record positive and negative findings and then use groups of findings to support your choice of interventions.
• After the crisis passes, reevaluate the patient to determine if interventions were adequate and appropriate.
  During an emergency, increase your efficiency by working closely with other staff members. For example, you can take a quick health history while another nurse begins an appropriate intervention.

Consider asking the following questions:
• When did the symptom first occur?
• Did it appear suddenly or gradually?
• How often does it occur?
• How long does it last?
• Does the symptom change over time (become more or less severe) or does it remain constant?
  Next, ask the patient to characterize precipitating, aggravating, and alleviating factors, such as exercise, changes in position, environmental conditions, or medications, that have an effect on

his chief complaint. Also ask the patient if he has noticed any associated signs and symptoms, such as sore throat, congestion, noisy or shallow respirations, hoarseness, gagging or choking, chest tightness with breathing, or pain and discomfort.

Timesaving tip: If your patient is experiencing pain or discomfort, have him rate the intensity on a scale of 1 to 10. Record his response. This scale helps you understand the patient's perception of the current problem and provides a basis for assessing prior and subsequent episodes.

Avoid asking leading questions during the interview. However, encourage the patient to give complete, precise answers. For instance, a response of "2 or 3 times an hour" reveals more about the frequency of a symptom than "off and on all day." For further information, see Chapter 2, Assessing chief complaints.

Past illnesses
Find out if the patient has any disorder that can affect the respiratory system or influence his recovery. Consider asking the following questions:
• Have you ever had asthma or emphysema?
• As a child, did you have infantile eczema, atopic dermatitis, or allergic rhinitis?
• Do you have any allergies?
• Have you received influenza or pneumococcal vaccinations?
• Have you received treatment for chronic sinus infection, recurrent bronchitis, or repeated episodes of pneumonia?
• Have you been diagnosed as having sarcoidosis, diabetes mellitus, or heart failure?
• Have you ever suffered a traumatic injury to the chest (such as a gunshot wound) or an injury that required surgery?
• What medications (prescription and nonprescription) are you taking at this time?

Family history
By taking a thorough family history, you can discover if your patient is at risk for hereditary or infectious respiratory disorders. Ask if any immediate relatives (parents, siblings, children) have cancer, sickle cell anemia, heart disease, diabetes, or a chronic illness, such as asthma, cystic fibrosis, or emphysema. If an immediate relative has one of these disorders, ask for information about the patient's maternal and paternal grandparents, aunts, and uncles. Ask the patient if anyone in his household or at work has an infectious disease, such as influenza or tuberculosis.

Lifestyle factors
When exploring the patient's lifestyle, look for factors that can influence the patient's disorder and his method of dealing with the problem.

Ask about the patient's daily activities, personal habits, diet, interpersonal relationships, mental status, occupational history, and work, community, and home environments. Consider asking the following questions:
• Do you smoke cigarettes? If so, when did you start and how many cigarettes do you smoke each day?
• Did you smoke in the past?
• Do you work with hazardous materials? If so, do you use protective devices while on the job?
• Does your job cause stress?
• Can you describe your eating habits? (Poor nutritional habits may increase the patient's risk of respiratory infection.)

Also, because the incidence of pulmonary disorders related to acquired immunodeficiency syndrome is increasing, you should ask about sexual practices, drug use, or other high-risk behaviors that may place the patient at risk.

Coping patterns
Assess the patient's stress management techniques and his ability to cope with respiratory illness. Consider asking the following questions:
• Has your illness caused you to make drastic alterations to your lifestyle?
• How have you coped with crises in the past?

Assessment TimeSaver

Respiratory examination checklist

Rely on your observation skills as you examine the patient's face, neck, skin, nails, and mucous membranes during the respiratory assessment. Also, measure the patient's vital signs. When you examine the thorax, you'll use all of your assessment skills — inspection, palpation, percussion, and auscultation. Follow this checklist to quickly determine important respiratory assessment findings.

General appearance
☐ age
☐ weight
☐ ease of breathing
☐ position

Vital signs
☐ temperature
☐ blood pressure
☐ pulse rate and rhythm
☐ respiratory rate and rhythm

Skin, nails, and mucous membranes
☐ color
☐ nail thickness and clubbing
☐ peripheral edema

Thorax
☐ structural deformities
☐ muscles of ventilation
☐ retractions
☐ symmetry
☐ costal angle
☐ tracheal position
☐ tenderness
☐ masses
☐ respiratory excursion
☐ tactile fremitus
☐ resonance
☐ diaphragmatic excursion
☐ breath sounds
☐ voice resonance

• Do you feel your current coping strategies are helping or hindering your progress?
• Are you having trouble coming to terms with your illness?

Use your assessment of the patient's coping patterns to determine his teaching needs. Does he understand his diagnosis? Is he willing to accept changes in his lifestyle? How important is good health to him? Is he willing to work to improve his health? If the patient isn't ready or willing to accept change, he's unlikely to respond to teaching.

Physical examination
Your next step is to perform a physical examination. Using a systematic sequence of assessment techniques will help ensure that you don't miss an important finding, even if you're rushed.

However, if your patient is acutely ill and requires emergency intervention, you'll need to remain flexible in your approach. (See *Respiratory examination checklist.*)

Before you begin, make sure that you have all the necessary equipment, including a stethoscope with a diaphragm and a bell, a felt-tip pen, a ruler, and a tape measure. Perform the physical examination in a quiet, well-lit room that ensures privacy. Adjust the thermostat, if necessary; cool temperatures may alter the patient's skin temperature and color, heart rate, and blood pressure.

Begin your assessment by observing the patient's general appearance. Then perform your examination, which includes measuring the patient's vital signs, observing his nail beds and skin, and assessing his face, neck, and chest.

General appearance

Look at the patient, noting his body type, overall health, and muscle composition. Is he well developed, well nourished, and alert? Does his appearance coincide with his given age? Also note his posture, gait, movements, and hygiene. Watch for nasal flaring, which may indicate respiratory distress (more commonly seen in infants).

Timesaving tip: Save time by making general observations about the patient's appearance as you take the health history. Then you need only confirm these observations quickly at the beginning of the physical examination.

Measure and record the patient's height and weight. These measurements will help guide treatment, determine medication dosages, and direct nutritional counseling. Also, cachectic and emaciated patients have a higher risk for respiratory infections than well-nourished patients.

Observe how easy or difficult the patient's breathing appears to be. How many words can he say with each breath? Observe the patient's posture as you speak with him. Patients often assume a tripod position (resting the elbows or arms on the knees, tables, or the arms of chairs) to ease breathing. If breathing seems difficult, explore the issue further during the chest examination.

Vital signs

The patient's vital signs — temperature, blood pressure, pulse rate, and respirations — provide baseline data for your respiratory assessment. Deviations from normal may signal changes in the patient's respiratory status.

Temperature

Take the patient's temperature. An elevation in body temperature often indicates infection. If the infection involves the lungs, it can impair the diffusion of gases between the lungs and the bloodstream. An increase in temperature also causes tissue metabolic rates to increase, resulting in an increased demand for oxygen. At temperatures above 100.6° F (38.1° C), the combination of impaired diffusion and increased oxygen demand stresses the body's ability to meet respiratory needs.

Make sure that you obtain an accurate reading. When using an oral thermometer, be aware that you may obtain a false-low reading if the patient has trouble keeping his lips closed, is receiving humidified oxygen, or is tachypneic (respirations greater than 20 breaths/minute). In these circumstances, use a rectal thermometer or a thermometer placed in the ear to ensure an accurate reading.

Blood pressure

Your patient's blood pressure may be normal, elevated, or depressed depending on his physical status and ability to compensate for existing respiratory difficulty. In acute respiratory distress, blood pressure is normal or slightly elevated initially as a compensatory mechanism; during decompensation, blood pressure falls.

Pulse rate

If your patient is experiencing hypoxemia (low blood oxygen level), his pulse rate may increase to 90 beats/minute in response to sympathetic stimulation. Other possible reasons for an elevated pulse rate include exertion, anxiety, and smoking.

An irregular pulse rate may reflect the presence of a cardiac arrhythmia, such as atrial fibrillation (common in patients with chronic respiratory problems), premature atrial contractions (a common response to hypoxia), or premature ventricular contractions. If you detect an irregular, thready, or weak pulse, assume that tissue and pulmonary perfusion has diminished.

Respiratory rate and pattern
Normal respiratory rates vary with age: For a resting adult, 20 respirations/minute or less is normal; for an active infant, up to 50 respirations/minute may be normal. To determine respiratory rate, count the number of respirations (inspiration and expiration) for 1 minute. If your patient has periodic or irregular breathing, monitor respirations for several minutes to ensure an accurate rate. Keep in mind that respiratory rate also changes in response to recent activity.

If your patient exhibits apnea, note the duration of the apneic periods. Note any other abnormal respiratory patterns, such as tachypnea or bradypnea. Alert the doctor if you suspect an alteration in the patient's breathing pattern. (See *Understanding respiratory patterns.*)

Assessing the skin and nails
Inspect the patient's skin for peripheral oxygenation. Cyanosis (a dusky or bluish skin tint) indicates a decrease in the amount of oxygen carried by arterial blood.

Distinguishing between central cyanosis and peripheral cyanosis is important. Central cyanosis results from hypoxemia and affects all organs. It may be caused by right-to-left cardiac shunting or a pulmonary disease. Central cyanosis may appear on the skin or mucous membranes of the mouth and lips or in other highly vascular areas, such as the earlobes, tip of the nose, or nail beds.

Peripheral cyanosis is caused by vasoconstriction, vascular occlusion, or reduced cardiac output. Peripheral cyanosis may appear on the earlobes, tip of the nose, nail beds, or fingertips. However, it does not affect mucous membranes.

If your patient has dark skin, you may find it difficult to detect central cyanosis. For these patients, inspect the oral mucous membranes and lips for a pale gray color, rather than the characteristic bluish tinge. Also, the patient's facial skin may appear pale gray or ashen.

Look for the presence of peripheral edema. Check the lower extremities of patients who can sit in a chair or walk. Check the lumbar area of the back in patients who are bedridden. Hypoxemia causes pulmonary vasoconstriction, which may result in right-sided heart failure (cor pulmonale) and peripheral edema. Low serum albumin levels due to poor nutrition may also cause peripheral edema.

Next, assess the patient's nail beds and toes for clubbing or abnormal enlargement. Clubbing is caused by chronic tissue hypoxia and is distinguished by nail thinning and an abnormal angle at the base of the nail on fingers and toes. (See *Recognizing clubbed fingers,* page 11.)

Assessing the thorax
Place the patient in semi-Fowlers position, if possible. Expose the patient's chest and observe which muscles of ventilation are used. Note the type and depth of respirations.

Look for signs that the patient is using accessory muscles during breathing. Normal breathing requires only the diaphragm and external intercostal muscles. Observe the sternocleidomastoid, scalene, and trapezius muscles in the patient's shoulders and neck to see if he's using these accessory muscles during inspiration. Hypertrophy of the accessory muscles may indicate that they are being used to ease breathing (especially in elderly patients). Be aware, however, that hypertrophy may be normal in well-conditioned athletes. Also, patients using accessory muscles often assume a tripod position (resting

Understanding respiratory patterns

Your patient's respiratory patterns provide you with important clues to his respiratory status and overall condition. Learn to recognize them.

Eupnea (normal)
The normal respiratory rate and rhythm is 12 to 20 breaths/minute for adults and teenagers, 20 to 30 breaths/minute for children ages 2 to 12, and 30 to 50 breaths/minute for infants. Occasional deep breaths occur 2 to 3/minute.

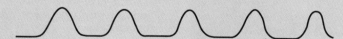

Tachypnea
This respiratory pattern is marked by an increased, regular rate of above 20 breaths/minute. If tachypnea occurs with fever, the rate increases by about 4 breaths/minute for each degree (Fahrenheit) above normal.

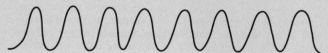

Bradypnea
Bradypnea refers to decreased, regular respirations of below 10 breaths/minute. This respiratory pattern is normal during sleep. Bradypnea may also occur with respiratory decompensation, metabolic disorders, or conditions that depress the brain's respiratory control center.

Hyperpnea
These deeper-than-normal respirations occur at a normal rate.

(continued)

Understanding respiratory patterns *(continued)*

Apnea
This respiratory pattern is marked by absent respirations. Apnea may be periodic and may occur with high-flow oxygen therapy.

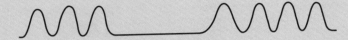

Biot's
These faster and deeper than normal respirations are marked by abrupt pauses and breaths of unequal depth. They may occur with spinal meningitis or other central nervous system conditions.

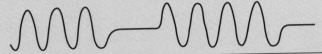

Cheyne-Stokes
In this respiratory pattern, faster and deeper than normal respirations are followed by slower respirations over a 30- to 170-second period. The pattern alternates with periods of apnea lasting 20 to 60 seconds.

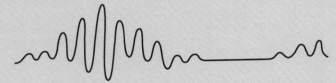

Kussmaul's
These respirations are faster and deeper than normal and continue without pause at over 20 breaths/minute in adults. Breathing sounds labored, with deep breaths that resemble sighs. This respiratory pattern may occur with renal failure or metabolic acidosis.

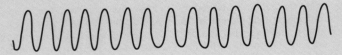

Recognizing clubbed fingers

To assess for chronic tissue hypoxia, check the patient's fingers for clubbing. Normally, the angle between the fingernail and the point where the nail enters the skin is about 160 degrees. Clubbing occurs when that angle increases to 180 degrees or more, as shown on right. With uncertain findings, double-check by asking the patient to place the first phalanges of each forefinger together, as shown in the sketches.

Normal, concave nail bases create a small, diamond-shaped space when the forefingers are placed together. Clubbed fingers are convex at the nail bases and touch without leaving a space when placed together.

Normal fingers

Clubbed fingers

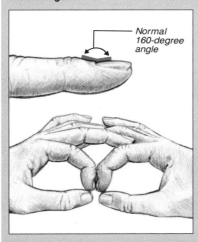

Normal 160-degree angle

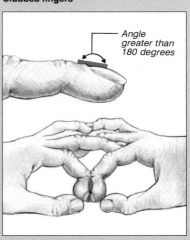

Angle greater than 180 degrees

the hands on the knees or the arms of a chair) to ease breathing.

Next, assess the patient's method of ventilation by placing the patient in the supine position and exposing the patient's chest and abdominal walls. Female patients may exhibit thoracic breathing — an upward and outward motion of the chest. Male patients may exhibit abdominal breathing, which uses the abdominal muscles. Patients with COPD may exhibit pursed-lip breathing, which prevents small airway collapse during exhalation.

Ask the patient to breath normally as you assess for shallow chest wall expansion (hypopnea) or unusually deep chest wall expansion (hyperpnea).

Keep in mind that observation alone is often inaccurate in determining the adequacy of normal breathing. An arterial blood gas (ABG) analysis is the most reliable way to assess adequacy of ventilation.

Assessing the posterior thorax

You will usually assess the posterior
thorax first and move to the anterior
thorax.

Inspection

Structural deformities in the posterior
thorax that may alter ventilation include an anteroposterior spine (kypho-
sis) and a lateral and anteroposterior
curvature of the spine (kyphoscoliosis).
These deformities can compress one
lung while allowing an overexpansion
of the other lung, eventually leading to
respiratory dysfunction. Acute changes
in the thoracic wall from trauma, such
as fractured ribs or a flail chest (fractures of two or more ribs in two or
more places), also alter ventilation by
allowing uneven chest expansion.

Palpation

Identify bony structures and landmarks, such as the first thoracic verte-
bra and the inferior scapular tips and
medial borders of both scapulae. Document the position of all abnormalities
in relation to these landmarks. For example, identify the first thoracic verte-
bra and then count the number of spi-
nous processes from this landmark to
the abnormality. The inferior scapular
tips and medial borders of both scapulae define the margins of the upper and
lower lung lobes posteriorly. Evaluate
abnormalities, such as the use of accessory muscles or complaints of pain,
and palpate for respiratory excursion
and tactile fremitus as well.

Percussion

Perform percussion in a quiet environment. Systematically percuss the posterior thorax according to the appropriate sequence. (See *Percussing the thorax.*) Percussion over a healthy lung
elicits a resonant sound — loud, long,
low-pitched, and hollow. However,
during your assessment you may hear a

variety of percussion notes. (See *Interpreting percussion notes,* page 14.)

Posterior percussion should sound
resonant to the level of T10. Hyperresonance may result from pneumothorax or overinflation of the lung;
dullness may result from tissue consolidation, as in pneumonia or atelectasis.

Auscultation

The pattern for auscultating the posterior thorax is the same as for the percussion sequence. Tell the patient to
breathe slowly and deeply, but caution
him against breathing too deeply or
rapidly.

Auscultate for bronchovesicular
breath sounds (heard over the interscapular area) and vesicular breath
sounds (heard in the suprascapular and
infrascapular areas). Note any absent,
decreased, or adventitious breath
sounds. For example, bronchovesicular
sounds auscultated in the periphery of
the lungs are adventitious breath
sounds. If you hear crackles and rhonchi (also adventitious breath sounds),
instruct the patient to cough, and then
listen again to see if they clear with
coughing.

Diaphragmatic excursion

Evaluate the movement of the patient's
diaphragm by measuring diaphragmatic excursion. Normal diaphragmatic excursion is 1¼″ to 2¼″ (3 to 6 cm).
Failure of the diaphragm to contract
downward may indicate paralysis or
muscle flattening due to COPD.
COPD may also cause the diaphragm
position to be lower at rest (expiration).
(See *Measuring diaphragmatic excursion,* page 15.)

Assessing the anterior thorax

When examining the anterior thorax,
note the location of any abnormalities
in terms of their proximity to the imag-
inary lines on the midsternum, mid-

Percussing the thorax

When percussing a patient's thorax, you should always:
• secure a quiet environment
• use mediate percussion, following the same sequence
• compare sound variations from one side to the other.

This helps ensure consistency and makes it easier to avoid overlooking important findings. In a respiratory assessment, you will usually percuss the posterior thorax first and then percuss the anterior and lateral thorax. Auscultation follows the same sequence as percussion.

Posterior thorax
To percuss the posterior thorax, progress in a zigzag fashion from the suprascapular to the interscapular to the infrascapular areas, avoiding the spinal column and the scapulae, as shown.

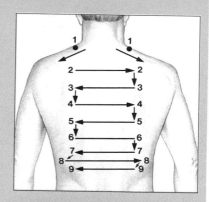

Anterior thorax
To percuss the anterior thorax, place one of your hands over each lung apex in the supraclavicular area. Then proceed downward, moving from side to side at 1½" to 2" (4- to 5-cm) intervals.

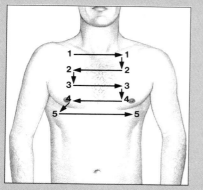

Lateral thorax
To percuss the lateral thorax, start at the axilla and move down the side of the rib cage, percussing between the ribs, as shown.

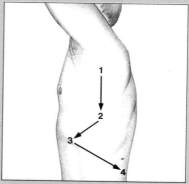

Interpretation

Interpreting percussion notes

You'll hear a variety of percussion notes during your assessment. Use these guidelines to characterize the notes and interpret their meaning.
• *Resonance:* low-pitched, moderate to loud, hollow. Heard over a normal lung.
• *Hyperresonance:* low-pitched, loud, booming. Heard over an emphysematous lung or a pneumothorax.
• *Tympany:* high-pitched, loud, musical or drumlike. Heard over an abdomen distended with air.
• *Dullness:* high-pitched, soft, thudlike. Normally heard over the heart and liver; also heard over pleural effusion or a neoplasm.
• *Flatness:* high-pitched, soft, extremely dull. Normally heard over the sternum; also heard over an atelectatic lung.

clavicular, midaxillary and anterior and posterior axillary lines.

Inspection
Inspect for structural deformities, such as a concave or convex curvature of the anterior chest wall over the sternum. Concave sternal depression (funnel chest [pectus excavatum]), and convex curvature (pigeon chest [pectus carinatum]) are two defects that can hinder breathing by preventing full chest expansion. COPD or the normal aging process may cause the rounded chest wall commonly called barrel chest.

Inspect between and around the ribs for retractions of soft tissues. Look for abnormalities in skin color, alterations in muscle tone, scars from surgery or trauma, or other visible abnormalities.

Note the angle between the ribs and the sternum at the xiphoid process.

This is the costal angle. In a normal adult, the costal angle is less than 90 degrees. An angle exceeding 90 degrees may signify that the chest wall is chronically expanded, as in barrel chest.

Inspect the anterior chest for symmetry of movement. Place the patient in the supine position; then stand at the foot of the bed and carefully observe the patient's chest as he breathes quietly and deeply. Look for equal expansion of the chest wall. Any exhibition of paradoxical movement — an area of the chest wall that collapses abnormally during inspiration and expands abnormally during expiration — indicates a loss of normal chest wall function. Paradoxical movement is common after trauma or improperly administered chest compression during cardiopulmonary resuscitation (CPR).

Unilateral absence of chest movement may be due to bronchial obstruction, a collapsed lung caused by air or fluid in the pleural space, or prior surgical removal of the lung on that side. Delayed chest movement may indicate congestion or consolidation of the underlying lung.

Palpation
By carefully palpating the trachea and the anterior thorax, you can detect abnormalities of the skin and underlying structures, areas of pain, and chest asymmetry.

First, palpate the trachea for position. Palpation may reveal that the trachea deviates from the midline. This may be due to atelectasis, thyroid enlargement, or pleural effusion. Also, a tumor or pneumothorax (collapsed lung) may displace the trachea to one side.

Next palpate the thorax for tenderness or abnormal masses. Gentle palpation should not cause pain. If the patient complains, assess the location, radiation, and severity of the pain. (Attempt to determine the cause by palpating the anterior chest. Disorders such as intercostal muscle strain, irritation of the nerves covering the xiphoid process, or inflammation of the cartilage connecting the bony ribs to the sternum [costochondritis] can cause pain during palpation and inspiration, causing the patient to breathe shallowly to reduce his discomfort. Palpation will not worsen pain caused by cardiac or pulmonary disorders, such as angina or pneumonia.) Be especially careful to palpate any areas that appeared abnormal during your general observation. Document any unusual findings, such as masses, crepitus, skin irregularities, or painful areas.

If palpation produces a crackly sound (similar to the sound of crumpling cellophane), suspect subcutaneous emphysema and immediately report your findings to the doctor. This characteristic sound indicates that air is leaking into the subcutaneous tissue from a breach in the respiratory system.

Next, gently palpate the costal angle. When palpating this area, remember that the region around the xiphoid process contains many nerve endings and care must be taken to avoid causing pain. If internal intercostal muscles are used to assist breathing, they will eventually pull the chest cavity upward and outward. If this has occurred, the costal angle will be greater than 90 degrees.

Next, place your hands on the lower rib cage (one hand on each side) with the palms down and palpate for the extent and symmetry of respiratory excursion as the patient takes a deep breath. Absent or delayed chest movement during respiratory excursion may indicate complete or partial obstruction of the airway or lung, diaphragmatic dysfunction on the affected side, or prior surgical removal of the lung.

Finally, palpate for tactile fremitus. Ask the patient to speak a resonant

Measuring diaphragmatic excursion

First instruct the patient to take a deep breath and hold it while you percuss down the right side of the posterior thorax. Begin at the lower border of the scapula and continue until the percussion note changes from resonance to dullness, which identifies the location of the diaphragm. Using a washable, felt-tip pen, mark this point with a small line.

Then instruct the patient to take a few normal breaths. Ask him to exhale completely and hold it while you percuss again to locate the point where the resonant sounds become dull. Mark this point with a small line.

Repeat this entire procedure on the left side of the posterior thorax. Remember that the diaphragm usually sits slightly lower on the left side than on the right side.

Next, using a tape measure or ruler, measure the distance between the two marks on each side of the posterior thorax, as shown here. The distance between these two marks reflects diaphragmatic excursion.

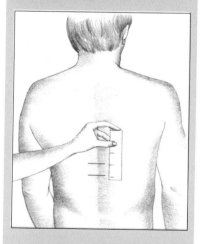

Palpating for tactile fremitus

Use the following steps to assess for tactile fremitus:
• Place your open palm flat against the patient's chest without touching the chest with your fingers.
• Ask the patient to repeat a resonant phrase, such as "ninety-nine," as you systematically move your hand over his chest from the central airways to the lung periphery and back. Always proceed in a systematic manner from the top of the suprascapular, interscapular, infrascapular, and hypochondriac areas (areas found from the 5th to 10th intercostal spaces to the right and left of midline).
• Repeat this procedure on the posterior thorax. You should feel vibrations of equal intensity on either side of the chest.

Understanding your findings
Fremitus usually occurs in the upper chest, close to the bronchi, and feels strongest at the second intercostal space on either side of the sternum. Little or no fremitus should occur in the lower chest. The intensity of the vibrations varies according to the thickness and structure of the patient's chest wall as well as the patient's voice intensity and pitch.

overinflated lungs, reduce tactile fremitus. Conditions that cause consolidation (alveoli become filled with cellular exudate), such as pneumonia, increase tactile fremitus. A grating feeling may signify a pleural friction rub. (See *Palpating for tactile fremitus*.)

Percussion
Percuss the anterior and lateral thorax over the intercostal spaces. Avoid percussing over bones, such as the manubrium, sternum, xiphoid process, clavicles, ribs, vertebrae, or scapulae.

To percuss the anterior chest, have the patient sit with his hands resting at his sides. Using a systematic sequence, percuss and compare sounds produced on one side to the sounds produced on the other side. Percussion of the anterior chest should produce resonance from below the clavicle to the fifth intercostal space on the right (where dullness occurs close to the liver) and to the third intercostal space on the left (where dullness occurs near the heart).

Next, percuss the lateral chest to obtain information about the left upper and lower lobes and about the right upper, middle, and lower lobes. Then repeat the percussion sequence on the right side. Percussion of the lateral chest should produce resonance to the sixth or eighth intercostal space.

Hyperresonance and dullness are the most common abnormal findings. Hyperresonance may result from air in the pleural space, which may be caused by pneumothorax or overinflation of the lung (common in emphysema). Dullness may result from a consolidation, possibly due to pneumonia or atelectasis. Flatness over the lung bases (with the patient sitting upright) indicates pleural effusion, masses, or hemothorax.

Auscultation
Auscultate the thorax to detect normal and abnormal breath sounds. Use the

phrase, such as "ninety-nine" or "blue moon." The patient's vocalization should produce vibrations of equal intensity on both sides of the chest. Normally, vibrations occur in the upper chest, close to the bronchi, and then decrease and disappear toward the periphery of the lungs.

Conditions that restrict air movement, such as pneumothorax, lung tumor, pleural effusion, or COPD with

Assessment TimeSaver

Recognizing normal breath sounds

Breath sound	Location	Characteristics	Respiration phase
Tracheal sounds	Over the trachea	Harsh, discontinuous	Equally audible during inspiration and expiration
Bronchial sounds	Over the manubrium	High-pitched, discontinuous	Prolonged during expiration
Bronchovesicular sounds	Over the upper one-third and to each side of the sternum (anterior), interscapular area (posterior)	Medium-pitched, continuous	Equally audible during inspiration and expiration
Vesicular sounds	Over the lung periphery	Low-pitched, continuous	Prolonged during inspiration

diaphragm of the stethoscope. Tell the patient to breathe slowly and deeply through his mouth (breathing through the nose may alter your findings). Explain that breathing too deeply or too rapidly can cause dizziness.

Following the same sequence you used for percussion, systematically auscultate the anterior and lateral thorax, first for normal breath sounds and then for abnormal breath sounds. Begin at the upper lobes and then move down the chest. Auscultate a point on one side of the chest and then move to the same point on the other side, comparing your findings. Always assess one complete breath (inspiration and expiration) at each point.

To assess the right middle lung lobe, auscultate breath sounds laterally at the fourth to the sixth intercostal spaces. (The sequence for auscultation is the same as the sequence for percussing the lateral chest.) Although difficult to assess (especially in female patients with large breasts), the right middle lobe is a common site of aspiration

pneumonia and, therefore, requires particular attention.

Classify normal and abnormal breath sounds according to location, intensity, characteristic sound, pitch (tone), and duration during both inspiration and expiration. When describing specific sounds, identify the quality using specific terms, such as *high-pitched* or *harsh*. (See *Recognizing normal breath sounds*.)

Adventitious breath sounds may be caused by fluid within alveoli, opening of compressed alveoli, secretions in small or large airways, narrowed airways, or pleural membrane inflammation. Certain adventitious breath sounds, including crackles, wheezes, rhonchi, subcutaneous emphysema, mediastinal crunch, and pericardial and pleural friction rubs, may appear in any lung lobe. (See *Assessing abnormal breath sounds*, page 18.)

Finally, identify the inspiratory and expiratory phase of normal and abnormal breath sounds, and determine whether the sound occurs during inspiration, expiration, or both. To do so,

Assessing abnormal breath sounds

Type	Description	Location	Cause
Crackles	Light crackling, popping, nonmusical sound, like hairs being rubbed together; further classified by pitch: high, medium, or low	Anywhere; heard in lung bases initially, usually during inspiration; also in dependent lung portions of bedridden patients. If crackles clear with coughing, they're not abnormal.	Air passing through moisture, especially in the small airways and alveoli (in pulmonary edema). Also, by alveoli "popping open" (in atelectasis)
Wheezes	Whistling sound; can be described as sonorous, bubbling, moaning, musical, sibilant and rumbling, crackling, or groaning	Anywhere; heard during inspiration or expiration. If wheezes clear with coughing, they may originate in the trachea or larger upper airways.	Fluid or secretions in the large airways or in airways narrowed by mucus, bronchospasm, or tumor
Rhonchi	Bubbling, gurgling sound	Central airways; heard during inspiration and expiration	Air passing through fluid-filled airways, as in upper respiratory tract infection
Pleural friction rub	Superficial squeaking or grating sound, like pieces of sandpaper being rubbed together	Lateral lung field; heard during inspiration and expiration (with patient in upright position)	Inflamed parietal and visceral pleural linings rubbing together
Grunting	Grunting noise	Central airways; heard during expiration in children and occasionally in adults with chronic obstructive pulmonary disease	Physiologic retention of air in lungs to prevent alveolar collapse
Stridor	Crowing noise	Trachea; heard during inspiration	Forced movement of air through edematous upper airway. In adults, laryngoedema, as in allergic reaction or smoke inhalation; laryngospasm, as in tetany; postextubation

place one hand on the patient's chest wall during auscultation. If the sound occurs as the thorax expands, it's part of inspiration; if it occurs as the thorax contracts, it's part of expiration.

To assess voice resonance, auscultate in the usual sequence while the patient repeats the term "ninety-nine." Normally, the patient's voice sounds muffled and indistinct; louder medially and softer in the lung periphery. Whispered pectoriloquy (distinct, understandable words) is indicative of consolidation of lung tissue, which may result from such conditions as a lung tumor, pneumonia, or pulmonary fibrosis.

Diagnostic tests

The results of diagnostic testing complete the objective data base. Together with the health history and physical examination findings, they form a profile of your patient's condition. One of the main diagnostic tests used to detect or monitor respiratory disorders is the chest X-ray.

Chest X-ray

In this test, X-rays penetrate the chest and produce images on specially sensitized film. Because pulmonary tissue is radiolucent, foreign bodies, infiltrates, fluids, tumors, and other abnormalities appear as densities (white areas) on the chest film. A chest X-ray is most useful when compared with a patient's previous films, allowing a radiologist to detect changes. Chest X-rays are used to detect pneumonia, pneumothorax, pulmonary edema, pleural effusion, and atelectasis. Acutely ill patients may undergo a series of chest X-rays to monitor the course of illness and the effectiveness of treatment and to detect complications.

By themselves, chest films may not provide definitive diagnostic information. For example, they may not reveal mild to moderate obstructive pulmonary disease. But they can show the location and size of lesions and can be used to identify structural abnormalities that influence ventilation and diffusion. Examples of abnormalities visible on X-ray images include pneumothorax, fibrosis, atelectasis, and infiltrates. (See *Recognizing abnormal chest X-ray findings,* page 20.)

Other diagnostic tests

The list below reviews the other diagnostic tests commonly ordered for patients with known or suspected respiratory problems.

• ABG analysis helps evaluate gas exchange in the lungs by measuring the partial pressures of arterial oxygen and carbon dioxide and the pH of arterial blood.

• Complete blood count (CBC) measures the blood's ability to transport oxygen by analyzing red blood cell and hemoglobin content. White blood cell and differential content may indicate possible respiratory infection.

• Sputum analysis detects viral, bacterial, and fungal respiratory infection through Gram staining and culturing. Cytology may reveal atypical or cancerous lung cells. (See *Types of sputum tests,* page 21.)

• Pulmonary function tests measure various lung volumes and capacities and help evaluate ventilation and the extent of dysfunction, diagnose obstructive or restrictive lung disease, and assess the effectiveness of respiratory therapy.

• Bronchoscopy, which permits direct inspection of the trachea and bronchi through a flexible fiber-optic or rigid bronchoscope, can be used to detect bleeding, to obtain a biopsy of a tumor or other lesion, or to remove foreign bodies, mucus plugs, or excess secretions.

• Radionuclide lung scans are performed to evaluate perfusion or ventilation. A perfusion lung scan involves injecting the patient with a radioactive contrast medium and scanning the area of radioactivity to evaluate blood flow to the lungs. This test is used to diagnose and evaluate pulmonary emboli. In a ventilation lung scan, the patient breathes in a mixture of radioactive gas. Scanning allows for the detection of ventilation abnormalities.

Recognizing abnormal chest X-ray findings

Anatomic area	Appearance	Abnormality	Possible respiratory causes
Trachea	Visible midline in the anterior mediastinal cavity; translucent; tubelike	• Deviation from midline	• Tension pneumothorax, atelectasis, pleural effusion
Heart	Visible in the left anterior mediastinal cavity; solid appearance from blood contents; edges may be clear in contrast to the surrounding air density of the lung	• Shift • Hypertrophy of right heart • Cardiac borders obscured by stringy densities	• Atelectasis • Cor pulmonale • Cystic fibrosis
Mediastinum (mediastinal shadow)	Visible as a space between the lungs; shadowy appearance that widens at the hilum	• Deviation to the nondiseased side; deviation toward the diseased side by traction • Gross widening	• Pleural effusion, fibrosis, or collapsed lung • Neoplasms, mediastinitis, cor pulmonale
Ribs	Visible as thoracic cavity encasement	• Break or misalignment • Widening of intercostal spaces	• Fractured sternum or ribs • Emphysema
Hila (lung roots)	Visible where bronchi join the lungs; appear as small, white, bilateral densities	• Shift to one side • Accentuated shadows • Atelectasis	• Emphysema, pulmonary abscess
Mainstem bronchus	Visible to about 1" (2.5 cm) from hila; translucent; tubelike	• Spherical or oval density	• Bronchogenic cyst
Bronchi	Usually not visible	• Visible	• Bronchial pneumonia
Lung fields	Usually not visible throughout, except for fine white areas from the hila	• Visible • Irregular, patchy densities	• Atelectasis • Resolving pneumonia, silicosis, fibrosis
Hemidiaphragm	Rounded, visible; right side about ³⁄₈" to ³⁄₄" (1 to 2 cm) higher than left side	• Elevation of diaphragm • Flattening of diaphragm • Unilateral elevation of either side	• Pneumonia, pleurisy, acute bronchitis, atelectasis • Asthma, emphysema • Unilateral phrenic nerve paresis

Types of sputum tests

Four types of laboratory tests may be performed on a sputum specimen to identify an infecting organism or abnormal cells: Gram stain, acid-fast stain, culture and sensitivity testing, and cytologic testing.

Gram stain
This test differentiates gram-positive bacteria from gram-negative bacteria. Gram-positive bacteria retain a blue stain after decolorization. Gram-negative bacteria lose the blue stain but counterstain red with safranine. This permits rapid identification of bacteria and indicates if the specimen is representative, as evidenced by many white blood cells (WBCs) and few epithelial cells. If oral contamination has occurred, few WBCs and many epithelial cells will be present. This test is used to identify the organism that causes tuberculosis.

Acid-fast stain
This test helps rapidly identify *Mycobacterium* organisms, which retain carbolfuchsin stain after treatment with an acid-alcohol solution. This test provides early presumptive diagnosis of tuberculosis.

Culture and sensitivity testing
In culture and sensitivity testing, the growth and isolation of microbes are initiated in a laboratory setting to positively identify microbes and to determine their vulnerability to specific antibiotics. The test helps diagnose lower respiratory infection or confirm an earlier presumptive diagnosis.

Cytologic (exfoliative) testing
This test is used to help identify tumors and other abnormal cells, to help diagnose and type malignant pulmonary lesions, and to identify granulomas, inflammation, and other benign conditions.

• Thoracic computed tomography (CT) scanning provides a three-dimensional image of the lungs and is used to evaluate masses, lesions, pleural fluid, and pneumothorax. It can help differentiate structures of varying densities that are in close proximity.
• Magnetic resonance imaging (MRI) is used to study fluid-filled soft tissues and to evaluate lung structure and blood flow. MRI has limited indications for respiratory problems, but it can be useful in distinguishing vascular from nonvascular structures in the hilum and mediastinum because it shows these tissues in greater detail than either X-rays or CT scans.

• Pulmonary angiography permits visualization of the pulmonary circulation so that blood flow abnormalities can be detected. During this test, a contrast dye is injected through a catheter that is inserted into the patient's pulmonary artery (or one of its branches), and a series of X-rays are taken, which track the dye as it flows through the pulmonary vascular tree.
• A percutaneous aspiration biopsy of a lung lesion is performed when a patient has a suspected malignant tumor, an unidentified pulmonary infection, or an unexplained pulmonary process. Fluid or tissue specimens obtained from this procedure are sent to the laboratory for microbiologic, histologic,

cytologic, and immunologic evaluation.

• Thoracoscopy permits direct visualization of the lung and pleural space through a small scope placed in a 1″ (2.5-cm) incision in the chest wall. Instruments may be placed through two other small incisions to perform procedures such as lung biopsies and resections and to treat lesions and recurrent pneumothoraces. There are less complications with thoracoscopy than with open lung biopsy and thoracotomy.

Nursing diagnosis

The next step of the nursing process — nursing diagnosis — describes the patient's actual or potential response to a health problem. As you formulate a nursing diagnosis, review your assessment data for patterns that indicate specific problems. Consider asking yourself the following questions:

• What are the patient's signs and symptoms?

• Which assessment findings are abnormal for this patient?

• Are there a cluster of findings that suggest a specific respiratory problem?

• How do the patient's behavior patterns and environment affect his respiratory health?

• Is the patient at risk for other respiratory problems?

• Does the patient understand his health status?

• What is the patient's response to his respiratory problem? Is he willing and motivated to change his state of health?

When formulating nursing diagnoses, use the NANDA taxonomy that fits your patient or, if necessary, create your own. To foster greater accuracy, you should also write an etiology, or "related to" statement, for each nursing diagnosis. The etiology should include conditions or circumstances that contribute to the development or continuation of the diagnosis, such as environmental, physiologic, psychological, cultural, or spiritual influences identified during assessment. Examples of "related to" statements include:

• Fatigue related to recurrent dyspnea

• Anxiety related to perceived threat of death secondary to respiratory distress

• Pain related to persistent cough

• High risk for aspiration related to depressed cough reflex

• Hopelessness related to lack of support systems

• Health seeking behaviors (smoking cessation) related to father's cancer diagnosis

• Impaired social interaction related to effects of long-term hospitalization.

Chapters 4 through 10 contain common nursing diagnoses for many respiratory disorders. Keep in mind, however, that diagnostic statements must be tailored to your patient's individual circumstances and needs. Each patient responds differently, and your nursing diagnoses should never become so standardized that they fail to reflect the individual needs of each patient under your care.

Developing individual diagnoses for each respiratory patient can be difficult. You can make this task easier and save time by becoming familiar with the most frequently used nursing diagnoses. (See *Common nursing diagnoses in respiratory care*.)

Ineffective airway clearance

This nursing diagnosis refers to the patient's inability to clear secretions or obstructions from the respiratory tract. Defining characteristics of ineffective airway clearance include adventitious breath sounds, such as crackles, rhonchi, stridor, or wheezes; changes in rate or depth of respirations; cough (productive or nonproductive); cyanosis; dyspnea; and tachypnea.

Common nursing diagnoses in respiratory care

Certain nursing diagnoses can be used frequently to describe the response patterns of respiratory patients. This list identifies and defines these diagnoses.

Activity intolerance • Insufficient physiologic or psychological energy to endure or complete required or desired daily activities

Altered cardiopulmonary tissue perfusion • Decrease in cellular nutrition and respiration caused by reduced capillary perfusion

Altered nutrition: Less than body requirements • Nutritional intake that is insufficient to meet metabolic needs and that results in unhealthful weight loss

Anxiety • Vague uneasy feeling of nonspecific or unknown origin

High risk for aspiration • State of being at risk for GI or oropharyngeal secretions, food, or fluids entering the tracheobronchial passages

Ineffective airway clearance • Inability to clear secretions or obstructions from the respiratory tract

Ineffective breathing pattern • Patient's inspiration or expiration pattern does not lead to adequate lung inflation or deflation

Dysfunctional ventilatory weaning response • Patient cannot adjust to lowered levels of mechanical ventilator support, thus interrupting and prolonging the weaning process

Fatigue • Overwhelming sense of exhaustion and decreased capacity for physical and mental work

Impaired gas exchange • Decreased passage of oxygen, carbon dioxide, or both between the alveoli of the lungs and the vascular system

Impaired verbal communication • Decreased or absent ability to use or understand language to express needs or feelings

Health seeking behaviors • State in which a patient in stable health actively seeks ways to alter personal health habits or the environment to move toward a higher level of health

Inability to sustain spontaneous ventilation • Inability to maintain breathing adequate to support life

Knowledge deficit • Inadequate understanding of information or an inability to perform skills needed to practice health-related behaviors

Pain • Patient experiences and reports severe discomfort or an uncomfortable sensation.

Ineffective airway clearance may be caused by increased quantity or tenaciousness of secretions (as with asthma, COPD, congestive heart failure [CHF], pneumonia, or lung cancer) or by decreased ability to cough effectively (as with cerebrovascular accident [CVA], chest trauma, COPD, or neuromuscular diseases).

Related factors may include fatigue, tracheobronchial infection, upper or lower airway obstruction or pooling (stasis) of secretions, trauma, pain, and perceptual or cognitive impairment.

Ineffective breathing pattern

This nursing diagnosis describes a state in which the patient's inspiration, expiration, or both, fails to provide adequate lung inflation or deflation. Defining characteristics of an ineffective breathing pattern include accessory muscle use, altered chest excursion, altered depth of respiration, abnormal ABG levels, cough, cyanosis, dyspnea, increased anteroposterior diameter, fremitus, nasal flaring, pursed-lip breathing (prolonged expiration phase), shortness of breath, tachypnea, and the use of the tripod position for breathing.

Ineffective breathing pattern may be associated with disorders that result in pain (such as chest wall injury, pericarditis, pleural effusion, pleurisy, pneumonia, pneumothorax, pulmonary embolus, or rib or vertebral fractures) or that increase the work or effort of breathing (such as COPD or neuromuscular diseases). This diagnosis also may apply when the patient's condition causes muscle fatigue during respiration, such as in anemia, COPD, cirrhosis, CHF, metabolic acidosis, and pulmonary edema.

Impaired gas exchange

This nursing diagnosis refers to a state in which there is decreased movement of oxygen, carbon dioxide, or both between the alveoli and the vascular system. Signs and symptoms of impaired gas exchange include anxiety, arrhythmias, confusion, cyanosis, decrease in mental acuity, dyspnea, inability to move secretions, irritability, somnolence, and tachycardia. Diagnostic tests reveal abnormal ABG levels and hypoxemia, with or without hypercapnia.

Impaired gas exchange may be associated with any pulmonary disease or with high-altitude sickness, carbon monoxide poisoning, drug overdose, neurologic trauma, and neuromuscular disease.

Other nursing diagnoses

Although your primary focus will be the patient's respiratory problems, you will also identify associated problems that need attention. For example, the patient may feel stress about his illness and his need for hospitalization. The patient may experience symptoms that include sleeplessness, anger toward the staff, and an inability to make decisions. You would identify this cluster of symptoms as *ineffective individual coping.* By identifying this problem and incorporating it into your plan of care, you can help the patient and his family members learn to cope with the illness, which, in turn, enhances compliance and recovery.

The health history may indicate that the patient has experienced anorexia and a loss of 20 lb (9 kg) since becoming ill. You formulate the nursing diagnosis *altered nutrition: less than body requirements, related to anorexia.* By clearly identifying the problem, you can select interventions that help to improve the patient's nutritional status, prevent respiratory complications such as infection, and speed recovery. Other examples of possible diagnoses include *activity intolerance, fatigue, health seeking behaviors,* and *pain.*

Patient teaching is a vital component of providing care for the respiratory patient. You may need to teach your patient about diagnostic procedures or the proper use of prescribed medications. Your teaching may focus on encouraging lifestyle changes to reduce respiratory risk factors in the patient's environment. *Knowledge deficit* is the diagnosis used most frequently to document learning needs. Because this diagnosis is so broad, you should include a carefully worded etiology to ensure that the patient's specific needs are clearly stated.

Planning

The next step of the nursing process involves creating a plan of action that will direct your patient care toward achieving specific goals. This step includes writing a plan of care to serve as a record of your nursing diagnoses, expected patient outcomes, nursing interventions, and evaluation data.

Early in the planning process, you will need to determine priorities for nursing care. Using your nursing diagnoses, you'll need to determine which problems require immediate attention and which can wait. Always give the highest priority to problems that pose immediate safety risks, and then address health-threatening and psychosocial concerns.

To save time and create a plan of care that is meaningful and attainable, enlist the help of staff members who are familiar with the patient. Be sure to involve your patient in the planning process. Ask what problems are most important to him. (These may differ from the problems you perceive as priorities.) A patient with a respiratory disorder is more likely to comply with treatment if you take time to learn his priorities. If, for example, your patient has a history of chronic respiratory distress, you may be most concerned about impaired gas exchange and possible respiratory arrest. The patient, however, may disclose that he is upset because his increasing shortness of breath has interfered with his work, social life, or sexual activity. (See *Setting priorities for nursing diagnoses in respiratory care,* pages 26 and 27.)

Establishing patient outcomes
Next you'll need to establish patient outcomes — measurable goals derived from the patient's nursing diagnoses. A patient outcome should describe a behavior or result that is to be achieved within a specific time frame. (Target dates help motivate the patient and help you keep the patient on schedule for discharge.)

You'll use patient outcomes to evaluate the effectiveness of nursing care; therefore, they should be realistic. For a patient with severe chronic obstructive pulmonary disease (COPD) with activity intolerance, an expected outcome may be to walk 10′ (3 m) before becoming short of breath prior to discharge. However, for a young, otherwise healthy patient with pneumonia, an expected outcome might be to return to normal activity and exercise tolerance within 3 weeks after discharge.

The success of your plan of care depends on accurate documentation of patient outcomes. Outcome statements that are vague, hard to measure, or unrealistic may invalidate a plan that is otherwise accurate and useful. When choosing patient outcomes, consider asking the following questions:
• What behavior will show that the patient has reached the specific goal?
• Which criteria will be used to measure the behavior (how much, how long, how far)?
• Under what conditions should the behavior occur?
• What is a realistic target time frame for the behavior?

For example, if your patient's nursing diagnosis is *ineffective breathing pattern related to retained secretions,* appropriate outcome statements might include the following:
• Patient will maintain a respiratory rate of 20 to 30 breaths/minute during hospitalization.
• His ABG levels will return to baseline within 24 hours.
• He will report an absence of dyspnea at rest within 24 hours.
• He will report an absence of dyspnea when ambulating in room within 48 hours.
• His chest X-ray will indicate full lung expansion within 24 hours.

Developing interventions
After establishing patient outcomes, you'll develop nursing interventions that will help the patient achieve those outcomes. Information obtained during your assessment of such factors as

Setting priorities for nursing diagnoses in respiratory care

As you plan care for your patient with a respiratory disorder, you'll need to establish priorities. Consider the significant assessment findings underlying your nursing diagnoses and address problems in the following order: life-threatening problems, health-threatening problems, and psychosocial concerns.

Consider this example.

Subjective data

Your new patient, Mrs. Dalton, a 34-year-old computer programmer, has a pulmonary embolism — an acute obstruction of the pulmonary vasculature by a dislodged thrombus, usually from the leg veins. You must quickly establish priorities for her nursing care to prevent deterioration of her condition, promote recovery, and help her improve her long-term health status.

Mrs. Dalton is being admitted to a monitored bed on your unit. During your initial assessment, you learn she has had right calf pain and swelling off and on for the past 2 weeks. She attributed the pain to bumping her leg on her desk at work and did not seek help until she developed sudden left lateral chest pain, shortness of breath, and fatigue.

Two years ago, Mrs. Dalton had an episode of thrombophlebitis of the right leg that required hospitalization. Otherwise, she has been healthy. She has never had surgery or been pregnant. She is allergic to sulfa drugs and takes oral contraceptives. She was warned never to take oral contraceptives again after her previous episode of thrombophlebitis; however, she felt it was the most convenient method of birth control and restarted 6 months ago. She has a sedentary job and gets little exercise. She does not smoke. She reports severe, stabbing, left lateral chest pain that worsens with deep breathing and coughing.

Objective data

Your examination of Mrs. Dalton reveals the following:

- general appearance — sitting upright with right hand splinting left side
- height, 5'7"; weight, 185 lb (84 kg)
- oral temperature, 100.6° F (87.8° C)
- blood pressure, 90/54 mm Hg; pulse rate, 92 beats/minute; regular pulse rhythm
- respirations, 32 breaths/minute and shallow
- warm, dry skin with no cyanosis
- clear breath sounds except for faint pleural friction rub left midaxillary line at seventh intercostal space.

Diagnostic test findings

- Chest X-ray shows left pleural effusion and left lower lobe wedge-shaped infiltrate.
- Arterial blood gas (ABG) levels show a partial pressure of arterial oxygen of 80 mm Hg, a partial pressure of arterial carbon dioxide of 32 mm Hg, and a pH of 7.52.
- Lung scan shows perfusion defect left lower lobe.

Assessment findings

Your assessment findings suggest that Mrs. Dalton has compromised respiratory function due to her pulmonary embolus, causing tachypnea, tachycardia, hypotension, and pleural effusion. Her use of oral contraceptives, sedentary lifestyle, and mild trauma she had to her leg all enhanced clotting and caused a deep vein thrombosis that eventually broke off and traveled to her pulmonary artery and smaller pulmonary vessels.

Mrs. Dalton's continued use of oral contraceptives and failure to report signs of deep vein thrombosis suggest

Setting priorities for nursing diagnoses in respiratory care *(continued)*

a lack of knowledge or denial. You also can tell by her words and appearance that she is in pain, which is contributing to her anxiety and may be further impairing respiration.

Setting priorities
The area of greatest concern is Mrs. Dalton's compromised respiratory status. Pulmonary emboli cause ventilation-perfusion mismatch leading to poor oxygenation of the blood. Also, pain and apprehension lead to increased but shallow respirations that cause a blowing off of too much carbon dioxide (respiratory alkalosis). You'll want to prevent respiratory failure and shock, two life-threatening complications. Therefore, you plan to carefully and frequently monitor Mrs. Dalton's vital signs and oxygenation status (through observation, ABG analysis, and pulse oximetry) to quickly detect deterioration in her condition.

Your next priority is to make Mrs. Dalton more comfortable by supporting her upright positioning with pillows and by providing pain medication, as prescribed. Because pain is impairing respiration further, relieving pain will help increase oxygenation and encourage compliance with therapy.

After addressing these immediate concerns, you plan to teach Mrs. Dalton to identify which behaviors have put her at risk for a pulmonary embolus to help avoid recurrence.

Nursing diagnosis
When writing a plan of care for Mrs. Dalton, you select the following nursing diagnoses in order of priority:
• Impaired gas exchange related to perfusion defect and rapid, shallow respirations
• Pain related to pulmonary embolus
• Knowledge deficit related to lack of awareness of risk factors for pulmonary embolism.

Additional care
Now that you have set priorities for Mrs. Dalton's problems, you can set goals and implement care. If you succeed in preventing life-threatening complications, you will have time to address all of Mrs. Dalton's needs.

your patient's age, emotional status, any physical and mental impairments, developmental and educational levels, environment, and cultural values is helpful. Talk with the patient and his family members. The more you know about the patient, the easier it will be to formulate appropriate interventions. For example, when developing an exercise program for a patient with COPD, it would be inappropriate to include bicycle riding if he has severe osteoarthritis of the knee.

Write your intervention in precise detail. Include how and when to perform the intervention (including supplies or equipment) as well as any special instructions. Examples of clearly stated interventions include the following:
• Assist patient OOB in chair for ½ hour b.i.d.
• Teach patient diaphragmatic pursed-lip breathing by 12/16/93.
• Encourage patient to perform coughing and deep-breathing exercises using splinting techniques before surgery. Turn q 2 hours (odd) as specified on turning schedule.

When writing interventions, clearly state the necessary action so they can be continued or modified by other nurses in your absence. Also, to ensure cooperation, make sure that the patient and his family members understand each intervention.

Implementation

During the fourth step of the nursing process, you put your plan of care into action. During this phase you'll have direct and prolonged contact with the patient. You'll also coordinate and direct the activities of other health care team members.

Treatment of respiratory disorders has become increasingly dependent on new technologies. You must be familiar with the proper use of specialized equipment, such as mechanical ventilators, oxygen administration systems, pulse oximeters, and suctioning equipment. In addition, the complex nature of many respiratory disorders and the patient's anxiety and other psychological responses require an extensive knowledge base as well as highly developed organizational and communication skills.

Implementation encompasses many tasks, so it's important to use your time effectively. Use your plan of care to help you organize your day and manage your time wisely. As you document your interventions, note changes in the patient's condition, new problems, the status or resolution of old problems, the patient's responses to treatments or medications, and the patient's family members' responses to your interventions. The following is a brief review of nursing interventions you may need to implement during your care of a patient with a respiratory disorder.

Therapeutic interventions
These interventions are geared toward alleviating the effects of illness or restoring optimal function. Major therapeutic interventions for acute respiratory conditions include:
• intubation (airway maintenance)
• mechanical ventilation
• administration of supplemental oxygen
• suctioning of secretions.

Other common therapeutic interventions include:
• administering medications, such as bronchodilators, corticosteroids, antibiotics, expectorants, and anticholinergics
• performing pulmonary hygiene measures, such as postural drainage and percussion
• adjusting ventilatory support devices, such as a phrenic nerve pacer or a noninvasive ventilator (either negative pressure or positive pressure via mask)
• promoting coughing, deep breathing, and use of incentive spirometer.

Emergency care
In a respiratory emergency, such as complete airway obstruction, you may need to intervene immediately by clearing the obstructed airway (if necessary) and initiating cardiopulmonary resuscitation (CPR). If you're not successful and you have appropriate equipment on hand, you may need to help the doctor remove a foreign object (if it's the cause of the obstruction) with a bronchoscope, Magill forceps, or suctioning equipment. As a last resort, you may need to help the doctor perform an emergency cricothyrotomy or percutaneous transtracheal catheter ventilation. If the obstruction is caused by an anaphylactic reaction, you may need to initiate emergency treatment for anaphylaxis.

Monitoring
Periodic or continuous evaluation of your patient's respiratory status and response to therapy is just as important as the initial assessment. Depending on the condition, patients with respiratory disorders should be monitored for signs and symptoms of respiratory distress, hypercapnia, and hypoxia. Breath sounds, breathing pattern, and pulmonary pressures should also be evaluated. In many cases, you'll also monitor the following:
- pulmonary function studies
- arterial blood gas (ABG) levels
- pulse oximetry values
- end-tidal carbon dioxide, tidal volume, and vital capacity
- complete blood count (CBC)
- electrocardiogram (ECG)
- cardiac status (for arrhythmias)
- adverse effects and blood levels of drugs
- sputum and culture and sensitivity reports
- lactic acid and albumin levels
- leukocyte and lymphocyte counts.

You'll also need to periodically evaluate other indicators of your patient's health, such as temperature, pulse rate, blood pressure, respirations, skin hydration, intake and output, daily weight, and mental status.

Patient teaching
Teaching can help the patient with a respiratory disorder maintain his health and avoid future problems. Many of your lessons will focus on providing the patient and his family members with information about the respiratory condition, including:
- symptoms to report to the doctor
- possible complications
- factors that may precipitate an acute respiratory emergency
- techniques (breathing, coughing, relaxation) that may be used to maintain an adequate baseline condition.

The patient may also need to be taught about drug therapy, oxygen therapy, and mechanical ventilation, including proper care, cleaning, and maintenance of oxygen and inhalation equipment that is to be used at home. Other possible teaching topics include stopping smoking, improving physical fitness, ensuring good nutrition, and relieving depression and anxiety. During hospitalization for pulmonary surgery, teaching focuses on reviewing preoperative and postoperative procedures, techniques, equipment, and care. A lung cancer patient should be taught about the type of treatment he will receive. This is commonly done by a doctor or nurse specializing in cancer treatment.

Preoperative care
Preoperative nursing measures may include evaluation of the patient's risk factors, current respiratory status, and general nutrition and state of hydration. Interventions may also include enforcing food and fluid restrictions; obtaining necessary diagnostic test information; establishing baseline pulmonary function studies, ECG readings, and vital signs; establishing an I.V. line; providing teaching regarding preoperative and postoperative care; offering reassurance; providing sedation; and providing respiratory treatments and medications to improve pulmonary status before surgery.

Postoperative care
Postoperative interventions may include checking dressings for signs of bleeding or infection, changing dressings, assessing vital signs and level of consciousness, providing analgesics, providing ventilator support, maintaining chest tube drainage, and communicating with family members. Postoperative nursing care may also involve preparing to administer oxygen if ABG analysis reveals hypoxemia; monitor-

ing hemodynamic status, including central venous pressure, pulmonary artery pressure, and pulmonary artery wedge pressure; placing the patient in semi-Fowler's position for comfort; and encouraging the use of an incentive spirometer to prevent postoperative atelectasis.

Emotional support

You may plan and implement interventions to enhance your patient's emotional well-being. For example, you can support the patient who is grieving the loss of respiratory health and function by establishing a trusting relationship and setting aside time to listen to his concerns. By regularly expressing concern for the patient's health, you can help him combat feelings of helplessness or worthlessness.

A trusting relationship also promotes patient compliance to therapeutic interventions and allows the patient to resume his usual role more easily upon discharge. For patients who are coping poorly with their respiratory disorder, you may need to provide a referral for psychological counseling. Family members may also need help in adjusting to changes in the patient and the increased demands that these changes may place on them.

Preparation for discharge

By preparing the patient for discharge, you can help to make the transition from the hospital to the home safe and smooth and ensure continued quality of care. Patients with chronic respiratory disorders, for example, may have to adjust to mechanical ventilation, oxygen therapy, inhalation devices, lifestyle restrictions, and long-term care.

Preparation for discharge may include:

• reinforcing the teaching plan
• reviewing the disorder (including possible complications)

• reviewing medications (including adverse effects), oxygen therapy (including instructions for use and care of equipment), ventilation or inhalation equipment (including instructions for use and care), deep-breathing and coughing techniques, and nutrition and activity guidelines
• reminding the patient when to return for follow-up appointments and diagnostic tests
• providing a referral to a pulmonary rehabilitation program, home health care agency, or medical equipment supplier
• contacting a homemaking service or consulting the community health nurse to arrange follow-up visits.

Discharge planning for the patient who has had major pulmonary surgery may include instructing the patient and family members to observe the chest tube insertion site for signs of inflammation, teaching the patient about wound care (including dressing changes) and signs of respiratory infection, and advising the patient to report persistent or new drainage and signs of infection to the doctor.

Evaluation

During evaluation, the last step in the nursing process, you judge the effectiveness of nursing care and gauge your patient's progress toward expected outcomes. The evaluation process begins as soon as you implement a plan of care and continues until the patient is discharged or all of the goals are met. Evaluating the patient gives you a chance to:

• determine if original assessment findings still apply
• uncover complications
• validate the appropriateness of nursing diagnoses, expected patient outcomes, and interventions

• analyze patterns or trends in your patient's care and his responses to care
• assess his response to all aspects of care, including medications, changes in diet and activity, procedures, unusual incidents or problems, and patient teaching
• determine how closely care conforms with established standards
• measure the effectiveness of your care
• assess the performance of other health care team members
• discover opportunities to improve the quality of care.

Evaluation is an ongoing activity that overlaps other phases of the nursing process; therefore, your evaluation findings may trigger a new cycle of assessment, nursing diagnosis, planning, implementation, and further evaluation.

To ensure a successful evaluation, keep an open mind. Never hesitate to consider new patient data or to revise previous judgments. Remember, no plan of care is perfect. In fact, you should anticipate revising the plan of care during the course of treatment.

Reassessment

Reassessing the patient's condition is the basis for evaluation. You'll reassess the patient at regular intervals, depending on his status and your hospital's policy. You may not need to complete a multisystem physical assessment again; just focus on areas identified in the nursing diagnosis. You'll also reassess the patient any time his status changes unexpectedly.

Next, compare reassessment data with criteria established in the patient outcomes documented in your plan of care. As you analyze reassessment data, consider asking the following questions:
• Do the data support the expected outcomes?

• Has the patient's condition improved, deteriorated, or stayed the same?
• Have new complications developed?
• Which outcomes were achieved? Which were partially achieved? Which were not achieved?

If you find that your expected outcomes have not been met by the projected dates, you must assess factors that might be interfering with progress. Consider all possible reasons that a patient may not be able to achieve a desired outcome. Below are some examples:
• The purpose and goals of the plan of care aren't clear.
• The expected outcomes aren't realistic in light of the patient's condition.
• The plan of care is based on incomplete or inaccurate assessment data.
• Nursing diagnoses are inaccurate.
• The nursing staff experienced conflicts with the patient or medical staff.
• Staff members didn't follow the plan of care.
• Interventions were not documented in detail, resulting in confusion or inconsistency.
• The patient failed to carry out activities outlined in the plan of care.
• The patient's condition changed or complications developed.

Writing evaluation statements

Evaluation statements provide a method for documenting the patient's response to care. These statements indicate whether expected outcomes were achieved and list the evidence supporting your conclusions.

The importance of clearly written evaluation statements can't be overemphasized. Documentation of patient outcomes is necessary to substantiate the rationales for nursing care and to justify the use of nursing resources. You'll record your evaluation statements in your progress notes or on the revised plan of care, according to your hospital's documentation policy.

Writing clear, concise evaluation statements is easy if you wrote precise patient outcome statements during the planning phase of care. The patient outcome statements provide a model for evaluation statements. For example, possible evaluation statements for the nursing diagnosis *ineffective airway clearance related to thick copious secretions* include:
• Patient achieves respiratory rate of 32 at rest without stridor.
• He performs coughing and deep-breathing exercises every ½ hour following use of incentive spirometer.
• He produces about 30 ml thick purulent sputum 2 to 4 times/hour.
• He tolerates oral intake without gagging or aspirating.
• He expresses understanding that hydration, coughing and deep-breathing techniques, and monitoring of respirations and sputum are needed to maintain good airway clearance.
• During auscultation, harsh crackles clear with coughing, except left lower lobe.

Modifying the plan of care
During evaluation, you may discover that the plan of care needs to be modified. If patient outcomes have been achieved, make sure that you record the date the outcome was achieved and if any nursing diagnosis has been resolved. Revise other outcome statements as necessary and determine which nursing interventions need to be revised or discontinued. If outcomes are not met or a change in the patient's condition has occurred, you may need to assign new priorities to existing nursing diagnoses or add new diagnoses. The same is true for interventions.

Like all steps of the nursing process, evaluation is ongoing. Continue to assess, diagnose, plan, implement, and evaluate for as long as you care for the patient.

CHAPTER 2

Exploring chief complaints

In respiratory disorders, the most common chief complaints include chest pain, dyspnea, cough, hemoptysis, chills, fatigue, fever, and wheezing. By fully investigating your patient's chief complaint and associated signs and symptoms, you can form a diagnostic impression of his problem and guide your subsequent care.

Chest pain

Besides cardiovascular disorders, chest pain most often results from conditions that affect the pleurae and lungs. At first, a pulmonary cause may be difficult to identify. The reason? Most pulmonary causes of chest pain are localized and pleuritic and may be mistaken for anginal pain. The pain may be steady or intermittent and mild or acute; it may range from a sharp shooting pain to a dull, aching feeling. (See *Causes of chest pain.*)

If your patient reports chest pain, take a health history and perform a physical examination according to the guidelines below.

History of the symptom
To better characterize your patient's chest pain, consider asking the following questions:
• When did the pain begin?
• Did it arise suddenly or build gradually? Is it more severe now than when it started?
• Is the pain constant or intermittent? If intermittent, how often does it occur and how long does it last? Is it occurring more frequently now than when it started?
• Where is the pain located? Does it radiate to other areas?
• Have you had this type of pain before?
• How would you describe the pain? Is it, for example, dull and aching, sharp and stabbing, or a sensation of "tightness"?
• On a scale of 1 to 10 (with 10 being the most severe), how severe is the pain?
• Do particular movements or activities (such as breathing, coughing, or exertion) precipitate or intensify the pain or its frequency?
• What relieves the pain? Does it stop or lessen if you rest or change position? Have any over-the-counter medications helped?

Associated findings
Note whether the patient has experienced any of the following signs or symptoms:
• abdominal pain
• anxiety
• chest wall trauma
• chills
• cough (possibly with blood-tinged sputum)
• dyspnea
• fever
• headache
• hemoptysis
• muscular pain (particularly backache)
• night sweats
• pleural friction rub
• rapid, shallow breathing
• sputum production (note the color, volume, and consistency)
• use of accessory muscles.

Previous conditions
Consult with the patient, members of his family, or members of the health care team to determine if the patient has a history of any of the following conditions or risk factors:
• alcohol use
• cancer
• chest trauma
• chronic cardiac or pulmonary disease
• connective tissue disease

Causes of chest pain

Chest pain may occur in the following disorders: asthma, bronchitis, coccidioidomycosis, interstitial lung disease, Legionnaires' disease, lung abscess, lung cancer, pleurisy, pneumonia, pneumothorax, tuberculosis, and pulmonary embolism. Chest pain associated with respiratory disorders may be caused by inflammation of the pleura (pleuritic chest pain), mucous membranes of the trachea or mainstem bronchi, or costochondral junctions; spasms of chest wall muscles; and gastroesophageal reflux.

Asthma
Life-threatening asthma attacks can cause diffuse, painful chest tightness. A dry cough and mild wheezing may accompany pain and may progress to a productive cough, audible wheezing, and severe dyspnea.

Bronchitis
Acute bronchitis produces burning chest pain or a sensation of substernal tightness. A dry cough that worsens and becomes productive in time may cause increased chest pain.

Coccidioidomycosis
In this disorder, pleuritic chest pain is accompanied by a nonproductive cough, fever, rash, or headache.

Interstitial lung disease
As this disorder progresses, the patient may experience pleuritic chest pain, which may be accompanied by progressive dyspnea, crackles (sounding like cellophane), a nonproductive cough, fatigue, weight loss, finger clubbing, or cyanosis.

Legionnaires' disease
Legionnaires' disease causes pleuritic chest pain accompanied by malaise, headache and, possibly, diarrhea; anorexia; diffuse myalgia; general weakness and, within 12 to 24 hours, sudden high fever and chills.

Lung abscess
Pleuritic chest pain develops insidiously. Pain is accompanied by a pleural friction rub and a productive cough that raises copious amounts of purulent, foul-smelling, blood-tinged sputum.

Lung cancer
Chest pain in lung cancer is often described as an intermittent aching deep within the chest. If the tumor has metastasized to the ribs or vertebrae, the pain becomes localized, continuous, and gnawing.

Pleurisy
Located in the lower and lateral aspects of the chest, pleuritic chest pain is typically unilateral and sharp and reaches maximum intensity within hours of onset. Factors that aggravate the pain include deep breathing, coughing, and thoracic movement.

Pneumonia
This disorder produces pleuritic chest pain that's aggravated by deep breathing. Pain is typically accompanied by fever, shaking chills, and a dry cough that becomes productive over time.

Pneumothorax
This life-threatening disorder causes sudden, severe, sharp chest pain. The pain is commonly unilateral (rarely localized) and increases with chest movement. When the pain is central and radiates to the neck, it may mimic myocardial infarction (MI).

Pulmonary embolism
This disorder produces substernal pain or a choking sensation. Typically, the patient first experiences a sudden

(continued)

Causes of chest pain *(continued)*

onset of dyspnea with intense angina-like or pleuritic pain, which may be aggravated by deep breathing and thoracic movement.

Tuberculosis
Tuberculosis patients may experience pleuritic chest pain with fine crackles occurring after coughing.

Nonrespiratory causes
Chest pain may also be caused by an-gina, MI, pericarditis, dissecting aortic aneurysm, blastomycosis, actinomycosis, cholecystitis, esophageal spasm, gastroesophageal reflux, hiatal hernia, peptic ulcer disease, gastritis, and pancreatitis. The symptom may also result from rib fracture, muscle strain, thoracic outlet syndrome, costochondritis, anxiety, herpes zoster, mediastinitis, sickle cell crisis, or Chinese restaurant syndrome (related to the metabolism of monosodium glutamate).

• exposure to coal dust or other irritants (occupational or residential)
• GI problems
• thrombophlebitis or deep vein thrombosis
• unusual amount of activity with arm and chest muscles.

Drug history
Note any past or current use of the following drugs:
• cocaine (may precipitate myocardial infarction)
• oral contraceptives (may predispose the patient to thrombophlebitis and pulmonary embolism)
• procainamide or hydralazine (rarely may lead to pericarditis)
• theophylline preparations, alcohol (may increase gastroesophageal reflux).

Physical examination
Assess the patient's vital signs, including temperature, blood pressure, respiratory rate and depth, and pulse rate and rhythm. Then examine him according to the steps described below.

Inspection
• Observe the patient's general appearance. Note his personal hygiene, nutritional status, level of consciousness, level of comfort, and any restlessness.
• Inspect the skin for cyanosis.
• Observe the neck for tracheal deviation, distended veins, and the use of accessory muscles for breathing.
• Inspect the abdomen for abdominal breathing.
• Observe the chest for asymmetrical expansion and sternal, intercostal, or supraclavicular retractions.

Palpation
• Palpate the skin for temperature and diaphoresis.
• Check the neck for tracheal deviation and subcutaneous crepitation.
• Palpate the chest for tactile fremitus and any areas of tenderness.

Percussion
• Percuss the lung fields for dullness or hyperresonance.

Auscultation
• Listen over the lungs for a pleural friction rub, crackles, rhonchi, wheez-

ing, diminished or absent breath sounds, bronchophony and egophony, amphoric breath sounds, and decreased vocal fremitus.
• Auscultate the heart for murmurs or gallops.

Dyspnea

A sensation of difficult or uncomfortable breathing, dyspnea varies considerably in its severity. In fact, its severity often bears little relation to that of the underlying disorder.

Dyspnea may develop slowly or suddenly, but an insidious onset is most common. It may subside quickly or persist for years. (See *Causes of dyspnea,* pages 38 and 39.)

If your patient complains of dyspnea, take a health history and perform a physical examination according to the guidelines below.

History of the symptom
To better characterize the patient's dyspnea, consider asking the following questions:
• When did you first feel short of breath?
• Did your shortness of breath start suddenly or gradually?
• Is it constant or intermittent? If intermittent, how often does it occur and how long does it last?
• Have you had similar episodes in the past? How does this episode compare with past episodes (on a scale of 1 to 10, with 1 being "less" and 10 being "much worse")?
• Are the episodes precipitated or aggravated by a specific activity?
• Does dyspnea occur when you're active or while you're resting?
• Does the feeling get better or worse in different positions? Which ones?

• How do you ease the discomfort? Have you used any medications or inhalers?

Associated findings
Note whether the patient has experienced any of the following signs or symptoms:
• anxiety
• chest pain
• fever
• nausea or vomiting (possible aspiration)
• persistent cough
• profuse sweating
• rhinitis
• sore throat
• sputum production
• undue fatigue
• weakness or light-headedness (may indicate hyperventilation)
• wheezing.

Previous conditions and treatments
Consult with the patient, members of his family, or members of the health care team to determine if the patient has a history of any of the following conditions, treatments, or risk factors:
• aspiration of a foreign body or gastric contents
• asthma
• cardiac or chronic obstructive pulmonary disease
• deep vein thrombophlebitis or varicose veins
• emotional stress
• exposure to known or suspected allergens
• a hip or leg fracture
• occupational or environmental exposure to irritants (for example, smoke, coal dust, or other respirable particulates)
• pneumothorax
• recent cardiopulmonary resuscitation, subclavian cannulation, or mechanical ventilation

(Text continues on page 40.)

Causes of dyspnea

Dyspnea is caused by lack of oxygen (hypoxemia), increased work of breathing, and altered ventilatory mechanics. Dyspnea occurs in the following respiratory disorders: adult respiratory distress syndrome (ARDS), aspiration of a foreign body, asthma, cor pulmonale, emphysema, flail chest, inhalation injury, lung cancer, pleural effusion, pneumonia, pneumothorax, pulmonary edema, pulmonary embolism, and tuberculosis.

ARDS
Acute dyspnea is the most common first complaint in this disorder, a life-threatening form of noncardiogenic pulmonary edema. As the syndrome progresses, dyspnea may be accompanied by restlessness, anxiety, decreased mental acuity, tachycardia, and crackles and rhonchi in both lung fields. Severe ARDS can also produce signs of shock, such as hypotension and cool, clammy skin.

Aspiration of a foreign body
Acute dyspnea marks this life-threatening condition and may be accompanied by paroxysmal intercostal, suprasternal, and substernal retractions. Other signs and symptoms may include use of accessory muscles, inspiratory stridor, tachypnea, decreased or absent breath sounds, asymmetrical chest expansion, anxiety, cyanosis, diaphoresis, and hypotension.

Asthma
Attacks of acute dyspnea characterize this chronic disorder. Dyspnea may be accompanied by wheezing, a nonproductive cough, use of accessory muscles, nasal flaring, intercostal and supraclavicular retractions, tachypnea, tachycardia, diaphoresis, prolonged expiration, flushing or cyanosis, and apprehension.

Cor pulmonale
Chronic dyspnea is common in this disorder. Typically, dyspnea begins gradually during exertion and then becomes progressively worse until it also occurs when the patient is at rest. Other common signs include a chronic productive cough, wheezing, tachypnea, distended neck veins, dependent edema, and hepatomegaly.

Emphysema
This chronic disorder gradually causes progressive exertional dyspnea. The patient will usually have a history of smoking or occupational exposure to a respiratory irritant. Accompanying signs and symptoms typically include barrel chest, hypertrophy of accessory muscles, diminished breath sounds, anorexia, weight loss, malaise, tachypnea, pursed-lip breathing, and prolonged exhalation.

Flail chest
Multiple rib fractures cause sudden dyspnea accompanied by paradoxical chest movement, severe chest pain, hypotension, tachypnea, tachycardia, and cyanosis. Bruising and decreased or absent breath sounds may be detected over the affected side.

Inhalation injury
Dyspnea may develop suddenly or gradually (over several hours) after inhalation of chemicals or hot gases. Other signs and symptoms may include hoarseness, a persistent cough, sooty or bloody sputum, oropharyngeal edema, crackles, rhonchi, and wheezing. The patient often exhibits thermal burns, singed nasal hairs, and orofacial burns and may develop signs of respiratory distress.

Causes of dyspnea *(continued)*

Lung cancer
In late-stage cancer, dyspnea develops slowly and becomes progressively worse. Associated findings may include fever, hemoptysis, a productive cough, wheezing, clubbing, chest pain, and a pleural friction rub.

Pleural effusion
In this disorder, dyspnea develops slowly and becomes progressively worse. Accompanying signs may include a nonproductive cough, dullness on percussion, tachycardia, tachypnea, and weight loss. You may also note decreases in chest expansion, tactile fremitus, and breath sounds.

Pneumonia
Dyspnea occurs suddenly and is usually accompanied by fever, shaking chills, pleuritic chest pain that worsens with deep inspiration, and a productive cough. The patient may experience cyanosis, fatigue, headache, myalgia, anorexia, abdominal pain, crackles, rhonchi, tachycardia, tachypnea, and diaphoresis.

Pneumothorax
This life-threatening disorder causes acute dyspnea accompanied by sudden, stabbing chest pain, which may radiate to the arms, face, back, or abdomen. Other signs and symptoms may include anxiety, restlessness, a reduction in blood pressure, a dry cough, cyanosis, decreased vocal fremitus, tachypnea, tachycardia, tympany, decreased or absent breath sounds on the affected side, asymmetrical chest expansion, splinting, and use of accessory muscles. *Tension pneumothorax* is usually accompanied by tracheal deviation, increased severity of anxiety, restlessness, and decreased blood pressure.

Pulmonary edema
In this life-threatening disorder, acute dyspnea may be preceded by signs of congestive heart failure (CHF), such as distended neck veins and orthopnea. Other signs may include cough (dry or producing copious pink, frothy sputum), tachycardia, tachypnea, crackles in both lung fields, an S_3 gallop, oliguria, a thready pulse, hypotension, diaphoresis, cyanosis, and marked anxiety.

Pulmonary embolism
Acute dyspnea usually accompanied by sudden pleuritic chest pain characterizes this life-threatening disorder. Associated findings may include tachycardia, a low-grade fever, tachypnea, cough (dry or producing blood-tinged sputum), a pleural friction rub, crackles, diffuse wheezing, dullness on percussion, decreased breath sounds, diaphoresis, restlessness, and acute anxiety. Signs of shock, such as hypotension and cool, clammy skin, may accompany massive embolism.

Tuberculosis
Dyspnea commonly occurs with chest pain, crackles, and a productive cough. Other findings may include night sweats, fever, anorexia and weight loss, vague dyspepsia, palpitations during mild exertion, and dullness on percussion.

Additional causes
Other causes of dyspnea include interstitial pulmonary fibrosis, arrhythmias, CHF, myocardial infarction, shock, amyotrophic lateral sclerosis, Guillain-Barré syndrome, myasthenia gravis, poliomyelitis, anemia, sepsis, and anxiety or panic attacks, especially when accompanied by hyperventilation.

• recent exposure to fire, steam, super-heated air, or fumes from burning chemicals or synthetic materials
• recent pregnancy
• an upper respiratory tract infection.

Drug history

Find out which medications the patient is taking, and ask about any known drug allergies. Drugs that may produce dyspnea include:
• antibiotics and drugs that can cause an anaphylactic reaction (especially penicillins and cephalosporins)
• drugs that may cause bronchospasm, such as acetylcysteine, adenosine, aspirin and aspirin-related agents (for example, naproxen, a nonsteroidal anti-inflammatory drug), beta blockers (atenolol, metoprolol, and propranolol), and cholinergics
• drugs that may cause left ventricular dysfunction resulting in dyspnea, such as beta blockers (atenolol, metoprolol, and propranolol), calcium channel blockers (diltiazem, nifedipine, and verapamil), and negative inotropic agents (flecainide, procainamide, and quinidine)
• drugs that may cause pulmonary fibrosis resulting in dyspnea, such as amiodarone, bleomycin, busulfan, melphalan, and nitrofurantoin.

Dyspnea may also occur during withdrawal from corticosteroid therapy if the respiratory condition being treated exacerbates.

Physical examination

Assess the patient's vital signs, including temperature, blood pressure, respiratory rate and depth, and pulse rate and rhythm. Then examine the patient according to the steps described below.

Inspection

• Observe the patient for personal hygiene, nutritional status, and level of comfort.

• Check the patient's respirations, noting their rate and depth. Look for abnormal respiratory patterns and signs of difficult breathing, such as grunting, pursed-lip exhalation, flared nostrils, intercostal retractions during inhalation and bulging on exhalation, and stridor during inhalation. Also note whether the patient takes frequent deep breaths or sighs (hyperventilation may cause a sensation of not getting enough air).
• Look for signs of chronic dyspnea, such as hypertrophy of accessory muscles (particularly shoulder and neck muscles).
• Observe for peripheral edema, finger clubbing, barrel chest, and distended neck veins.
• Inspect for oropharyngeal edema, singed nasal hairs, orofacial burns, prolonged capillary refill time, chest bruising, and ascites.
• Note the color, consistency, amount, and odor of any sputum.
• Inspect for asymmetrical chest expansion.

Palpation

• Gently palpate the neck for tracheal deviation.
• Palpate the chest for decreased diaphragmatic excursion, subcutaneous crepitation, and decreased tactile fremitus.
• Palpate the skin for diaphoresis.

Percussion

• Percuss over both lungs. Note any hyperresonance, tympany, or dullness.

Auscultation

• Auscultate the lungs for crackles, rhonchi, wheezing, decreased or absent unilateral breath sounds, egophony, bronchophony, decreased vocal fremitus, and a pleural friction rub.
• Listen over the heart for tachycardia, a pericardial friction rub, and abnor-

mal sounds or rhythms, such as ventricular or atrial gallop.

Nonproductive cough

A noisy, forceful expulsion of air from the lungs that's free of sputum or blood, a nonproductive cough represents one of the most common complaints of patients with respiratory disorders. What's more, a nonproductive cough that turns productive is a classic sign of progressive respiratory disease.

Normally, the cough reflex serves as a protective mechanism that clears airway passages. The reflex may be activated by a mechanical, chemical, thermal, inflammatory, or psychogenic stimulus. Or it may result from external pressure caused, for example, by subdiaphragmatic irritation or a mediastinal tumor. Some individuals cough voluntarily as a nervous habit.

If the patient has paroxysms of coughing, the cough may become more frequent and progressively worse. Persistent nonproductive coughing can cause damage, such as airway collapse or alveoli or bleb rupture.

An acute cough occurs spontaneously and is typically self-limiting. A cough that persists longer than 30 days is considered to be chronic and may have many causes. (See *Causes of a nonproductive cough,* pages 42 and 43.)

If your patient reports a persistent nonproductive cough, take his health history and perform a physical examination according to the guidelines below.

History of the sign
To better understand your patient's nonproductive cough, consider asking the following questions:
• When did your cough start? Do you experience bouts of coughing? How frequently do you cough? (*Note:* Patients commonly are unaware of the frequency or severity of a cough. Family members can often provide more accurate information.)
• Does the cough get worse at night or when you lie down? Is it worse first thing in the morning? During a particular activity?
• What factors aggravate it? What factors alleviate it?
• How would you characterize the sound of your cough (harsh, brassy, dry, hacking)?
• Do you have chest pain when you cough? If so, where does the pain occur? Does it radiate?

Associated findings
Note whether the patient has experienced any of the following signs or symptoms:
• activity intolerance
• chest pain or tightness
• dyspnea
• fatigue
• symptoms of upper respiratory infection (such as a stuffy or runny nose, ear congestion, sore throat, headache, or postnasal drip)
• weight loss
• wheezing.

Previous conditions and treatments
Consult with the patient, members of his family, or members of the health care team to determine if the patient has a history of any of the following conditions, treatments, or risk factors:
• allergies (especially to pets, dust, food, or pollen)
• chronic cardiovascular or pulmonary disease
• exposure to cigarette smoke (smoking or living or working with someone who does)

(Text continues on page 44.)

Causes of a nonproductive cough

Respiratory disorders that may cause a nonproductive cough include airway occlusion, asthma, atelectasis, chronic bronchitis, bronchogenic carcinoma, interstitial lung disease, laryngeal cancer, Legionnaires' disease, lung abscess, pleural effusion, pneumonia, pneumothorax, pulmonary edema, and pulmonary embolism.

Airway occlusion
Partial occlusion of the upper airway leads to sudden onset of dry, paroxysmal coughing. The patient typically gags, wheezes, and becomes hoarse. You may also note stridor, tachycardia, and decreased breath sounds.

Asthma
An acute attack of asthma often begins with a nonproductive cough and mild wheezing that progresses to severe dyspnea, audible wheezing, chest tightness, and a cough that produces thick mucus. Associated signs and symptoms may include apprehension, rhonchi, prolonged exhalations, intercostal and supraclavicular retractions on inhalation, use of accessory muscles, flaring nostrils, tachypnea, tachycardia, diaphoresis, and flushing or cyanosis.

Atelectasis
In this disorder, deflating lung tissue stimulates cough receptors, causing a nonproductive cough. Associated findings may include pleuritic chest pain, anxiety, dyspnea, tachypnea, and tachycardia. The patient may have cyanotic and diaphoretic skin and decreased breath sounds, and his chest may be dull on percussion. You may also note inspiratory lag, substernal or intercostal retractions, decreased vocal fremitus, and tracheal deviation toward the affected side.

Bronchogenic carcinoma
Early indicators of this disorder include a chronic nonproductive cough, dyspnea, vague chest pain and, occasionally, wheezing.

Interstitial lung disease
This disorder typically produces a nonproductive cough and progressive dyspnea. Other signs and symptoms may include central cyanosis, finger clubbing, fine crackles, fatigue, variable chest pain, tachycardia, tachypnea, and weight loss.

Laryngeal cancer
A mild nonproductive cough accompanied by minor throat discomfort and hoarseness is an early sign of laryngeal cancer. As the disease progresses, the patient may experience dysphagia, dyspnea, cervical lymphadenodopathy, stridor, and earache.

Legionnaires' disease
A nonproductive cough follows a prodrome of malaise, headache and, possibly, diarrhea, anorexia, diffuse myalgia, and general weakness. Later, the cough produces sputum that's mucoid, mucopurulent and, possibly, tinged with blood.

Lung abscess
A nonproductive cough is an early sign of this disorder. Other early signs and symptoms include weakness, dyspnea, and pleuritic chest pain and may include diaphoresis, fever, headache, malaise, fatigue, crackles, decreased breath sounds, anorexia, and weight loss. Later, the cough produces copious sputum that's purulent, foul-smelling and, possibly, tinged with blood.

Pleural effusion
A nonproductive cough is common in pleural effusion. Other signs and symp-

Causes of a nonproductive cough *(continued)*

toms include dyspnea, pleuritic chest pain, decreased chest motion, a pleural friction rub, tachycardia, and tachypnea. You may note flatness on percussion, decreased or absent breath sounds, and decreased tactile fremitus.

Pneumonia

Bacterial pneumonia usually starts with a dry, hacking, painful cough that rapidly progresses to a productive cough. Other findings include shaking chills, headache, high fever, dyspnea, pleuritic chest pain, tachypnea, tachycardia, grunting respirations, nasal flaring, decreased breath sounds, fine crackles, rhonchi, and cyanosis. When assessing the chest, you may note dullness on percussion. If consolidation is present, you'll note egophony, bronchophony, and bronchial breath sounds.

In mycoplasmal pneumonia, a harsh, barking, nonproductive cough typically begins 2 to 3 days after the onset of malaise, headache, and sore throat. Paroxysmal coughing can result in substernal chest pain. Fever is common; however, the patient doesn't appear seriously ill.

Viral pneumonia causes a nonproductive, hacking cough and the gradual onset of malaise, headache, anorexia, and a low-grade fever.

A nonproductive cough accompanied by fever and dyspnea may develop insidiously in *Pneumocystis carinii* pneumonia, an opportunistic infection often seen in patients with acquired immunodeficiency syndrome.

Pneumothorax

This life-threatening disorder may cause a dry cough, but signs and symptoms of respiratory distress (such as severe dyspnea, tachycardia, tachypnea, and cyanosis) are more common.

Pulmonary edema

Early signs and symptoms include a dry cough, dyspnea on exertion, paroxysmal nocturnal dyspnea, orthopnea, tachycardia, tachypnea, dependent crackles, and ventricular gallop. In severe pulmonary edema, respirations become rapid and labored with diffuse crackles, and the patient's cough produces frothy, bloody sputum.

Pulmonary embolism

This life-threatening disorder may produce a dry cough, although a cough that produces blood-tinged sputum is more common. Other common findings include dyspnea, pleuritic or anginal chest pain, a low-grade fever, and tachycardia. Less common findings include massive hemoptysis, chest splinting, and leg edema. If the embolus is large, you may note cyanosis, syncope, distended neck veins, a pleural friction rub, diffuse wheezing, dullness on percussion, and decreased breath sounds.

Additional causes

A nonproductive cough may be caused by a common cold, sarcoidosis, chronic sinusitis, acute tracheobronchitis, coccidioidomycosis, hypersensitivity, laryngitis, esophageal achalasia, esophageal diverticula, esophageal occlusion, gastroesophageal reflux, thoracic aortic aneurysm, Hodgkin's disease, mediastinal tumor, psittacosis, or pericardial effusion.

Angiotensin-converting enzyme inhibitors and inhalation of various drugs (such as bronchodilators, inhaled corticosteroids, cromolyn sodium, and pentamidine) can cause coughing. Treatments such as suctioning, incentive spirometry, and bronchoscopy may also stimulate coughing.

• GI problems, such as indigestion, heartburn, vomiting, or epigastric pain
• recent exposure to smoke or irritating fumes or chemicals
• recent upper respiratory tract infection, surgery, or trauma
• suctioning, incentive spirometry, or bronchoscopy.

Drug history

Find out which medications the patient is taking (including over-the-counter ones), and ask about any known drug allergies. Ask about recent changes in the schedule or dosage of prescribed drugs. Note any past or current use of the following drugs:
• angiotensin-converting enzyme inhibitors (captopril, enalapril, lisinopril, quinapril, and ramipril)
• those that are inhaled and could irritate the bronchial mucosa, such as inhaled bronchodilators (albuterol, ipratropium, and metaproterenol), inhaled corticosteroids (beclomethasone and triamcinolone), cromolyn sodium, and pentamidine.

Physical examination

Assess the patient's vital signs, including temperature, blood pressure, respiratory rate and depth, and pulse rate and rhythm. Then examine the patient according to the steps described below.

Inspection

• Observe the patient's general appearance, personal hygiene, nutritional status, and level of consciousness. Note any discomfort, restlessness, or agitation.
• Inspect the skin for pallor, sweating, or flushing. Assess the skin, nail beds, and mucous membranes for cyanosis.
• Examine the patient's fingers for clubbing and lower extremities for edema.
• Inspect the nose and throat for congestion, inflammation, drainage, or signs of infection.

• Inspect the neck and abdomen for signs of accessory muscle use. Examine the chest for retractions or abnormal chest wall motion.

Palpation

• Palpate the neck for tracheal deviation and for enlarged lymph nodes.
• Palpate the chest for excursion and vocal fremitus.

Percussion

• Percuss the chest for dullness, tympany, or flatness.

Auscultation

• Auscultate the lungs for abnormal, adventitious, or absent or diminished breath sounds. Also listen for a pleural friction rub.
• Auscultate the heart for murmurs or gallops.

Productive cough

A productive cough clears airways of accumulated secretions that normal mucociliary action fails to remove. In most cases, it's a reflexive response to stimulation of the airway mucosa. A productive cough may contain sputum, blood, or both. The color, consistency, amount, and odor of the sputum provides important clues about the patient's condition.

A productive cough usually results from a respiratory disorder, such as an acute or a chronic infection that causes inflammation, edema, and increased mucus production in the airways. However, it can also result from inhalation of allergenic or irritating substances or foreign bodies. In fact, the most common cause of chronic productive coughing is cigarette smoking, which produces mucoid sputum.

Many patients fail to understand the significance of a chronic productive cough and put off seeking medical attention until an associated problem, such as dyspnea, hemoptysis, chest pain, weight loss, or recurrent respiratory infection, develops. This delay can have serious consequences because productive coughing can signal several life-threatening disorders, such as lung cancer or tuberculosis. (See *Causes of a productive cough,* pages 46 to 48.)

If your patient reports a productive cough, take his health history and perform a physical examination according to the guidelines below.

History of the sign
To better understand the nature of the patient's productive cough, consider asking the following questions:
• How long have you had this cough? Does it seem to be getting worse or better?
• How often do you have bouts of coughing? Do coughs occur singly or in spasms? (*Note:* Patients commonly are unaware of the frequency or severity of a cough. Family members can often provide more accurate information.)
• Can you describe the color and tenacity of your sputum? Does it have an odor? Does it contain blood?
• Do you cough up a lot of sputum each day? Is your cough most productive in the morning?
• Is coughing precipitated or aggravated by a particular activity or position?
• How would you describe the sound of your cough (hacking, brassy)?
• Have you experienced any chest pain when you cough? If so, where is the pain located?

Associated findings
Note whether the patient has experienced any of the following signs or symptoms:
• chest pain
• dyspnea
• fatigue

• fever
• sinus congestion or postnasal drip
• weight loss
• wheezing.

Previous conditions
Consult with the patient, members of his family, or members of the health care team to determine if the patient has a history of any of the following conditions or risk factors:
• alcohol or drug abuse
• allergies
• chronic cardiovascular or pulmonary disease
• cigarette smoking
• human immunodeficiency virus (HIV) infection or a high risk for HIV infection
• recent exposure to respirable irritants, such as smoke, toxic fumes, or asbestos.

Drug history
Find out which medications the patient is taking (including over-the-counter ones), and ask about any known drug allergies. Ask about any recent changes in the schedule or dosage of prescribed drugs. Expectorants and bronchodilators may induce a productive cough. Note any past or current use of the following drugs:
• ammonium chloride
• bronchodilators (albuterol and metaproterenol)
• calcium iodide
• guaifenesin
• potassium iodide
• terpin hydrate.

Physical examination
Assess the patient's vital signs, including temperature, blood pressure, respiratory rate and depth, and pulse rate and rhythm. Then examine the patient according to the steps described on pages 48 and 49.

(Text continues on page 48.)

Causes of a productive cough

Respiratory disorders that may cause a productive cough include aspiration pneumonitis, asthma, bronchiectasis, chemical pneumonitis, chronic bronchitis, Legionnaires' disease, lung abscess (ruptured), lung cancer, pneumonia, pulmonary edema, pulmonary embolism, pulmonary emphysema, pulmonary tuberculosis, silicosis, and tracheobronchitis.

Aspiration pneumonitis
The patient typically has a cough that produces pink, frothy and, possibly, purulent sputum. Associated signs and symptoms include marked dyspnea, fever, tachypnea, tachycardia, wheezing, and cyanosis.

Asthma
In a severe (possibly life-threatening) attack of asthma, the patient's cough may produce tenacious mucoid sputum and mucus plugs. The attack typically starts with a dry cough and mild wheezing and then progresses to severe dyspnea, audible wheezing, chest tightness, and a productive cough. Other findings may include apprehension, prolonged exhalation, intercostal and supraclavicular retraction on inhalation, use of accessory muscles, rhonchi, crackles, nasal flaring, tachypnea, tachycardia, diaphoresis, and flushing or cyanosis.

Bronchiectasis
Chronic coughing produces copious, mucopurulent sputum with characteristic layers: the top is frothy, the middle is clear, and the bottom is dense with purulent particles. Halitosis is common and the patient's sputum may smell foul or overwhelmingly sweet. Associated findings include hemoptysis, persistent coarse crackles, wheezing, rhonchi, dyspnea on exertion, weight loss, fatigue, malaise, weakness, and recurrent fever. Finger clubbing is a late sign.

Chemical pneumonitis
This disorder causes coughing that produces purulent sputum. Other findings may include dyspnea, wheezing, orthopnea, fever, malaise, crackles, laryngitis, or rhinitis. Examination may reveal irritation of mucous membranes of the conjunctivae, throat, and nose. Signs and symptoms may intensify for 24 to 48 hours after exposure and then resolve. However, if the disorder is severe, symptoms may recur 2 to 5 weeks later.

Chronic bronchitis
In chronic bronchitis, a chronic, productive cough occurs on most days for at least 3 months a year for 2 consecutive years. The cough produces mucoid sputum that may become purulent, blood-tinged, or foul-smelling with infection. Coughing occurs most often when the patient is lying down or when he gets up after sleeping. Paroxysmal coughing may occur during exercise. Other signs and symptoms may include prolonged exhalation, use of accessory muscles, barrel chest, tachypnea, cyanosis, wheezing, dyspnea on exertion, scattered rhonchi, and coarse crackles (precipitated by coughing).

Legionnaires' disease
A dry cough that develops during the initial 48 hours eventually produces scant sputum, which is mucoid and nonpurulent and may be streaked with blood. Other early signs and symptoms include high fever, chills, malaise, fatigue, weakness, anorexia, and diffuse myalgia. Many patients also have pleuritic chest pain, headache, tachypnea, tachycardia, nausea, vomiting, dyspnea, crackles, mild temporary am-

Causes of a productive cough *(continued)*

nesia, disorientation, confusion, flushing, mild diaphoresis, and prostration.

Lung abscess (ruptured)
The cardinal sign of a ruptured lung abscess is a cough that produces copious amounts of purulent, foul-smelling, and possibly blood-tinged sputum. The cough may be accompanied by diaphoresis, anorexia, finger clubbing, weight loss, weakness, fatigue, fever, chills, dyspnea, headache, malaise, pleuritic chest pain, halitosis, inspiratory crackles, and tubular or amphoric breath sounds over the abscess. Percussion of the chest may reveal dullness on the affected side; however, if a large cavity remains after the abscess drains, the percussion note may be hyperresonant.

Lung cancer
A chronic cough that produces small amounts of purulent or mucopurulent blood-streaked sputum is an early sign of bronchogenic carcinoma. A cough associated with bronchioalveolar cancer produces large amounts of frothy sputum. Other signs and symptoms may include dyspnea, anorexia, fatigue, weight loss, chest pain, fever, diaphoresis, wheezing, and finger clubbing.

Pneumonia
The characteristics of the patient's cough depend on the underlying cause of his pneumonia. Bacterial pneumonia causes a dry cough that later becomes productive. Coughing associated with pneumococcal pneumonia may produce rust-colored sputum. In *Klebsiella* pneumonia, the cough may produce "brick red" or "currant jelly" sputum. In staphylococcal pneumonia, the sputum may be salmon-colored; in streptococcal pneumonia, it's mucopurulent. Mycoplasmal

pneumonia may cause a cough that produces scant, blood-flecked sputum; however, a nonproductive cough that starts 2 to 3 days after the onset of malaise, headache, fever, and sore throat is most common. Paroxysmal coughing causes substernal chest pain.

Pulmonary edema
In severe pulmonary edema, coughing produces frothy, bloody sputum. Early signs of this disorder include a dry cough, dyspnea on exertion, and paroxysmal nocturnal dyspnea that progresses to orthopnea. Other early signs and symptoms include fever, fatigue, tachycardia, tachypnea, dependent crackles, and ventricular gallop. As respiration becomes rapid and labored, the patient develops diffuse crackles, a productive cough, increased tachycardia and, possibly, arrhythmia. The patient's pulse becomes thready, his blood pressure falls, and his skin becomes cold, clammy, and cyanotic.

Pulmonary embolism
This life-threatening disorder can cause a productive or nonproductive cough. When productive, the cough yields blood-tinged sputum. Often, severe dyspnea is the first symptom of pulmonary embolism. Dyspnea may be accompanied by anginal or pleuritic chest pain. Other common signs include marked anxiety, a low-grade fever, tachycardia, tachypnea, and diaphoresis. Less common signs include massive hemoptysis, chest splinting, leg edema, cyanosis (with a large embolus), syncope, distended neck veins, a pleural friction rub, diffuse wheezing, crackles, chest dullness on percussion, decreased breath sounds, and evidence of circulatory collapse.

(continued)

Causes of a productive cough *(continued)*

Pulmonary emphysema
Patients with pure emphysema experience very little coughing or none at all. If present, the cough is dry. If the patient also has chronic bronchitis or an acute infection, the cough may be productive. Associated findings may include weight loss, use of accessory muscles, tachypnea, grunting pursed-lip exhalations, diminished breath sounds, dyspnea on exertion, rhonchi, barrel chest, and anorexia.

Pulmonary tuberculosis
In this disorder, a mild to severe productive cough may be accompanied by hemoptysis, malaise, dyspnea, and pleuritic chest pain. Sputum may be scant and mucoid or copious and purulent. Nights sweats, fatigue, weight loss, and amphoric breath sounds are common. Percussion may reveal dullness. Palpation after coughing may reveal increased tactile fremitus.

Silicosis
A productive cough with mucopurulent sputum is an early sign in silicosis. Other signs and symptoms include dyspnea on exertion, tachypnea, weight loss, fatigue, weakness, and recurrent respiratory infection. Auscultation reveals end-inspiratory fine crackles at the lung bases.

Tracheobronchitis
Initially, inflammation causes onset of a nonproductive cough. The cough becomes productive as secretions increase. Sputum may be mucoid, mucopurulent, or purulent. Other findings include chills, a sore throat, a slight fever, muscle and back pain, and substernal tightness. The patient typically has rhonchi and wheezes and may have crackles. Severe tracheobronchitis may cause fever and bronchospasm.

Additional causes
Although rare, a productive cough may be caused by fungal infections such as actinomycosis, blastomycosis, and psittacosis. Treatments and diagnostic testing for pulmonary disorders may aggravate a productive cough. Expectorants and bronchodilators may increase sputum production and contribute to a productive cough.

Inspection
• Observe the patient's general appearance, personal hygiene, nutritional status, and level of consciousness. Note any discomfort, restlessness, or agitation. Also note whether he looks older than his given age.
• Inspect the skin for cyanosis.
• Examine the patient's mouth and nose for congestion, drainage, or inflammation. Note his breath odor; halitosis may suggest pulmonary infection.
• Assess for the use of accessory muscles and for retractions.
• Examine the patient's chest for symmetry.

Palpation
• Palpate the skin for diaphoresis and temperature.
• Palpate the chest for respiratory excursion, symmetry, and vocal and tactile fremitus.

Percussion
• Percuss the chest for dullness, tympany, or flatness and diaphragmatic excursion.

Auscultation

• Auscultate the lungs for abnormal or diminished breath sounds, wheezing, crackles, rhonchi, and a pleural friction rub. If abnormal, auscultate for egophony and bronchophony.

Hemoptysis

An ominous and frightening sign, hemoptysis is the expectoration of blood or bloody sputum from the lungs or tracheobronchial tree. It can range from mild (blood-streaked sputum) to severe (frank, red and frothy bleeding that may be life-threatening).

Common causes of hemoptysis include chronic bronchitis, bronchogenic carcinoma, or bronchiectasis; however, the sign can accompany inflammatory, infectious, cardiovascular, or coagulation disorders or, rarely, ruptured aortic aneurysm. In approximately 15% of patients, the cause is unknown. *Massive hemoptysis* most commonly results from lung cancer, bronchiectasis, active tuberculosis, or cavitary pulmonary disease brought on by necrotic infections or tuberculosis. (See *Causes of hemoptysis,* pages 50 and 51.)

If your patient is expectorating large amounts of blood, anticipate emergency endotracheal intubation and suctioning. As time permits, take the patient's health history and perform a physical examination according to the guidelines below.

History of the sign

To better understand the patient's hemoptysis, consider asking the following questions:

• When did you begin coughing up blood?
• Have you experienced similar episodes in the past?
• How often do you cough up blood? How much blood is produced? (Help the patient quantify the amount by suggesting measurements, such as a teaspoon, a tablespoon, or half of a cup.)
• Are you coughing up more blood now than in the past?
• Are the episodes becoming more frequent?

Associated findings

Note whether the patient has experienced any of the following signs or symptoms:

• chest, neck, or abdominal pain (ask about characteristics and location)
• dysphagia
• dyspnea
• fever
• hoarseness
• increased sputum production
• nausea
• vomiting.

Previous conditions and treatments

Consult with the patient, members of his family, or members of the health care team to determine if the patient has a history of any of the following conditions, treatments, or risk factors:

• a bleeding disorder
• cardiovascular disease
• chest trauma
• cigarette smoking (ask how long the patient has smoked and how much)
• a hip or leg fracture
• pneumonia
• prolonged bed rest
• pulmonary disease
• a recent flulike syndrome, including headache, anorexia, fever, chills, weakness, and weight loss
• recent invasive pulmonary procedures (such as bronchoscopy, laryngoscopy, or lung biopsy)
• thrombophlebitis or varicose veins.

Drug history

Find out which medications the patient is taking (including over-the-counter ones), and ask about any known drug

Causes of hemoptysis

Respiratory disorders that may cause hemoptysis include bronchiectasis, chronic bronchitis, laryngeal cancer, lung cancer, lung abscess, pulmonary edema, pulmonary embolism with infarction, pulmonary hypertension, pulmonary tuberculosis, and silicosis.

Bronchiectasis
In this disorder, hemoptysis results from inflamed bronchial surfaces and eroded bronchial blood vessels. The patient may expectorate blood-tinged sputum or blood; the sputum may be copious, foul-smelling, and purulent. The patient may have a chronic cough, coarse crackles, fever, weight loss, fatigue, weakness, malaise, and dyspnea on exertion. Finger clubbing is a late sign.

Chronic bronchitis
A common first sign in this disorder is a productive cough that lasts 3 or more months and eventually produces blood-streaked sputum. Massive hemorrhage is unusual. Other common signs and symptoms include dyspnea, prolonged exhalation, wheezing, scattered rhonchi, use of accessory muscles, barrel chest, and tachypnea.

Laryngeal cancer
Hemoptysis typically follows hoarseness, which occurs early in the disorder. Other findings may include dysphagia, dyspnea, stridor, cervical lymphadenopathy, and neck pain.

Lung abscess
Coughing in lung abscess typically produces large amounts of purulent, foul-smelling sputum. In about half of all patients, the sputum is blood-streaked because of bronchial ulceration, necrosis, and granulation tissue. Other common signs and symptoms include fever, chills, diaphoresis, anorexia, weight loss, headache, weakness, dyspnea, pleuritic or dull chest pain, and finger clubbing. Auscultation reveals tubular or cavernous breath sounds and crackles. Percussion reveals dullness on the affected side; however, if a large cavity remains after the abscess drains, the percussion note may be hyperresonant.

Lung cancer
Recurring hemoptysis caused by ulceration of the bronchus is an early sign of lung cancer. The expectoration may range from blood-streaked sputum to blood. Related findings include a productive cough, dyspnea, fever, anorexia, weight loss, and wheezing. Chest pain is a late symptom.

Pulmonary edema
Severe pulmonary edema, both cardiogenic and noncardiogenic, commonly causes frothy, blood-tinged, pink sputum. Other signs and symptoms include severe dyspnea, orthopnea, gasping, anxiety, cyanosis, diffuse crackles, ventricular gallop, and cold, clammy skin. Less common signs include tachycardia, lethargy, cardiac arrhythmias, tachypnea, hypotension, and a thready pulse.

Pulmonary embolism with infarction
Hemoptysis is a common finding in this life-threatening disorder. Massive hemoptysis is less common. Early symptoms typically include dyspnea and anginal or pleuritic chest pain. Other signs include tachycardia, tachypnea, a low-grade fever, and diaphoresis. Examination reveals decreased breath sounds, a pleural friction rub, crackles, diffuse wheezing, dullness on percussion, signs of circulatory collapse (a weak, rapid pulse; hypotension), signs of cerebral ischemia (transient loss of consciousness, seizures), and signs of hypoxemia (restlessness, hemiplegia, and other focal neurologic deficits).

Causes of hemoptysis *(continued)*

Pulmonary hypertension
Common signs and symptoms, which typically develop late is this disorder, include hemoptysis, dyspnea on exertion, and fatigue. The patient may experience pain on exertion that's similar to anginal pain and that may radiate to the neck but not to the arms. Other findings include arrhythmias, syncope, cough, and hoarseness.

Pulmonary tuberculosis
Sputum tinged or streaked with blood is common in tuberculosis. Massive hemoptysis may occur in advanced cavitary tuberculosis. Accompanying signs and symptoms may include a chronic productive cough, fine crackles after coughing, dyspnea, dullness on percussion, increased tactile fremitus, amphoric breath sounds, night sweats, malaise, fatigue, fever, anorexia, weight loss, and pleuritic chest pain.

Silicosis
Initially, this chronic disorder causes a productive cough with mucopurulent sputum. In time, the sputum becomes blood-streaked and massive hemoptysis may occur. Other findings may include fine, end-inspiratory crackles at lung bases, dyspnea on exertion, tachypnea, weight loss, fatigue, and weakness.

Additional causes
Hemoptysis may be associated with pulmonary involvement in systemic lupus erythematosus, Wegener's granulomatosis, tracheal trauma, thrombocytopenia, or disseminated intravascular coagulation. Also, lung or airway injury from bronchoscopy, laryngoscopy, mediastinoscopy, or lung biopsy can cause bleeding and hemoptysis. On rare occasions, an aortic aneurysm ruptures into the tracheobronchial tree, causing hemoptysis and sudden death. Drugs that may be associated with hemoptysis include anticoagulants and aspirin.

---

allergies. Note any past or current use of the following drugs:
* anticoagulants
* aspirin
* oral contraceptives.

Physical examination
Assess the patient's vital signs, including temperature, blood pressure, respiratory rate and depth, and pulse rate and rhythm. Then examine the patient according to the steps described below.

Inspection
* Observe the patient's general appearance and level of consciousness. Look for signs of restlessness, anxiety, lethargy, stupor, or coma. Be prepared to intervene if a change in the patient's condition warrants emergency measures.

* Examine the patient's nose, mouth, and pharynx for sources of bleeding. For example, check for poor oral or dental hygiene or gingivitis. Note the color, consistency, amount, and odor of sputum.

* Observe the rate and depth of the patient's respirations. Note whether he is having difficulty breathing. Record any change in his normal respiratory pattern.

* Observe the chest for abnormal movement, use of accessory muscles, and retractions. Note any distention of neck veins.

• Inspect the skin for lesions, pallor, or central or peripheral cyanosis.

Palpation
• Palpate the patient's chest, noting any asymmetry, tenderness, respiratory excursion, fremitus, or abnormal pulsations. If the patient has a history of trauma, carefully palpate for tracheal deviation and note any edema.
• Palpate the skin for diaphoresis.

Percussion
• Percuss the lungs for flatness, dullness, hyperresonance, or tympany.

Auscultation
• Auscultate all lung fields for quality and intensity of breath sounds. Listen for crackles, rhonchi, and wheezing.
• Auscultate the heart for murmurs, gallops, bruits, and a pleural friction rub.

Chills

Extreme, involuntary muscle contractions, chills are accompanied by fever and characteristic paroxysms of violent shivering and teeth-chattering. They tend to arise suddenly and often herald infection.

Certain neoplastic conditions may also cause chills. Some disorders, such as pneumococcal pneumonia, produce a single, shaking chill. Other pneumonias produce intermittent chills with recurring high fever. (See *Causes of chills.*)

If your patient reports chills, take his health history and perform a physical examination according to the guidelines below.

History of the sign
To better characterize the patient's chills, consider asking the following questions:

• When did your latest episode of chills begin?
• Have you had similar episodes in the past? How long does each episode last?
• Are episodes isolated or do they recur? How often do they recur?
• Have fever and sweating accompanied your chills?

Associated findings
Note whether the patient has experienced any of the following signs or symptoms:
• chest pain
• dyspnea
• fatigue
• fever
• headache
• malaise
• myalgia
• productive cough.

Previous conditions
Consult with the patient, members of his family, or members of the health care team to determine if the patient has a history of any of the following conditions or risk factors:
• allergies
• exposure to someone with a respiratory infection, such as pneumonia or influenza
• human immunodeficiency virus (HIV) infection or a high risk for HIV infection
• a recent or chronic infection
• a recent fever for which he took aspirin.

Drug history
Find out which medications the patient is taking (including over-the-counter ones), and ask about any known drug allergies. Note any past or current use of amphotericin B.

Physical examination
Assess the patient's vital signs, including temperature, blood pressure, respiratory rate and depth, and pulse rate

Causes of chills

Respiratory disorders that may cause chills include Legionnaires' disease, lung abscess, and pneumonia.

Legionnaires' disease
Within 12 to 48 hours after onset of this disease, the patient suddenly develops chills and a high fever. Prodromal signs and symptoms often include malaise, headache, diarrhea, anorexia, diffuse myalgia, and weakness. An initially nonproductive cough progresses to a cough that produces mucoid or mucopurulent sputum, and hemoptysis may occur. Other signs and symptoms may include nausea, vomiting, confusion, mild, temporary amnesia, pleuritic chest pain, dyspnea, tachypnea, crackles, tachycardia, and skin that's flushed and mildly diaphoretic.

Lung abscess
In addition to chills, lung abscess causes fever, sweating, pleuritic chest pain, dyspnea, finger clubbing, weakness, headache, malaise, anorexia, weight loss, and a cough that produces large amounts of sputum that's purulent, foul-smelling, and often bloody.

Pneumonia
A single shaking chill suggests the sudden onset of pneumococcal pneumonia; other pneumonias characteristically cause intermittent chills. In all pneumonias, related findings may include fever, a cough that produces bloody sputum, pleuritic chest pain, dyspnea, tachypnea, tachycardia, cyanosis, and diaphoresis. Occasionally, aches, anorexia, fatigue, and headache are present. Examination may reveal bronchial breath sounds, crackles, rhonchi, increased tactile fremitus, and grunting respirations.

Nonrespiratory causes
Chills may be caused by localized bacterial infections, such as pelvic inflammatory disease, pyelonephritis, septic arthritis, sinusitis, and otitis media. Generalized infections (such as bacteremia, septic shock, and influenza) and tick-borne diseases (such as malaria and Rocky Mountain spotted fever) also cause chills. Chills can result from lymphomas, transfusion reactions, and some drugs, such as amphotericin B.

and rhythm. Then examine the patient according to the steps described below.

Inspection
• Obtain a rectal or aural temperature for accuracy.
• Inspect the skin for cyanosis or pallor.
• Observe the neck, chest, and abdomen for signs that the patient is using accessory muscles.

Palpation
• Palpate the chest for tenderness, respiratory excursion, and tactile fremitus.
• Palpate the skin for diaphoresis.

Percussion
• Percuss the chest for dullness caused by consolidation.

Auscultation
• Auscultate the lungs for abnormal breath sounds, crackles, rhonchi, egophony, and bronchophony.

Fatigue

Fatigue is a feeling of excessive tiredness, lack of energy, or exhaustion accompanied by a strong desire to rest or sleep. This common symptom differs from weakness, which reflects muscle involvement, but may occur with it.

Fatigue represents a normal response to overexertion, prolonged emotional stress, and sleep deprivation. However, it can also be a nonspecific symptom of a psychological or physiologic disorder — especially viral infections and endocrine, cardiovascular, or neurologic disease. In pulmonary disorders, fatigue results from an insufficient supply of oxygen to meet metabolic demands and may be expressed as an intolerance to activity. (See *Causes of fatigue*.)

If your patient complains of fatigue, take his health history and perform a physical examination according to the guidelines below.

History of the symptom

To better characterize your patient's fatigue, consider asking the following questions:
- How long have you felt tired?
- Is your fatigue constant or intermittent?
- What precipitates or aggravates your fatigue? What relieves it?
- Does your fatigue limit your activities? How much activity can you tolerate before becoming tired?

Associated findings

Note whether the patient has experienced any of the following signs or symptoms:
- anxiety or restlessness
- cyanosis
- dyspnea
- loss of consciousness
- nausea or vomiting
- pain or discomfort
- palpitations
- periodic weakness
- persistent cough
- tachypnea.

Causes of fatigue

Respiratory disorders that cause fatigue include chronic obstructive pulmonary disease (COPD) and pulmonary hypertension.

COPD

The earliest and most persistent symptoms of COPD are progressive fatigue and dyspnea. Other signs may include a chronic cough that's unusually productive, weight loss, barrel chest, cyanosis, and slight dependent edema.

Pulmonary hypertension

Patients with pulmonary hypertension are easily fatigued and typically experience dyspnea on exertion and, possibly, syncope. As the disease progresses, dyspnea may occur at rest. If the patient also has right ventricular failure, edema, ascites, neck vein distention, and hepatomegaly may be evident.

Nonrespiratory causes

Fatigue is a common nonspecific sign for many disorders, including endocrine, neuromuscular, and cardiovascular disease, as well as depression, anxiety, rheumatoid arthritis, systemic lupus erythematosus, renal failure, and infection. Fatigue may be caused by a variety of drugs, most notably antihypertensives and sedatives. In digitalis glycoside therapy, fatigue may indicate toxicity.

Previous conditions

Consult with the patient, members of his family, or members of the health care team to determine if the patient has a history of any of the following conditions or risk factors:

• congenital heart anomalies
• emotional stress
• hypertension
• a recent change in daily routine
• rheumatic fever.

Drug history

Find out which medications the patient is taking (including over-the-counter ones), and ask about any known drug allergies. Note any past or current use of the following drugs:

• antihypertensives
• carbamazepine (can cause somnolence)
• corticosteroids (from neuropathy)
• digitalis glycosides
• negative inotropic agents (flecainide, procainamide, and quinidine) if they cause left ventricular failure
• sedatives.

Physical examination

Assess the patient's vital signs, including temperature, blood pressure, respiratory rate and depth, and pulse rate and rhythm. Then examine the patient according to the steps described below.

Inspection

• Observe the patient's general appearance. Note any sign of distress or troubled breathing.
• Inspect the skin for signs of cyanosis.
• Inspect the chest for barrel chest or other deformities. Examine the chest, neck, and abdomen for signs that the patient is using accessory muscles.

Palpation

• Palpate the chest for respiratory excursion.
• Palpate peripheral pulses for rate, rhythm, and symmetry.

• Palpate the abdomen for ascites and hepatomegaly.

Percussion

• Percuss the chest for diaphragmatic excursion and hyperresonance or dullness.
• Percuss the liver for tenderness and enlargement.

Auscultation

• Auscultate the lungs for abnormal or adventitious breath sounds, crackles, rhonchi, and wheezing.
• Auscultate the heart for murmurs, gallops, or a pericardial friction rub.

Fever

This common sign can stem from a disorder affecting virtually any body system. In pulmonary disorders, fever usually reflects acute or chronic infection, neoplasm, or infarction. (See *Causes of fever,* page 56.)

If your patient has a fever, take his health history and perform a physical examination according to the guidelines below.

History of the sign

To better characterize your patient's fever, consider asking the following questions:

• When did your fever begin?
• How high did your temperature get?
• What steps have you taken to treat your fever?
• Does your fever recur? How soon?
• What is the daily pattern of temperature extremes?

Associated findings

Note whether the patient has experienced any of the following signs or symptoms:

• chest pain
• chills

Causes of fever

Respiratory disorders that may cause fever include bronchiectasis, Legionnaires' disease, lung abscess, lung cancer, pneumonia, pulmonary embolism with infarction, and tuberculosis.

Bronchiectasis
Recurrent fever and chills occur with a cough that produces copious, foul-smelling, mucopurulent sputum. The patient appears chronically ill and may exhibit weight loss, malaise, finger clubbing, and dyspnea. Auscultation reveals crackles and wheezes.

Legionnaires' disease
In this disorder, the patient experiences an unremitting fever that may reach 105° F (40.5° C). Prodromal signs and symptoms include diarrhea, anorexia, malaise, myalgia, weakness, headache, chills, and a persistent cough (dry, progressing to productive). Other findings may include nausea, vomiting, disorientation, confusion, pleuritic chest pain, tachypnea, dyspnea, crackles, bradycardia, and mild, temporary amnesia.

Lung abscess
Fever is a cardinal sign of lung abscess. Other signs and symptoms may include malaise, weight loss, chills, sweating, dyspnea, and chest pain. The patient's cough may produce bloody, purulent, or foul-smelling sputum.

Lung cancer
Fever appears late in the course of this illness along with a dry cough, dyspnea, and weight loss. Hoarseness, wheezing, chest or shoulder pain, hemoptysis, and weakness may also occur.

Pneumonia
Fever is accompanied by productive coughing, pleuritic chest pain, and shaking chills in most types of pneumonia. Sputum varies from mucoid and purulent in atypical and bacterial community-acquired pneumonias to thick, rusty, and bloody sputum in *Klebsiella* pneumonia. Examination reveals rapid, shallow respirations and crackles. Signs of consolidation (dullness on percussion, increased fremitus, bronchophony, and egophony) may be evident.

Pulmonary embolism with infarction
A low-grade fever often occurs after pulmonary embolism. Initial signs and symptoms of this disorder may include chest pain, dyspnea, tachycardia, and a cough that may produce blood-tinged sputum. Auscultation may reveal an S_3 gallop, crackles, and a pleural friction rub.

Tuberculosis
A low-grade fever and night sweats are characteristic of tuberculosis. These signs may be accompanied by fatigue, weight loss, anorexia, weakness, and a cough that may produce mucopurulent sputum. Auscultation reveals crackles.

Nonrespiratory causes
Fever is a common sign in infection, thyroid storm, heat exhaustion, and heatstroke as well as immunodeficiency, inflammatory, and neoplastic disorders. Fever may result from a hypersensitivity reaction to radiographic contrast media, drugs (such as barbiturates and phenytoin [in overdose]; antibiotics, methyldopa, procainamide, and quinidine; and phenothiazines [may impair central thermoregulation]), blood transfusions, or other agents.

- dyspnea
- fatigue
- headache
- hematemesis
- myalgia
- productive cough.

Previous conditions and treatments

Consult with the patient, members of his family, or members of the health care team to determine if the patient has a history of any of the following conditions, treatments, or risk factors:
- cancer
- chronic pulmonary disease
- human immunodeficiency virus (HIV) infection or high risk for HIV infection
- immunosuppressive therapy
- recent surgery
- tuberculosis.

Drug history

Find out which medications the patient is taking (including over-the-counter ones), and ask about any known drug allergies. Ask about recent changes in the schedule or dosage of prescribed medications. Note any past or current use of the following drugs:
- barbiturates, phenytoin (may cause fever in overdose)
- drugs associated with drug fever (antibiotics, methyldopa, procainamide, and quinidine)
- phenothiazines (may impair central thermoregulation).

Physical examination

Assess the patient's vital signs, including temperature, blood pressure, respiratory rate and depth, and pulse rate and rhythm. Then examine the patient according to the steps described below.

Inspection
- Observe the patient's general appearance, nutritional status, level of comfort, and level of consciousness.
- Examine the patient's mouth to assess dental hygiene. Inspect the skin for signs of cyanosis.
- Examine the neck, chest, and abdomen for signs of accessory muscle use.
- Inspect the sputum produced for color, consistency, amount, and odor.

Palpation
- Palpate the chest for tenderness and fremitus.
- Palpate the skin for diaphoresis.

Percussion
- Percuss the chest for dullness.

Auscultation
- Auscultate the lungs for abnormal breath sounds, crackles, wheezing, and a pleural friction rub.
- Auscultate the heart for gallops.

Wheezing

Also called sibilant rhonchi, these adventitious breath sounds can have a high-pitched, musical, squealing, creaking, or groaning quality. Wheezes that originate in the large airways can be heard by placing an ear over the chest wall or near the patient's mouth; wheezes that originate in smaller airways, by auscultating the anterior or posterior chest. The amount of discomfort caused by wheezes largely depends on the patient's perception. Unlike rhonchi, wheezes aren't cleared by coughing.

Wheezing is a common chief complaint in many pulmonary disorders — especially in asthma. Prolonged wheezing during expiration often results from shortened and narrowed bronchi caused by bronchospasm, mucosal thickening or edema, extrinsic pressure (as in tension pneumothorax or goiter), or partial obstruction from a tumor, foreign body, or secretions. Wheezing that occurs during inspiration typically reflects airway obstruction. (See *Causes of wheezing.*)

If your patient complains of wheezing, take his health history and perform a physical examination according to the guidelines below.

History of the sign
To better understand your patient's wheezing, consider asking the following questions:
- How long have you experienced wheezing?
- How often does it occur?
- How long does each episode last?
- What factors precipitate or aggravate your wheezing?
- Is it worse during exertion? Does rest help relieve it?
- Have you had similar episodes in the past? If so, how were they treated?
- What medications or other treatments are you currently using? Have they been effective?
- Do you have a cough? Is it constant or intermittent? Is it productive? Can you describe the sputum?
- Have you experienced any chest pain?

Associated findings
Note whether the patient has experienced any of the following signs or symptoms:
- anorexia
- chest pain (especially pleuritic pain)
- dyspnea
- fever
- weight loss.

Previous conditions and treatments
Consult with the patient, members of his family, or members of the health care team to determine if the patient has a history of any of the following conditions, treatments, or risk factors:
- allergic reaction
- aspiration of foreign body

- cancer
- chronic cardiovascular disease
- chronic pulmonary disease
- cigarette smoking
- recent exposure to fire, smoke, or other respirable irritants or toxic fumes
- recent surgery, illnesses, or trauma.

Drug history
Find out which medications the patient is taking (including over-the-counter ones), and ask about any known drug allergies. Ask about recent changes in the schedule or dosage of prescribed drugs. Note any past or current use of the following drugs:
- bisulfites (may be used in preservatives)
- drugs that can cause an anaphylactic reaction
- drugs that can cause bronchospasm (adenosine, beta blockers, and cromolyn sodium).

Physical examination
Assess the patient's vital signs, including temperature, blood pressure, respiratory rate and depth, and pulse rate and rhythm. Then examine the patient according to the steps described below.

Inspection
- Observe for signs of respiratory distress, such as nasal flaring, irritable or anxious behavior, audible wheezing, stridor, and rapid, shallow, or labored breathing.
- Inspect the skin for cyanosis or pallor.
- Examine the neck for distended neck veins or signs of accessory muscle use.
- Inspect the chest for asymmetrical motion, sternal or intercostal retractions, and any abnormal shape (for example, barrel chest).

Palpation
- Palpate the chest for respiratory excursion, fremitus, and tenderness.

Causes of wheezing

Respiratory disorders that may cause wheezing include acute chemical pneumonitis, aspiration of a foreign body, aspiration pneumonitis, asthma, bronchiectasis, chronic bronchitis, coccidioidomycosis, emphysema, lung cancer, inhalation injury, pulmonary edema, tension pneumothorax, and tuberculosis.

Acute chemical pneumonitis
In this disorder, mucosal injury causes increased secretions and edema, leading to wheezing, dyspnea, orthopnea, crackles, malaise, fever, and a cough that produces purulent sputum. The patient may also exhibit signs of conjunctivitis, pharyngitis, laryngitis, and rhinitis.

Aspiration of a foreign body
Partial obstruction of an airway by a foreign body produces a sudden onset of wheezing (possibly stridor), a dry, paroxysmal cough, gagging, and hoarseness. Other findings include tachycardia, dyspnea, decreased breath sounds and, possibly, cyanosis. If the foreign body is retained, inflammation, fever, pain, and swelling may result.

Aspiration pneumonitis
Wheezing may accompany tachypnea, marked dyspnea, cyanosis, tachycardia, fever, a productive (and eventually purulent) cough, and pink, frothy sputum.

Asthma
Wheezing, an early and cardinal sign of asthma, is heard at the mouth during exhalation. The patient typically has a cough that's dry initially and that later becomes productive with thick mucus. Other findings include apprehension, prolonged expiration, intercostal and supraclavicular retractions, rhonchi, accessory muscle use, nasal flaring, tachypnea, tachycardia, diaphoresis, and flushing or cyanosis.

Bronchiectasis
In bronchiectasis, production of excessive amounts of mucus may cause intermittent, localized, or diffuse wheezing. Wheezing may be accompanied by a cough that produces foul-smelling, mucopurulent sputum; hemoptysis; rhonchi; and coarse crackles. Other signs and symptoms may include weight loss, fatigue, weakness, dyspnea on exertion, fever, malaise, and halitosis. Finger clubbing may be a late sign.

Chronic bronchitis
Wheezing varies in severity, location, and intensity. Associated findings include prolonged exhalation, coarse crackles, scattered rhonchi, dyspnea, use of accessory muscles, barrel chest, tachypnea, edema, weight gain, cyanosis, and a productive cough.

Coccidioidomycosis
This disorder may cause wheezing and rhonchi accompanied by a cough, fever, chills, pleuritic chest pain, headache, weakness, malaise, anorexia, and macular rash.

Emphysema
Mild to moderate wheezing may be accompanied by dyspnea, malaise, tachypnea, diminished breath sounds, peripheral cyanosis, pursed-lip breathing, and anorexia. Other signs may include use of accessory muscles, barrel chest, and a chronic productive cough.

Lung cancer
Bronchial obstruction by a tumor may cause localized wheezing. Additional findings may include dyspnea, a productive cough, hemoptysis (beginning

(continued)

Causes of wheezing *(continued)*

as blood-tinged sputum and possibly progressing to massive hemorrhage), anorexia, and weight loss. The patient may also have upper extremity edema and chest pain.

Inhalation injury
Wheezing can accompany other early findings, including hoarseness, coughing, singed nasal hairs, orofacial burns, and soot-stained sputum. Later effects include crackles, rhonchi, and respiratory distress.

Pulmonary edema
Wheezing may accompany other common signs and symptoms, such as coughing, dyspnea on exertion, and paroxysmal nocturnal dyspnea that may progress to orthopnea. Examination typically reveals tachycardia, tachypnea, dependent crackles, and a diastolic gallop. Signs that accompany severe pulmonary edema include diffuse crackles; arrhythmias; hypotension; a thready pulse; rapid, labored respirations; a cough that produces frothy, bloody sputum; and cold, clammy, cyanotic skin.

Tension pneumothorax
Signs of this life-threatening disorder include wheezing, dyspnea, tachycardia, tachypnea, and the sudden onset of severe, sharp chest pain (often unilateral). Other common findings include a dry cough, cyanosis, use of accessory muscles, asymmetrical chest expansion, anxiety, and restlessness. Examination typically reveals subcutaneous crepitation, decreased vocal fremitus, tracheal deviation, and hyperresonance or tympany and diminished or absent breath sounds on the affected side.

Tuberculosis
In later stages of this disorder, fibrosis may cause wheezing. Other common findings include a productive cough, pleuritic chest pain, fine crackles, night sweats, anorexia, weight loss, fever, malaise, dyspnea, and fatigue. Examination reveals dullness on percussion, increased tactile fremitus, and amphoric breath sounds.

Nonrespiratory causes
Wheezing may be caused by anaphylaxis and airway compression due to goiter. Drugs associated with wheezing include bisulfites (may be used in preservatives), those that can cause an anaphylactic reaction, and those that can cause bronchospasm (adenosine, beta-adrenergic blockers, and cromolyn sodium).

- Palpate the neck for tracheal deviation.
- Palpate the skin for diaphoresis.

Percussion
- Percuss the chest for dullness, hyperresonance, and diaphragmatic excursion.

Auscultation
- Auscultate the lungs for absent or decreased breath sounds, crackles, rhonchi, and a pleural friction rub.
- Note the location of wheezes and whether they are present on inhalation or exhalation.

CHAPTER 3

Monitoring respiratory status

Monitoring can alert you to subtle yet significant changes in your patient's respiratory status. Types of monitoring include serial arterial blood gas (ABG) analyses, mixed venous oxygen saturation (SvO2) monitoring, pulse oximetry, bedside pulmonary function monitoring, and apnea monitoring.

ABG analysis

ABG analysis provides information on ventilation, oxygenation, and acid-base balance by measuring blood pH, partial pressure of oxygen in arterial blood (PaO_2), and partial pressure of carbon dioxide in arterial blood ($PaCO_2$). Blood pH reflects the blood's acid-base balance. PaO_2 indicates the amount of oxygen that the lungs deliver to the blood, and $PaCO_2$ indicates the lungs' capacity to eliminate carbon dioxide. ABG samples can also be analyzed for oxygen content, arterial oxygen saturation (SaO_2) level, and bicarbonate (HCO_3^-) content. (See *Interpreting ABG values.*)

ABG analysis is commonly ordered for patients who have chronic obstructive pulmonary disease, pulmonary edema, acute respiratory distress, adult respiratory distress syndrome (ARDS), myocardial infarction, or pneumonia. It's also performed during episodes of shock and following coronary artery bypass surgery, resuscitation from cardiac arrest, changes in respiratory therapy or status, and prolonged anesthesia. ABG analysis may be performed to guide treatment for metabolic disorders such as diabetic ketoacidosis.

Implementation

You can obtain an arterial sample through percutaneous puncture of the brachial, radial, or femoral artery or through an arterial line. Typically, a respiratory technician or a specially trained nurse collects the sample; however, a doctor usually collects femoral artery samples. Before attempting a radial puncture, you should perform Allen's test to assess the adequacy of the blood supply to the patient's hand. (See *Performing Allen's test,* page 64.)

Prepare the collection equipment by filling a plastic bag or basin with ice and following the procedure below to heparinize a 10-ml glass or plastic syringe with aqueous heparin (1:1,000):

• Attach a 20G needle to the syringe and open the ampule of heparin.
• Draw all the heparin into the syringe to prevent the sample from clotting.
• Hold the syringe upright and pull the plunger back slowly to the 7-ml mark. (Rotate the barrel as it fills to coat the inside of the syringe.)
• Slowly force the heparin toward the hub of the syringe, and expel all but about 0.1 ml of the heparin.
• To heparinize the needle, first replace the 20G needle with a 22G needle.
• Holding the syringe upright, tilt it slightly, and eject the remaining heparin. (Excess heparin in the syringe alters blood pH and PaO_2 values.)

While wearing gloves, clean the puncture site with povidone-iodine or alcohol sponges. Then palpate the artery with the index and middle fingers of one hand while holding the syringe over the puncture site with your other hand. Puncture a radial artery at a 30- to 45-degree angle; a brachial artery at a 60-degree angle. Watch for blood flowing into the syringe. Don't pull back on the plunger; arterial blood should enter the syringe automatically. Fill the syringe to the 5-ml mark.

To collect a sample from an arterial line, turn the line's stopcock so that the heparin flush solution is turned off. Withdraw at least 3 ml of blood and

Interpretation

Interpreting ABG values

Arterial blood gas (ABG) values provide important information about the efficiency of the patient's gas exchange and acid-base balance. You can also use ABG values to monitor the effects of respiratory interventions.

Although ABG measurement requires blood sampling, an invasive procedure that may cause pain (especially for patients without an arterial line), the information it provides allows a more thorough assessment of gas exchange.

Normal ABG values
- Blood pH: 7.35 to 7.45
- Partial pressure of oxygen in arterial blood (PaO_2): 80 to 100 mm Hg (decreases with age)
- Partial pressure of carbon dioxide in arterial blood ($PaCO_2$): 35 to 45 mm Hg
- Bicarbonate (HCO_3^-): 22 to 26 mEq/liter
- Arterial oxygen saturation (SaO_2): 95% to 100%.

Abnormal ABG values
ABG values such as those below indicate the following conditions:
- A pH higher than 7.45 (alkalosis) reflects a hydrogen ion (H^+) deficit.
- A pH lower than 7.35 (acidosis) reflects an H^+ excess.
- A PaO_2 greater than 100 mm Hg indicates more than adequate supplemental oxygen administration.
- A PaO_2 less than 80 mm Hg indicates hypoxemia (possibly resulting from pneumonia, pulmonary embolism, pulmonary infarction, chronic lung disease, pulmonary edema, pneumothorax, adult respiratory distress syndrome, or acute respiratory failure).

In patients older than 65, estimate the expected PaO_2 by subtracting half the patient's age from 105 mm Hg.
- A $PaCO_2$ greater than 45 mm Hg indicates possible hypercapnia (a decrease in the lungs' capacity to eliminate carbon dioxide).
- A $PaCO_2$ less than 35 mm Hg indicates respiratory alkalosis and hyperventilation.
- When PaO_2 decreases to below 60 mm Hg or $PaCO_2$ is greater than 50 mm Hg, emergency intervention is usually required.
- When HCO_3^- decreases to below 22 mEq/liter, a bicarbonate deficit may result that can cause metabolic acidosis. When HCO_3^- exceeds 26 mEq/liter, a bicarbonate excess may result that can cause metabolic alkalosis.
- An SaO_2 less than 97% may contribute to a low PaO_2 value.

---

discard it. Then draw 5 ml of blood into the syringe.

After collecting a percutaneous sample, press a gauze pad firmly over the puncture site for at least 5 minutes, or until the bleeding stops. If the patient is receiving anticoagulant therapy or has a blood dyscrasia, apply pressure to the puncture site for 10 to 15 minutes. If necessary, ask a coworker to hold the gauze pad in place while you prepare the sample for the laboratory. Don't ask the patient to hold the pad because if pressure is insufficient, a large, painful hematoma may form, hindering future punctures at that site.

Remove air bubbles from the syringe, and clean any blood that may have leaked from it. Cap the syringe, and label it with the patient's name and room number, the time and date of sample collection, and your signature. Finally, transport the syringe on ice to the laboratory.

Performing Allen's test

Before you collect a sample from the radial artery, you must assess collateral arterial blood supply by performing Allen's test.

• Begin by resting the patient's arm on a mattress or bedside stand. Have the patient clench his fist. Then, using your index and middle fingers, press for several seconds on the radial and ulnar arteries.

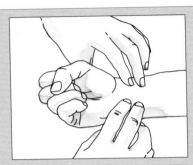

• While maintaining pressure, ask him to unclench his fist and hold his hand in a relaxed position. The palm will be blanched because pressure from your fingers impairs the normal blood flow.

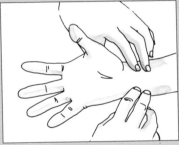

• Release pressure from the patient's ulnar artery. If the hand becomes flushed (indicating blood filling the vessels), you can safely proceed with a radial artery puncture. If the hand doesn't flush, perform this test on the other arm.

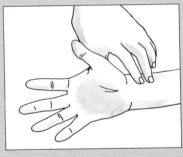

Nursing considerations
• If the patient is receiving supplemental oxygen, wait until therapy has been underway for at least 15 minutes before drawing arterial blood.
• Unless ordered to do otherwise, continue giving oxygen while collecting arterial samples. However, be sure to indicate on the laboratory request slip the amount and type of oxygen therapy the patient is receiving.
• If the patient isn't receiving supplemental oxygen, indicate that he's breathing room air.

• If the patient has just received a breathing or nebulizer treatment or if mechanical ventilator settings have just been changed, wait 20 minutes before drawing samples.

• If you use excessive force when attempting to puncture an artery, you risk advancing the needle through the opposite wall of the artery or touching the periosteum of a bone, causing the patient considerable pain. If this happens, slowly withdraw the needle a short distance and check for blood return. If blood does not enter the syringe, withdraw the needle completely and start with a new heparinized needle.

• Don't make more than two attempts to withdraw blood from the same site. Probing the artery may injure it and the radial nerve. Also, hemolysis will alter test results.

$S\bar{v}O_2$ monitoring

In this procedure, a fiber-optic thermodilution pulmonary artery (PA) catheter continuously monitors oxygen delivery to tissues and oxygen consumption by tissues. Impaired oxygen delivery, the result of such disorders as hemorrhagic shock, cardiogenic shock, adult respiratory distress syndrome, and sepsis, can be readily detected by monitoring mixed venous oxygen saturation ($S\bar{v}O_2$) before the oxygen-deficient tissues cause cardiac and respiratory failure. (See *Understanding $S\bar{v}O_2$ monitoring equipment,* page 66.)

$S\bar{v}O_2$ monitoring is also used to evaluate a patient's response to drug administration, endotracheal tube suctioning, ventilator setting changes, positive end-expiratory pressure, and changes in fraction of inspired oxygen. $S\bar{v}O_2$ usually ranges from 60% to 80%, with the normal value being 75%. (See

Interpreting $S\bar{v}O_2$ test results and waveforms, page 67.)

Implementation

Catheter insertion follows the same technique used with any thermodilution flow-directed PA catheter. After a PA catheter has been inserted and the $S\bar{v}O_2$ optical module has been set up and calibrated, confirm that the light intensity tracing on the graphic printout is within normal range. This ensures correct position and function of the catheter.

To monitor and document trends, record (on graph paper) the digital readout of $S\bar{v}O_2$ at least once per hour. Set the monitor's alarms to go off when $S\bar{v}O_2$ is 10% above or below the current reading.

If the intensity of the tracing is low, ensure that all connections between the catheter and oximeter are secure and that the catheter is patent and not kinked. If the tracing is damped or erratic, try to aspirate blood from the catheter to check for patency. If you can't aspirate blood, notify the patient's doctor (to replace the catheter). Also, check for a damped PA waveform, which indicates a wedged catheter. If the catheter is wedged, attempt to flush the line. Also, turn the patient from side to side and instruct him to cough. If the catheter remains wedged, notify the patient's doctor immediately.

If the intensity of the tracing is high, the catheter may be pressing against a vessel wall. Flush the line. If the tracing doesn't return to normal, notify the doctor (to reposition the catheter).

Nursing considerations

• Collect the initial $S\bar{v}O_2$ sample from the distal port of the PA catheter. Send it to the laboratory to compare the laboratory's $S\bar{v}O_2$ measurement with the measurement indicated by the fiber-optic catheter.

Understanding S$\overline{v}$O$_2$ monitoring equipment

The mixed venous oxygen saturation (S$\overline{v}$O$_2$) monitoring system includes:
• a flow-directed fiber-optic catheter with lumens for proximal or central venous pressure (CVP) monitoring, distal or pulmonary artery (PA) monitoring, and balloon inflation
• an optical module and cable
• a co-oximeter (monitor).

Connecting the equipment
For the S$\overline{v}$O$_2$ equipment to function properly, you must make the following connections:
• Connect the cardiac output computer connector to the cardiac output computer cable.
• Connect the distal lumen to an external PA pressure monitoring system.
• Connect the proximal (CVP) lumen to another monitoring system or to a continuous flow administration unit.
• Connect the optical module to the co-oximeter unit.

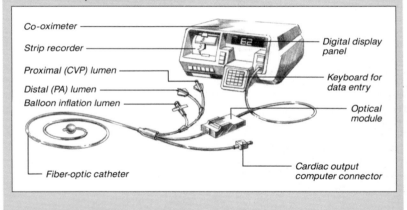

Co-oximeter
Strip recorder
Proximal (CVP) lumen
Distal (PA) lumen
Balloon inflation lumen
Fiber-optic catheter

Digital display panel
Keyboard for data entry
Optical module
Cardiac output computer connector

• If the catheter values and laboratory values differ by more than 4%, follow the manufacturer's instructions to enter the laboratory's S$\overline{v}$O$_2$ value into the co-oximeter.
• Recalibrate the monitor according to your hospital's policy (possibly every shift), every 24 hours, or whenever the catheter has been disconnected from the optical module.

• Be alert for thrombosis and infection, the major complications of S$\overline{v}$O$_2$ monitoring. *Thrombosis* can result from local irritation by the catheter. A heparin flush solution helps prevent this. Thromboembolism can occur if a thrombus breaks off and lodges in the circulatory system. Monitor the patient for signs and symptoms of *infection,* such as redness or drainage at the catheter site.

Interpretation

Interpreting S̄v̄O₂ test results and waveforms

A normal mixed venous oxygen saturation (S̄v̄O₂) waveform resembles a fairly steady line without peaks or valleys. S̄v̄O₂ may vary with activities such as suctioning or turning. Look for such trends as a steadily declining value or a sudden drop in S̄v̄O₂ that doesn't return to baseline with cessation of activity or maintenance of the catheter or monitor.

Decreased S̄v̄O₂

A declining S̄v̄O₂ or an S̄v̄O₂ less than 60% indicates impaired oxygen delivery, as indicated in the waveform at right. This occurs during hypoxemia and cardiac failure. Hypoxemia may result from obstructive or restrictive lung disease, pneumonia, respiratory failure in neuromuscular disorders, or suctioning. Shock, hemorrhage, arrhythmias, hyperthermia, shivering, or seizures may also reduce S̄v̄O₂.

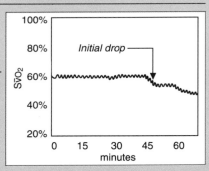

Increased S̄v̄O₂

An S̄v̄O₂ greater than 80% occurs with increased oxygen delivery, reduced oxygen demand, or diminished oxygen extraction by tissues. In the waveform at right, initiating positive end-expiratory pressure (PEEP) causes a rise in S̄v̄O₂, thereby allowing for a reduction in fraction of inspired oxygen (FIO_2).

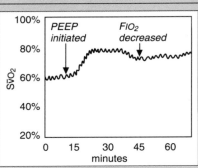

Special considerations

• To accurately assess the results of S̄v̄O₂ monitoring, consider analyzing hematocrit and hemoglobin levels and other factors that may indicate cardiac output changes.

• If S̄v̄O₂ decreases to less than 60%, or if it varies by more than 10% for 3 minutes or longer, reassess the patient.
• If S̄v̄O₂ doesn't return to baseline after appropriate nursing interventions, notify the doctor.

Pulse oximetry

A noninvasive procedure for monitoring arterial oxygen saturation (SaO_2), pulse oximetry, unlike arterial blood gas analysis, may be performed intermittently or continuously. Since pulse oximetry may be done continuously, it can alert you more quickly to perfusion abnormalities.

In pulse oximetry, a sensor containing a photodetector and light sources is placed on the finger, toe, nose, hand, ear, forehead, or temple. Two diodes send red and infrared light through a pulsating arterial vascular bed, like the one in the fingertip. The photodetector measures the relative absorption of red and infrared light within the vascular bed and then relays this data to a monitor, called a pulse oximeter, that displays the SaO_2 value with each heartbeat and shows the pulse rate measured at the sensor site. In this way, SaO_2 is calculated without interference from surrounding venous blood, skin, connective tissue, or bone. Some monitors also display a waveform, called a plethysmogram, and a pulse amplitude bar. (See *Preparing the patient for oximetry monitoring* and *Understanding pulse oximetry*.)

Types of sensors

Two types of sensors can be used — a transmission sensor or a reflectance sensor. A *transmission sensor,* the most common type, has the light sources and photodetector directly opposite one another. It's usually positioned on the patient's finger, toe, nose, hand, or ear. In a *reflectance sensor,* the light sources are adjacent to the photodetector. This type of sensor is placed on a flat surface, such as the forehead or temple.

Various kinds of sensors may be used, depending on the patient's age, size, and clinical condition and on the type of oximeter being used. These include:
• neonatal foot sensor
• infant toe sensor
• pediatric finger or toe sensor
• adult finger or toe sensor (for limited activity)
• adult finger-clip sensor
• adult nasal sensor (used during surgery or if cardiac output is decreased)
• ear sensor. (See *Choosing the correct pulse oximetry sensor,* page 70.)

Implementation

For adults, the finger and ear sensors are most commonly used.

Timesaving tip: If the patient has significantly reduced peripheral vascular pulsations or is taking a vasoactive drug, use a nasal sensor, which detects pulsations of the septal anterior ethmoidal artery.

Teaching TimeSaver

Preparing the patient for oximetry monitoring

Prepare the patient for oximetry monitoring by teaching him the following:
• Explain the monitoring technique to the patient.
• Tell him that the monitor will painlessly measure the amount of oxygen in his body on an ongoing basis.
• Mention how long the monitoring will last.
• Inform him where the sensor will be placed or, if possible, have him choose the site.
• Instruct the patient to avoid moving the sensor site excessively to ensure reliable findings.
• Tell him to report any discomfort at the site.
• Caution the patient and his family not to alter the alarm settings or volume.

Understanding pulse oximetry

The pulse oximeter allows noninvasive monitoring of a patient's arterial oxygen saturation (SaO_2) levels by measuring the absorption (amplitude) of light waves as they pass through areas of the body that are highly perfused by arterial blood. Oximetry is also used to monitor pulse rate.

A sensor containing a photodetector and light-emitting diodes is attached to the patient's body (shown here on the index finger). The diodes send red and infrared light beams through the perfused tissue. The sensor records the relative amount of each color absorbed by arterial blood and transmits the data to a monitor, which displays the information with each heartbeat. If the SaO_2 level or pulse rate varies from preset limits, the monitor emits visual and audible alarms.

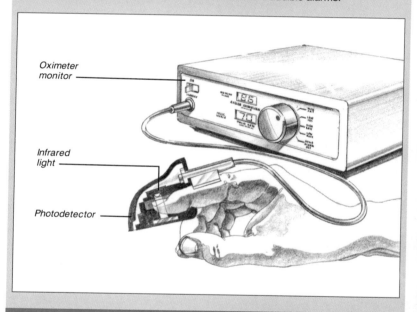

Oximeter monitor

Infrared light

Photodetector

Using a finger sensor

• Remove any false fingernails and nail polish from the test finger.

• Place the sensor over the patient's finger so that the light sources and the photodetector oppose each other.

• If the patient has long fingernails, position the probe perpendicular to the finger, if possible, or clip the fingernail.

• Turn on the power switch. If the device is working properly, a beep will sound, a display will light momentarily, and the pulse searchlight will flash. The SaO_2 and pulse rate displays will show stationary zeros. After four to six heartbeats, the SaO_2 and pulse rate displays will supply information with each beat, and the pulse amplitude in-

Choosing the correct pulse oximetry sensor

Selecting the right sensor can promote accurate pulse oximetry results. Weight limits for sensors overlap, which allows you to choose the most appropriate sensor. For example, you may need to use the pediatric sensor for a small adult. The choice of sensor also depends on the expected duration of monitoring, the patient's activity level, and concerns about infection.

Kind of sensor	Weight parameter	Position of sensor
Adhesive neonatal	Less that 6.6 lb (3 kg) or more than 88 lb (40 kg)	Neonate's foot or hand or adult's finger
Adhesive infant	2.2 to 44 lb (1 to 20 kg)	Infant's toe
Adhesive pediatric	22 to 110 lb (10 to 50 kg)	Index, middle, or ring finger, or toe
Adhesive adult	More than 66 lb (30 kg)	Index, middle, or ring finger, or toe
Adhesive adult nasal	More than 110 lb (50 kg)	Cartilaginous portion of the nose, just below the bridge
Adult finger-clip	More than 88 lb (40 kg)	Index, middle, or ring finger; don't place on toe
Earclip (not used on neonates or infants)	None	Earlobe
Reflectance	None	Forehead or temple

dicator will begin tracking the patient's pulse.

Using an ear sensor
• Massage the patient's earlobe for 10 to 20 seconds with an alcohol sponge. (Mild erythema indicates adequate vascularization.)
• Following the manufacturer's instructions, attach the ear probe to the patient's earlobe or pinna.
• Use an ear sensor stabilizer for prolonged testing or for testing during exercise. Be sure to establish good contact on the ear. (An unstable sensor may set off the low-perfusion alarm.) In a few seconds, an SaO_2 reading and a pulse waveform will appear on the oximeter screen.

• Leave the ear probe in place for 3 minutes or more, until readings stabilize at the highest point; or take three separate readings and average them.
• Revascularize the patient's earlobe before each reading.
• After the procedure, remove the sensor, turn off and unplug the unit, and clean the sensor by gently rubbing it with an alcohol sponge. (See *Factors affecting pulse oximetry results.*)

Nursing considerations
Normal SaO_2 levels range from 95% to 100% for healthy adults and children and from 93.8% to 100% within 1 hour after birth for healthy, full-term neonates. Lower levels may indicate hypoxemia, which warrants intervention. For such patients, follow hospital poli-

Factors affecting pulse oximetry results

Physiologic, environmental, mechanical, and other factors may affect pulse oximetry results. So, before concluding that abnormal results signal a perfusion problem, review this list of interfering factors.

Physiologic factors

Various physiologic factors may interfere with accuracy:
• An elevated bilirubin level may falsely lower arterial oxygen saturation (SaO_2) readings.
• Elevated carboxyhemoglobin or methemoglobin levels (which may occur in heavy smokers or urban dwellers) may falsely elevate SaO_2 readings.
• Certain I.V. substances, such as lipid emulsions and dyes, may prevent accurate readings.
• Poor perfusion (brought on by peripheral vascular disease or use of vasoconstrictive drugs, for example) may interfere with blood flow to the site, making it impossible to obtain a reading. If only small amounts of blood flow through the finger's arterial bed, the oximeter may fail to identify the arterial pulse and may not display the SaO_2 value. To prevent this problem, use a nasal sensor or place a reflectance sensor on the patient's forehead.
• Venous pulsations may interfere with accuracy. Normally nonpulsatile, venous blood may pulsate from right ventricular failure, a tight sensor, or any tourniquet-like effect. Because the oximeter responds to pulsating blood, it will detect both pulsating venous blood and pulsating arterial blood, producing a false SaO_2 value. Usually, you can avoid this problem by making sure that the sensor isn't fastened too tightly.
• Anemia may interfere with an accurate interpretation of SaO_2. Always double-check the patient's hemoglobin level. Even if he's anemic, with a hemoglobin value of 5 g/dl, the SaO_2 value may seem normal because the hemoglobin that's available to carry oxygen is fully saturated. Yet the patient may have insufficient oxygen to meet his metabolic needs. To correct this problem, be prepared to administer red blood cells or whole blood.

Environmental factors

Erroneous readings can result from excessive light from phototherapy, surgical lamps, direct sunlight, or bright ambient light. To compensate, cover the sensor with a sheet or towel.

Mechanical factors

Check the patient's vital signs. If they are sufficient to produce a signal, look for the following mechanical problems:
• *Poor connection.* Be sure the sensors are properly aligned and that wires are intact and fastened securely. Make sure that the pulse oximeter is plugged into a power source.
• *Equipment malfunction.* Ensure that the equipment is working properly by removing the sensor from the patient and testing it on yourself or another healthy person. Set alarm limits at 85% and 100% to test the instrument.
• *Poor skin contact.* Use fresh adhesive to apply an adhesive sensor.

Additional factors

Other factors can cause inaccurate readings.
• *Patient movement.* If the patient constantly moves the finger or toe to which the sensor is attached, the pulse oximeter may identify the motion as arterial pulsations. Reposition the sensor or use a different type of sensor.
• *Dark ear pigment.* Reposition the sensor and revascularize the site or use a finger sensor.

cy or the doctor's orders, which may include increasing oxygen therapy. If SaO_2 levels decrease suddenly, be prepared to resuscitate the patient immediately. Notify the doctor of any significant change in the patient's condition.

• To maintain a continuous display of SaO_2 levels, be sure the monitoring site is clean, dry, and protected from strong light.

• If the patient's skin is irritated by the adhesive used to keep the disposable sensor in place, reposition the sensor or replace it with a model that is held in place with a clip instead of with tape.

• Check for the following indications of circulatory impairment: blanching, coolness, and numbness of the skin.

• When monitoring continuously, rotate the sensor site every 4 hours.

• If an oximetry monitor is used on the same extremity as a blood pressure cuff, false-low readings may occur while blood pressure is being measured.

Bedside pulmonary function monitoring

Pulmonary function tests (PFTs) help assess the integrity and function of the airways, pulmonary vasculature, and pulmonary interstitium. A doctor may order PFTs to:

• evaluate ventilatory function through spirometric measurements

• determine the cause of dyspnea

• assess the effectiveness of therapies such as bronchodilators and steroids

• determine if a respiratory abnormality is associated with an obstructive or a restrictive disease

• evaluate the extent of dysfunction

• identify patients at risk for respiratory compromise.

Values for each PFT will vary according to an individual's body size. At the onset of testing, predicted values are calculated for each patient. Deviations from these values are then analyzed for patterns that suggest obstructive or restrictive lung disease or other pulmonary dysfunction. (See *Distinguishing between obstructive and restrictive pulmonary dysfunction.*)

Although comprehensive PFTs usually are performed in a pulmonary function laboratory, simpler bedside procedures are now available to monitor changes in the acutely ill patient. Bedside monitoring may include such measurements as tidal volume (VT), minute volume (MV), vital capacity (VC), maximal voluntary ventilation (MVV), maximal inspiratory and expiratory pressure (MIP, MEP), forced vital capacity (FVC), forced expiratory volume (FEV), forced expiratory flow (FEF), and peak expiratory flow (PEF).

Bedside monitoring supplements other procedures, such as arterial blood gas (ABG) analysis, chest X-rays, physical examination, and complete PFTs. Results help guide nursing care and therapy. The need for specific information, the type of equipment available, and the patient's ability to participate in testing determine which measurements are taken. (See *Interpreting pulmonary function tests,* pages 74 and 75.)

Equipment
The type of equipment used depends on the specific test. For example, PEF measurement requires a peak flow meter; MIP and MEP measurements require a pressure manometer; and VT, MV, VC, MVV, and expiratory flow rate measurements require a spirometer.

A spirometer measures the volume of inhaled and exhaled air. As the patient breathes, a spirogram — a tracing of changes in lung volume — may be recorded.

For some tests, additional equipment may include a mouthpiece, an

Distinguishing between obstructive and restrictive pulmonary dysfunction

Pulmonary function tests (PFTs) can help distinguish obstructive pulmonary impairment from restrictive pulmonary impairment.

Obstructive impairment
In obstructive impairment, PFTs reveal:
• reduced expiratory flow rates, including forced expiratory volume in 1 second, maximal breathing capacity, forced expiratory flow rate, and maximal midexpiratory flow rate
• increased residual volume, functional residual capacity, and the ratio of residual volume to total lung capacity.

Restrictive impairment
In restrictive impairment, PFTs reveal:
• diminished total lung capacity, inspiratory capacity, and vital capacity
• reduced or normal functional residual capacity, inspiratory reserve volume, expiratory reserve volume, residual volume, and tidal volume
• baseline flow rates
• decreased lung compliance.

airway adapter, and a noseclip. You also may need a pulse oximeter to determine the oxygen saturation of the patient's blood before or during testing.

Implementation
• Explain pulmonary function monitoring to your patient and his family, and answer all of their questions. (See *Explaining pulmonary function tests,* page 76.)
• Because patient cooperation, motivation, and effort can significantly affect test results, make sure he isn't too fatigued or sedated to follow directions.
• Have him refrain from smoking, eating heavy meals, and drinking beverages before testing to avoid interference with maximal breathing effort.
• Complete any bronchial hygiene procedures, including postural drainage and suctioning, before testing. Withhold bronchodilators, unless the doctor orders otherwise.
• If the patient is on a mechanical ventilator, position him in Fowler's or semi-Fowler's position. Otherwise, have him sit or stand, as the test requires. Make sure that he's comfortable.

• Gather all equipment. Obtain a flow sheet for immediate recording of measurements. If your patient is prone to oxygen desaturation, measure his SaO_2 value with a pulse oximeter before testing; if indicated, hyperoxygenate him.

Measuring V_T
Typically, you'll use a spirometer to measure VT.
• If the patient is on a mechanical ventilator, disconnect the ventilator. Then wait about 30 to 60 seconds to reestablish his normal respiratory pattern before measuring VT. To determine if he's becoming hypoxemic during testing, use a pulse oximeter.
• Attach the mouthpiece to the spirometer. Place a noseclip on the patient, and have him verify that he can't pass air through his nose. Then place the mouthpiece in his mouth.
• Ask the patient to breathe normally. After 10 breaths, note the volume on the spirometer. Divide this volume by 10 to obtain an average VT. Reconnect the patient to the ventilator when measurements are complete.

(Text continues on page 76.)

Interpretation

Interpreting pulmonary function tests

For any pulmonary function test (PFT), an abnormal value may indicate the need for additional testing. Be sure to consider the patient's age, weight, and diagnosis when interpreting bedside PFT results. Also consider the results along with arterial blood gas levels. Consider PFT results to be suspect if the patient grows fatigued or short of breath during testing. These results may not reflect the patient's actual expiratory potential.

Pulmonary function measurement	Method of calculation	Implications
Tidal volume (V_T) Amount of air inhaled or exhaled during normal breathing	Determine the spirographic measurement for 10 breaths; then divide by 10.	Decreased V_T may indicate restrictive disease and requires further testing, such as complete pulmonary function studies or a chest X-ray.
Minute volume (MV) Total amount of air breathed per minute	Multiply V_T by respiratory rate.	Normal MV can occur in emphysema; decreased MV may indicate other diseases, such as pulmonary edema.
Inspiratory reserve volume (IRV) Amount of air inspired after normal inspiration	Subtract V_T from inspiratory capacity.	Abnormal IRV alone doesn't indicate respiratory dysfunction; IRV decreases during normal exercise.
Expiratory reserve volume (ERV) Amount of air that can be exhaled after normal expiration	Obtain from direct spirographic measurement.	ERV varies, even among healthy people.
Residual volume (RV) Volume of air that's always in the lungs and can't be exhaled (must be measured indirectly)	Subtract ERV from functional residual capacity.	RV greater than 35% of total lung capacity after maximal expiratory effort may indicate obstructive pulmonary disease, such as emphysema or asthma.
Vital capacity (VC) Total volume of air that can be exhaled after maximum inspiration	Obtain from direct spirographic measurement, or add V_T, IRV, and ERV.	Normal or increased VC with diminished flow rates may indicate reduction in functional pulmonary tissue. Decreased VC with normal or increased flow rates may indicate diminished respiratory effort, impaired thoracic expansion, or limited diaphragmatic excursion.
Inspiratory capacity (IC) Total amount of air that can be inhaled after normal expiration	Obtain from direct spirographic measurement, or add IRV and V_T.	Decreased IC indicates restrictive pulmonary disease.

Interpreting pulmonary function tests *(continued)*

Pulmonary function measurement	Method of calculation	Implications
Functional residual capacity (FRC) Amount of air remaining in lungs after normal expiration	Measure using helium dilution technique, or add ERV, V_T, and IRV.	Increased FRC indicates overdistention of lungs, which may result from obstructive pulmonary disease.
Total lung capacity (TLC) Total volume of the lungs at peak inspiration	Add V_T, IRV, ERV, and RV; or FRC and IC; or VC and RV.	Low TLC indicates restrictive pulmonary disease; high TLC indicates overdistended lungs associated with obstructive pulmonary disease.
Forced vital capacity (FVC) Total amount of air that can be exhaled after maximum inspiration	Obtain from direct spirographic measurement at 1-, 2-, and 3-second intervals.	Decreased FVC indicates flow resistance in respiratory system from obstructive pulmonary disease, such as chronic bronchitis, emphysema, or asthma.
Forced expiratory volume (FEV) Volume of air expired in the 1st, 2nd, or 3rd second of FVC maneuver	Obtain from direct spirographic measurement; expressed as percentage of FVC.	Decreased FEV_1 and increased FEV_2 and FEV_3 may indicate obstructive pulmonary disease; diminished or normal FEV_1 may indicate restrictive pulmonary disease.
Maximal midexpiratory flow (MMEF) Average flow rate during middle half of FVC; also called forced expiratory flow	Calculate from the flow rate and the time needed for expiration of middle 50% of FVC.	Low MMEF indicates obstructive pulmonary disease.
Maximal voluntary ventilation (MVV) Greatest volume of air breathed per unit of time; also called maximum breathing capacity	Obtain from direct spirographic measurement.	Reduced MVV may indicate obstructive pulmonary disease; normal or diminished MVV may indicate restrictive pulmonary disease, such as myasthenia gravis.
Diffusing capacity for carbon monoxide (DLCO) Milliliters of carbon monoxide diffused per minute across the alveolocapillary membrane	Calculate from analysis of amount of carbon monoxide exhaled compared with amount inhaled.	Lowered DLCO in the presence of a thickened alveolocapillary membrane indicates interstitial pulmonary disease, such as pulmonary fibrosis.
Maximum inspiratory force (MIF) Muscles' ability to move a volume of air sufficient to maintain adequate ventilation	Obtain from direct measurement using an inspiratory force manometer that has a manifold with a hole that's occluded as the patient inhales.	MIF greater than -20 cm H_2O indicates sufficient ability of muscles to breathe spontaneously.

Teaching TimeSaver

Explaining pulmonary function tests

To help prepare the patient for pulmonary function tests, explain the following:

• He'll be asked to breathe a certain way for each test. For example, he may be asked to inhale deeply and exhale completely or to inhale quickly.

• He may receive an aerosolized bronchodilator and may then be asked to repeat one or two tests to evaluate the drug's effectiveness.

• An arterial puncture may also be performed during the test for arterial blood gas analysis.

• The test will proceed quickly if the patient follows directions, tries hard, and keeps a tight seal around the mouthpiece or tube to ensure accurate results.

• He mustn't smoke or eat a large meal for 4 hours before the test.

• He may experience dyspnea and fatigue during the test but will be allowed to rest periodically.

• He should inform the technician if he experiences dizziness, chest pain, palpitations, nausea, severe dyspnea, or wheezing. He should also report swelling or bleeding from the arterial puncture site and any paresthesia or pain in the affected limb.

commonly results from reduced oxygen reserve.)

• Attach the mouthpiece to the spirometer and instruct the patient to inhale as deeply as possible. Then insert the mouthpiece so his lips are sealed tightly around it. This helps prevent air leakage and ensures an accurate digital readout or spirogram recording.

• Press the button on the spirometer to reset the dial to zero. Ask the patient to exhale completely. Then read the measurement on the spirometer.

• Let the patient rest briefly. Then repeat the procedure twice to obtain three measurements.

Measuring MVV

Also called maximal breathing capacity, MVV refers to the total volume of air that can be exchanged in 1 minute with the patient's maximum voluntary effort. MVV reflects overall respiratory efficiency, including respiratory muscle status, lung compliance, airway resistance, and neurologic coordination.

• Attach the mouthpiece to the spirometer. Ask the patient to breathe into the spirometer as deeply and rapidly as possible over a specified period — usually 10, 12, or 15 seconds.

• Because there is some dead air space in the trachea, multiply the expired volume measurement by a factor of 6, 5, or 4, as indicated, to obtain MVV.

Measuring MIP

Representing maximal alveolar pressure during inspiration, MIP reflects inspiratory muscle strength and diaphragm function and helps assess a patient's readiness for weaning from mechanical ventilation. MIP also is called peak inspiratory pressure, negative inspiratory force, negative inspiratory effort, or peak inspiratory force.

• Make sure that the airway is free of secretions. If the patient is on a ventilator, disconnect it.

Calculating MV

Follow the procedure for measuring VT. Then multiply VT by the respiratory rate (breaths/minute) to obtain the patient's MV.

Measuring VC

Representing the greatest possible breathing capacity, VC is the amount of air that can be exhaled after maximum inspiratory effort. (VC is often measured in a patient with tachypnea because an increased respiratory rate

• Attach the inspiratory force meter or pressure manometer to the mouthpiece or airway adapter.

• Apply a noseclip to the patient, and have him verify that he can't pass air through his nose.

• Instruct the patient to exhale.

• With your thumb or fingertip, occlude the airway by covering the safety port on the inspiratory force meter or pressure manometer.

• Ask the patient to inhale as deeply as possible as you block his airway. As he does so, note the value on the pressure manometer.

Measuring MEP

Commonly used to determine respiratory muscle strength in patients with neuromuscular problems, the MEP measurement also evaluates coughing ability.

• Connect the pressure manometer to the mouthpiece; then place the mouthpiece in the patient's mouth.

• Put a noseclip on the patient, and have him verify that he can't pass air through his nose.

• Ask the patient to inhale as deeply as possible. Occlude the airway by closing the safety port or valve on the pressure gauge with your thumb or fingertip.

• Instruct the patient to exhale as deeply as possible as you block his airway. Note the value on the manometer; MEP is the maximal pressure produced for 2 or 3 seconds.

Calculating expiratory flow

Expiratory flow reflects three measurements — FVC, FEV, and FEF. FVC is the amount of air exhaled forcefully and quickly after maximal inspiration. FEV is the amount of air exhaled in the first, second, or third second of an FVC maneuver. FEF is the average flow rate during the middle of an FVC maneuver. All three measurements can be derived from the same

procedure, which uses a spirometer that produces a graphic reading.

• Plug in the spirometer and set the baseline time.

• If desired, allow the patient to practice the required breathing procedure with the breathing tube unhooked. After practicing, replace the tube and check the seal.

• Instruct the patient not to breathe through his nose. Apply a noseclip if he has trouble complying.

• Place the mouthpiece in the patient's mouth. Ask him to inhale deeply, then to exhale forcefully, quickly, and completely.

• Remove the mouthpiece promptly to prevent recording the patient's next inspiration.

• Read the measurement on the spirometer. This measurement is the FVC. To obtain the FEF, average the flow rate obtained over the course of the FVC procedure.

• Observe the recording on the spirometer to obtain the amount of FVC exhaled in 1, 2, or 3 seconds. This is the FEV, and the amounts recorded are denoted by FEV_1, FEV_2, and FEV_3, respectively.

• Let the patient rest briefly, and repeat the procedure two or three times to make sure that your measurements are accurate.

• After completing the procedure, discard the mouthpiece, remove the spirographic chart, and follow the manufacturer's instructions for cleaning and sterilizing the equipment.

Measuring PEF

PEF represents the highest flow rate attained during an FVC maneuver. Sometimes called maximal expiratory flow rate, this measurement helps determine the extent of obstructive disease or bronchospasm. When done before or after bronchodilator administration or respiratory therapy, it helps gauge therapeutic effectiveness.

• Attach the mouthpiece to the peak flowmeter.
• Have the patient sit up. Then instruct him to inhale as deeply as possible. Insert the mouthpiece and have him seal his lips tightly around it.
• Instruct the patient to exhale forcefully into the flowmeter in one short, sharp blast.
• Note the PEF reading on the dial, recorded in liters per second or minute.

Nursing considerations
• Try to schedule bedside PFTs during a quiet time when both you and the patient are free from distractions.
• Don't perform bedside pulmonary function monitoring immediately after a large meal (to prevent abdominal discomfort).
• If the patient wears dentures that fit poorly, remove them to prevent air leakage around the mouthpiece. If the dentures fit well, leave them in place to promote a tight seal.
• If the patient is likely to develop hypoxemia or difficulty breathing during measurement, provide oxygen before and after the test.
• Use of certain drugs, such as analgesics or bronchodilators, may produce misleading results. Withhold bronchodilators and other respiratory treatments, as ordered, before a test. If the patient receives a bronchodilator during the test, wait 4 hours before administering another dose.
• Encourage the patient during the test. This often helps patients exhale more forcefully. If the patient coughs during expiration, wait until his coughing subsides before repeating the measurement.
• For single-breath maneuvers, expect to repeat the test two or three times and record the highest value. Between measurements, have the patient rest and return him to the ventilator, if indicated.

• For serial testing, have the patient use the same position each time because variations in positioning may cause an inconsistent performance and unreliable results. Document the position along with test results.
• Take necessary measures to prevent infection — a crucial concern with bedside pulmonary function equipment. Use disposable components whenever possible. Follow your hospital's policy on handling used equipment.
• Document measurements on the patient's medical record, noting mechanical ventilator settings, bronchodilator administration, and patient positioning. Compare new values with previous results, including baseline measurements, and report significant variations to the doctor.
• Bedside PFTs usually are discontinued once the patient becomes stable or has been successfully weaned from a mechanical ventilator.
• Before the patient is discharged, provide appropriate teaching. If his condition warrants, teach him how to obtain PFT measurements at home to help assess disease progression and identify any need for more aggressive intervention.

Apnea monitoring

Commonly performed at the bedside, apnea monitoring provides an early warning of impending apneic episodes, documents the incidence and degree of apnea, and assesses the effectiveness of interventions.

In adults, apnea is defined as an absence of breathing lasting 10 seconds or longer. Apnea occurs in two distinct types: central and obstructive. Mixed apnea — a combination of central and obstructive apnea — also may occur.

In *central apnea,* the patient has no central respiratory output and therefore no respiratory effort. Central apnea is related to abnormal central nervous system functions that aren't fully understood.

In *obstructive apnea,* central respiratory output occurs but pharyngeal closure prevents airflow. Obstructive apnea may result from collapse of the compliant pharyngeal muscles, altered airway configuration caused by positioning, failure of smaller airways to remain patent, anatomic airway narrowing from fat or tissue edema, chronic inflammation caused by snoring, or increased upper airway resistance secondary to swelling or obstruction.

Many people normally experience brief periods of apnea during sleep. In *sleep apnea syndrome (SAS),* multiple episodes of obstructive or mixed apnea occur, accompanied by loud, repetitive snoring and daytime somnolence. Although definitions of SAS vary, the term usually refers to 30 or more periods of apnea per 7 hours of sleep or more than 5 such episodes per hour. SAS may cause problems ranging from mild to serious, including insomnia, daytime hypersomnolence, personality changes, cognitive dysfunction, arrhythmias, and laboratory test abnormalities (such as polycythemia, hypercapnia, and hypoxemia).

Among preterm infants, apneic episodes commonly are accompanied by bradycardia. Infantile apnea may result from an immature respiratory control center, respiratory center depression, failure of peripheral chemoreceptors to override hypoxemic depression of the respiratory center, reflex responses of the posterior pharynx and lungs, or airway obstruction related to positioning.

Equipment
Apnea monitoring usually requires a thoracic impedance monitor and chest electrodes. The monitor detects changes in thoracic impedance, which increases

Interpretation

Interpreting apnea monitoring findings

Normally, respirations are regular and rhythmic, without prolonged interruption. Therefore, consider frequent apnea a significant finding, especially when accompanied by other symptoms. The patient may need additional evaluation, including complete polysomnography assessment.

Apnea duration and frequency may be related to such treatments as drug therapy, continuous positive airway pressure, or surgery. As interventions change, note any improvement or deterioration in the patient's respiratory rate and pattern.

during inspiration and decreases during expiration. A respiratory amplifier displays the respiratory rate. Some monitors also display a respiratory waveform, whose amplitude reflects respiratory depth. (See *Interpreting apnea monitoring findings.*)

Implementation
Before the procedure, explain apnea monitoring to the patient and his family. (See *Explaining apnea monitoring,* page 80.) After teaching, take the following steps:
• Plug the power cable into a grounded electrical outlet, and wash your hands when done.
• Use alcohol pads to clean the patient's chest and abdomen at the sites where electrodes will be placed. Dry the skin thoroughly.
• Place electrodes on the patient's chest and abdomen, as the manufacturer directs. Attach the leadwires to the electrodes. Be sure to target areas where chest wall movement is greatest to help detect an adequate signal.

Teaching TimeSaver

Explaining apnea monitoring

To help prepare the patient for apnea monitoring, review these topics with him and his family members.
- Tell them that an electronic device will monitor the patient's breathing.
- Describe the monitoring procedure.
- Explain the application of the device and the information the monitor will display.
- Warn that the alarm settings must never be changed and the monitor never turned off.

• Turn on the monitor. Set the high and low respiratory rate alarms and adjust the apnea time period. Make sure that the alarm volume is audible and the printer (if available) is loaded with paper.

• Observe the respiratory rate, waveform, and heart rate displayed on the monitor. Document this information in the patient's medical record at least as often as you record routine vital signs. Report and document the presence and degree of any apneic episodes, including their time, frequency, and duration. Also document any associated bradycardia or other findings.

Nursing considerations

• When an apnea alarm sounds, first assess the patient, checking for bradycardia and other arrhythmias, cyanosis, and airway obstruction. Be prepared to ventilate and oxygenate the patient if he remains unresponsive to stimulation. Carefully assess airway adequacy and intervene as necessary to maintain patency.

• After correcting apnea, evaluate the patient for the underlying cause by thoroughly assessing his respiratory, neurologic, and metabolic status. If you suspect sepsis, obtain cultures and administer antibiotics, as ordered. Specific therapy aims to treat the underlying cause of apnea.

• If your patient has obstructive apnea, stay alert for airway obstruction during apnea monitoring. The chest wall may continue to move even though the airway is obstructed. Because the apnea monitor can't distinguish between effective and ineffective ventilation, a patient with unstable respiratory status may require additional monitoring, such as pulse oximetry.

• If artifact or poor signal quality triggers the apnea alarm, reassess the position and integrity of chest electrodes. If necessary, reposition or replace electrodes to enhance signal quality. Also replace any loose electrodes. Remove electrodes carefully, particularly if the patient has or may develop impaired skin integrity.

• Before discharge, teach the patient and his family how to use an apnea monitor at home, if indicated.

• Apnea monitoring usually is discontinued after testing has been completed or when apneic episodes decrease in frequency and duration to a clinically acceptable level. It also may be discontinued if the doctor orders an alternate form of respiratory monitoring.

CHAPTER

4

Caring for patients with acute respiratory disorders

Adult respiratory distress syndrome

A form of pulmonary edema, adult respiratory distress syndrome (ARDS) can quickly lead to acute respiratory failure. Sometimes difficult to recognize, ARDS nonetheless requires prompt diagnosis and treatment.

ARDS results from increased permeability of pulmonary membranes, which allows fluid to accumulate in the lung interstitium, alveolar spaces, and small airways. This causes the lung to stiffen, which impairs ventilation and reduces the oxygenation of pulmonary capillary blood. (See *What happens in ARDS.*)

Without prompt diagnosis and treatment, ARDS can result in death within 48 hours of onset. Even with technologic advances in monitoring and treatment, mortality remains at 40% to 60%. When the underlying cause is sepsis, neoplasm, renal failure, or nonpulmonary organ failure, mortality may be as high as 90%. Severe ARDS can lead to metabolic and respiratory acidosis and ensuing cardiac arrest. Most patients who recover from ARDS have little or no permanent lung damage. Some, however, develop pulmonary fibrosis and have permanent respiratory difficulties.

Causes

ARDS results directly or indirectly from injuries to the lung, which may be due to a variety of clinical conditions. (See *Causes of ARDS,* page 84.)

ASSESSMENT

Because ARDS can be fatal, you must recognize patients who may be at risk and assess them for early signs. Your assessment should include consideration of the patient's health history, physical examination findings, and diagnostic test results.

Health history

Your patient's recent health history usually indicates a risk factor that precipitates ARDS. In many instances, however, the precipitating condition (such as massive trauma) prevents the patient from answering any health history questions. In such cases, move on quickly to the physical examination.

Physical examination

ARDS progresses through four distinct phases. During your assessment, watch your patient for signs indicating a progression to ARDS. (See *Four phases of ARDS,* page 85.)

Diagnostic test results

The following tests may reveal factors that indicate possible ARDS:

• Arterial blood gas (ABG) analysis (performed with the patient breathing room air) shows a reduced partial pressure of oxygen in arterial blood (PaO_2), below 60 mm Hg, and a decreased partial pressure of carbon dioxide in arterial blood ($PaCO_2$), below 35 mm Hg. Although the patient may already be receiving oxygen, a decreased PaO_2 persists.

Timesaving tip: The hallmark of ARDS is refractory hypoxemia (an abnormal deficiency of oxygen in arterial blood) that's unresponsive to supplemental oxygen. The resulting blood pH usually reflects respiratory alkalosis.

As respiratory distress worsens, ABG values can show respiratory acidosis (rising $PaCO_2$, above 45 mm Hg), metabolic acidosis (declining bicarbonate ion levels, below 22 mEq/liter), and a declining PaO_2 despite oxygen therapy.

• Pulmonary artery catheterization helps confirm the presence of noncardiogenic pulmonary edema (by

What happens in ARDS

In adult respiratory distress syndrome (ARDS), capillary membrane permeability is enhanced. As a result, plasma and proteins leak from the capillaries into the interstitial spaces and alveoli (as indicated by the arrows), thereby reducing lung compliance and volume and inhibiting normal gas exchange.

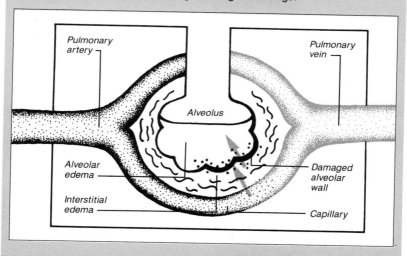

measuring the pulmonary artery wedge pressure [PAWP]). However, it does not identify the cause. PAWP values in ARDS are typically 12 mm Hg or less. Mixed venous oxygen saturation ($S\overline{v}O_2$) may be abnormal, reflecting tissue hypoxia.

• Serial chest X-rays taken early in ARDS show bilateral, fluffy infiltrates. In later phases, lung fields display a ground-glass appearance. Eventually, with irreversible hypoxemia, chest X-rays show "whiteouts" of both lung fields.

Differential diagnosis must rule out cardiogenic pulmonary edema, pulmonary vasculitis, and diffuse pulmonary hemorrhage. The following tests may be performed to determine the cause of ARDS:

• sputum analyses (including Gram stain and culture and sensitivity tests)
• blood cultures (to identify infectious organisms)
• toxicology tests (to screen for drug ingestion)
• serum amylase test (to rule out pancreatitis).

NURSING DIAGNOSIS

Common nursing diagnoses for a patient with ARDS include:

• Ineffective airway clearance related to excessive secretions and a weak or absent cough

FactFinder

Causes of ARDS

Many different conditions may lead to adult respiratory distress syndrome (ARDS).

Most common causes
- Sepsis
- Aspiration of gastric secretions
- Massive trauma

Less common causes
- Multiple blood transfusions
- Near drowning
- Diffuse parenchymal lung injuries
- Prolonged cardiopulmonary bypass
- Anaphylaxis
- Diffuse pneumonia (especially viral pneumonia, but also bacterial, fungal, mycoplasmal, and pneumocystic pneumonia)
- Disseminated intravascular coagulation
- Overdose of heroin, aspirin, ethchlorvynol, or other drugs
- Idiosyncratic drug reactions (to ampicillin and hydrochlorothiazide)
- Oxygen toxicity
- Inhalation of smoke or irritant gases, such as nitrous oxide, ammonia, or chlorine
- Leukemia
- Acute miliary tuberculosis
- Pancreatitis
- Thrombotic thrombocytopenic purpura
- Fat or air emboli (microemboli)
- Extensive burns
- Ionizing radiation
- Eclampsia
- Severe nervous system trauma from an extrathoracic injury
- Hepatic failure
- Flail chest

- Anxiety related to deteriorating health and possible impending death
- Impaired gas exchange related to pulmonary edema, ventilation-perfusion mismatch, and intrapulmonary shunting
- Altered nutrition: Less than body requirements, related to increased metabolic demand and lack of nutrients
- Inability to sustain spontaneous ventilation related to profound hypoxemia associated with injury to alveolocapillary membrane
- Decreased cardiac output related to inadequate fluid replacement, end-stage sepsis, or decreased preload caused by mechanical ventilation with positive end-expiratory pressure (PEEP)
- High risk for infection related to malnutrition, altered cell-mediated immunity, invasive monitoring and therapeutic devices, and accumulation of alveolar fluid.

PLANNING

Because ARDS is life-threatening, direct your nursing care toward clearing the patient's airways, easing his ventilation, and alleviating his anxiety.

Based on the nursing diagnosis *ineffective airway clearance,* develop appropriate patient outcomes. For example, your patient will:
- produce clear, thin mucus when coughing or through suctioning or postural drainage and percussion
- maintain clear or baseline breath sounds
- maintain ABG values within specified limits.

Based on the nursing diagnosis *anxiety,* develop appropriate patient outcomes. For example, your patient will:
- talk, write, or use nonverbal gestures to express feelings of anxiety
- use support systems and relaxation techniques to improve coping skills
- show evidence that anxiety is abated, either verbally or through behavior.

Four phases of ARDS

Adult respiratory distress syndrome (ARDS) occurs in four phases, each of which produces characteristic effects.

Phase 1
The patient appears normal and remains alert after the initial injury. He hyperventilates and has dyspnea on exertion. You may also find:
- high-normal respiratory and pulse rates
- diminished breath sounds
- chest X-ray that reveals clear or slightly congested lungs
- arterial blood gas (ABG) analysis that shows normal or slightly reduced partial pressure of carbon dioxide in arterial blood ($PaCO_2$), averaging 30 to 40 mm Hg
- decreased tissue perfusion.

Phase 2
The patient shows signs of subclinical respiratory distress, such as use of accessory muscles to breathe; a dry cough with thick, frothy sputum; and bloody, sticky secretions. You may also observe:
- anxiety and restlessness
- diaphoresis; cool, clammy skin on palpation
- tachypnea
- tachycardia
- elevated blood pressure
- basilar crackles on auscultation
- ABG analysis that reveals hypocapnia and hypoxemia that persists despite oxygen administration and $PaCO_2$ typically ranging from 25 to 30 mm Hg
- continued hyperventilation; possibly no change in chest X-ray.

Phase 3
The patient appears gravely ill and visibly struggles for air. You may also observe:
- severe dyspnea, tachypnea, and tachycardia with arrhythmias (usually premature ventricular contractions and ST-segment and T-wave changes)
- labile blood pressure
- decreased mentation
- pale, cyanotic skin
- productive cough
- crackles, rhonchi, and wheezing on auscultation (requiring intubation and ventilation)
- chest X-ray that shows pulmonary edema
- continued hyperventilation
- ABG analysis that shows further diminished $PaCO_2$ (20 to 35 mm Hg) and partial pressure of oxygen in arterial blood (50 to 60 mm Hg)
- intrapulmonary shunting that may involve 20% to 30% of the patient's cardiac output.

Phase 4
Now in acute respiratory failure, the patient has severe hypoxemia. Lacking spontaneous respirations, his mental status deteriorates and he may become agitated, then unresponsive. Because he can't continue to compensate by hyperventilating, his $PaCO_2$ increases, reflecting a marked reduction in the number of functioning alveolocapillary units. You may also find:
- bradycardia (less than 60 beats/minute) with arrhythmias and severe hypotension
- metabolic and respiratory acidosis
- cardiac output decreased by 50% to 60%
- pale, cyanotic skin
- chest X-ray that shows "whiteouts" of both lung fields

The patient is at risk for developing pulmonary fibrosis and for sustaining potentially fatal pulmonary damage.

Based on the nursing diagnosis *impaired gas exchange,* develop appropriate patient outcomes. For example, your patient will:
• maintain baseline PaO$_2$ (normal values range from 75 to 100 mm Hg)
• maintain baseline PaCO$_2$ (normal values range from 35 to 45 mm Hg)
• maintain arterial oxygen saturation of 95%
• maintain baseline breath sounds
• be successfully weaned from mechanical ventilation
• maintain baseline level of consciousness (LOC)
• show evidence of minimal or absent residual lung damage after recovery from ARDS
• demonstrate baseline peak inspiratory pressure (PIP).

Based on the nursing diagnosis *altered nutrition,* develop appropriate patient outcomes. For example, your patient will:
• maintain a positive nitrogen balance
• receive a specified daily caloric intake
• maintain or return to his target weight.

Based on the nursing diagnosis *inability to sustain spontaneous ventilation,* develop appropriate patient outcomes. For example, your patient will:
• maintain a respiratory rate within 5 breaths/minute of baseline
• maintain acceptable ABG levels
• indicate feeling comfortable, with no reports of pain, dyspnea, or fatigue
• not show signs of respiratory distress
• maintain acceptable pulmonary function test results before and after ventilator use.

Based on the nursing diagnosis *decreased cardiac output,* develop appropriate patient outcomes. For example, your patient will:
• maintain a stable fluid balance to avoid interstitial edema
• maintain body weight within an acceptable range

• achieve a heart rate within range of baseline and be free of arrhythmias
• maintain systolic blood pressure above 90 mm Hg and mean arterial pressure (MAP) above 80 mm Hg
• void more than 30 ml/hour of urine
• maintain S$\bar{v}$O$_2$ between 60% and 80%
• have warm, dry skin
• have normal PAWP, central venous pressure (CVP), and pulmonary artery pressure (PAP) readings
• maintain cardiac output, cardiac index, and systemic vascular resistance within specified ranges.

Based on the nursing diagnosis *high risk for infection,* develop appropriate patient outcomes. For example, your patient will:
• maintain body temperature within a specified range
• have clean, dry catheter insertion sites without erythema
• demonstrate an absence of pathogen growth as evidenced by cultures such as blood and sputum
• exhibit respiratory secretions that are clear, thin, and odorless.

IMPLEMENTATION

Adjust your nursing interventions to suit the patient's condition. He will need to be carefully monitored no matter which stage of ARDS he is in. Since ARDS is potentially fatal, communicate the importance of complying with the treatment. (See *Medical care of the patient with ARDS.*)

Nursing interventions
• Watch for and immediately report all respiratory changes in the patient at risk for ARDS. This is especially important during the first few days after onset, when the patient may appear to be improving. Early warning signs of ARDS are dyspnea, tachypnea, or hypoxemia that fails to respond to supplemental oxygen.

Treatments

Medical care of the patient with ARDS

Treatment for adult respiratory distress syndrome (ARDS) addresses the cause of the syndrome and focuses on halting the progression of life-threatening hypoxemia and respiratory acidosis.

Supportive care
Supportive care includes administering humidified oxygen through a tight-fitting mask, which allows for continuous positive airway pressure.

Another supportive measure is carefully managing the patient's fluid status to achieve baseline intravascular volume and to ensure adequate cardiac output and tissue perfusion without making pulmonary edema substantially worse. Using fluid challenges or diuretic therapy (depending on which direction pulmonary artery wedge pressure [PAWP] is taking) helps the patient maintain PAWP at 6 to 12 mm Hg. However, these therapies alone seldom fulfill the ARDS patient's ventilatory requirements. He usually needs intubation, mechanical ventilation, and positive end-expiratory pressure.

Drug therapy
When a patient with ARDS requires mechanical ventilation, drug therapy may be used to ease ventilation, to help decrease peak inspiratory pressure, and to minimize restlessness (thereby decreasing oxygen consumption and production of carbon dioxide). Prescribed drugs may include sedatives, narcotics, or neuromuscular blockers, such as vecuronium.

Electrolyte and acid-base imbalances must be addressed during therapy. When ARDS results from fatty emboli or a chemical injury, a short course of high-dose corticosteroids may help, if treatment is started early enough. Treatment with sodium bicarbonate may reverse severe metabolic acidosis.

Nonviral infections call for treatment with antibiotics.

Current research
Treatments under development include:
• prostaglandin E$_1$ to promote vasodilation and, possibly, to improve ventilation-perfusion mismatch
• exogenous surfactants
• a monoclonal antibody that may prevent white blood cells from adhering to the pulmonary endothelium
• extracorporeal membrane oxygenation, an aggressive treatment that allows lung bypass.

Timesaving tip: You can save time by obtaining ear or pulse oximetry measurements and spirometry measurements at the patient's bedside. These measurements can indicate the presence of hypoxemia and gross lung compliance.
• Frequently assess the patient's respiratory status throughout the course of ARDS. Note his respiratory rate, rhythm, and depth. Watch for dyspnea, nasal flaring, and accessory muscle use. Listen for adventitious or diminished breath sounds. Check for frothy sputum (indicating pulmonary edema). Evaluate the patient's LOC, noting confusion, anxiousness, agitation, or mental sluggishness.
• Monitor the patient's ABG levels frequently. Record the results of ABG analysis, oximetry, and mixed venous blood sampling, if available.

• Anticipate using mechanical ventilation when the patient's respiratory rate climbs above 30 breaths/minute and his PaO_2 falls below 55 mm Hg with a fraction of inspired oxygen of 21%; if his $PaCO_2$ rises; or if his cardiovascular status is unstable.

• Administer oxygen, as directed, to maintain positive airway pressure. Expect to use either continuous positive airway pressure or, more likely, mechanical ventilation with PEEP. (See *Using PEEP and CPAP.*)

• Maintain ventilator efficiency when using mechanical ventilation. Frequently check the accuracy of ventilator settings for specified delivery of oxygen, PEEP, tidal volume, respiratory rate, and other indices.

• Promptly drain condensation from the tubing (but away from the patient to avoid lavaging the patient's lungs).

• Begin PEEP as ordered, usually at 3 to 5 cm H_2O, and increase as ordered by small increments. Record the effects on the patient's cardiac output and ABG levels.

• Gradually reduce PEEP as the patient's condition improves. Never abruptly discontinue it; doing so could bring on an immediate alveolar collapse with hypoxemia.

• Assess lung compliance by monitoring PIP and static compliance values in mechanically ventilated patients. A PIP level above 40 cm H_2O may indicate worsening lung compliance, accumulated airway secretions, airflow blockage from kinked tubing, or incoordination of spontaneous and ventilator breaths from patient agitation.

• If PIP doesn't decrease after suctioning or after resolving mechanical problems, notify the respiratory therapist and the doctor.

• Give sedatives or anxiolytics as ordered to reduce restlessness and associated oxygen consumption. Monitor and record the patient's response to medication.

• Be alert for signs of complications induced by ARDS such as pulmonary hypertension, pulmonary fibrosis, and oxygen toxicity.

• Maintain an open airway by suctioning. Use a sterile, nontraumatic technique. Also use sterile technique for other invasive procedures.

• Use the closed tracheal suctioning system to suction mechanically ventilated patients. (See *Closed tracheal suctioning*, page 91.)

• Assist during a tracheotomy and provide tracheostomy care if necessary (if ARDS leads to long-term respiratory distress with prolonged ventilatory weaning).

• Check that the air or inhaled gas is adequately humidified to help liquefy tenacious secretions. Perform postural drainage and percussion to help mobilize secretions.

• Auscultate breath sounds after suctioning and performing postural drainage and percussion; note any changes. Also note the amount, color, and consistency of secretions and if any odor is evident.

• Look for any indications of infection — for example, an elevated white blood cell count, fever, redness and drainage at a catheter insertion site, or changes in wounds, incisions, or puncture sites.

• Care for indwelling line sites according to hospital protocol, using strict aseptic technique.

• Monitor serum electrolyte levels and correct imbalances as directed.

• Monitor the patient's cardiac output. Stay alert for signs of decreased cardiac output, such as tachycardia, decreased $S\overline{v}O_2$, hypotension, cool, clammy skin, decreased peripheral pulses, reduced urine output, and altered mentation.

• To maintain or restore adequate cardiac output, administer fluids and inotropic drugs as prescribed.

Using PEEP and CPAP

When mechanical ventilation fails to maintain an adequate partial pressure of oxygen in arterial blood (PaO_2), the patient may benefit from the addition of positive end-expiratory pressure (PEEP). PEEP applies positive pressure during expiration on a ventilator. When spontaneous respirations fail to maintain PaO_2, the patient may benefit from the use of continuous positive airway pressure (CPAP). CPAP applies positive pressure throughout the respiratory cycle during spontaneous breathing.

PEEP and CPAP prevent airway pressure from returning to zero, or atmospheric pressure. This, in turn, creates an intra-alveolar volume great enough to overcome the elastic forces of the lung, which helps reopen collapsed alveoli and prevents small airway closure at the end of expiration. Using PEEP or CPAP increases functional residual capacity (FRC) and substantially improves gas exchange. This, in turn, decreases intrapulmonary shunting and ventilation-perfusion mismatch, resulting in improved PaO_2.

Normal alveolus

FRC provides the volume that keeps the alveolus open for gas exchange. The dark to light shades within the capillary represent increasingly oxygenated blood, indicating adequate ventilation and perfusion.

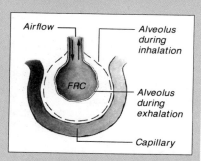

Airflow — Alveolus during inhalation

FRC

Alveolus during exhalation

Capillary

Deflated alveolus

Because less area is available for gas exchange, FRC significantly declines. The dark shading in the capillary indicates poorly oxygenated blood.

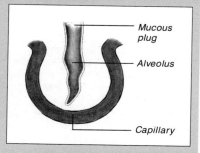

Mucous plug

Alveolus

Capillary

(continued)

Using PEEP and CPAP *(continued)*

Alveolar changes with PEEP or CPAP
The positive pressure exerted by
PEEP or CPAP keeps the alveolus expanded, increasing FRC. The shading
of the capillary indicates adequate ventilation and perfusion.

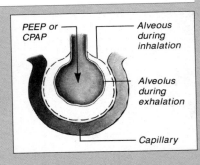

• Assess the patient's CVP, PAP, and
PAWP. Suspect reduced venous return
(possibly caused by fluid volume deficit or increased intrathoracic pressure
associated with mechanical ventilation
and PEEP) if any of these measurements is below normal.
• Closely monitor the patient's heart
rate and rhythm, blood pressure, and
vital signs. Watch for arrhythmias that
may result from hypoxemia, acid-base
disturbances, or electrolyte imbalances.
• Administer antiarrhythmics as prescribed.
• Control your patient's fluid status.
Titrate fluid replacements accurately
for adequate cardiac output, but avoid
overhydration, which may exacerbate
pulmonary edema.
• Establish a baseline weight to help
evaluate fluid status. Weigh the patient
daily, at the same time each day and
with the patient wearing the same
amount of clothing, and maintain strict
intake and output records.
• Closely monitor the patient's hemodynamic status. Determine the desired
hemodynamic parameters (usually a
PAWP of 6 to 12 mm Hg). Greater

pressures may indicate fluid overload,
necessitating diuretic therapy. PAWP
measurements below this range may
indicate inadequate intravascular fluid
volume. In this case, anticipate a fluid
challenge.
• Consider other assessment parameters when assessing fluid status, such as
CVP, PAP, urine output, serum and
urine electrolyte values, and osmolality
values.
• Reposition the patient frequently to
decrease atelectasis and to prevent
complications of immobility.
• Report any signs indicating that the
patient's condition is deteriorating,
such as hypotension, increased secretions, elevated temperature, or worsening ABG values.
• Monitor the patient's nutritional intake. If requested, administer tube
feedings or parenteral nutrition using a
flow-control device.
• Plan your patient care to allow periods of uninterrupted sleep. For best results, arrange for alternate periods of
rest and activity.
• Help keep the patient's joints mobile
by performing passive range-of-mo-

Closed tracheal suctioning

An alternative to conventional suctioning, closed tracheal suctioning allows you to suction the patient without interrupting mechanical ventilation and positive end-expiratory pressure therapy. It offers the advantage of containing the patient's secretions and is faster than open suctioning.

Equipment

The closed tracheal suctioning apparatus consists of a catheter in a sleeve that attaches to the ventilator circuitry as it joins the endotracheal or tracheostomy tube. Once attached, the catheter system can remain in place for 24 hours, reducing the risk of secondary infection during frequent suctioning.

Procedure

To use the closed tracheal suctioning system, follow these steps:

• Remove the tip protector and attach the control valve to the wall suction unit. The valve for activating suction pressure has a locked position to prevent it from being accidentally activated by the patient.

• Turn on the wall suction, depress the thumb control valve, and set the wall suction to the desired level.

• Attach the T-piece to the ventilator tubing and the endotracheal or tracheostomy tube. Keeping the T-piece parallel with the patient's chin, guide the bidirectional catheter into the left lung by rotating the catheter clockwise toward the one o'clock position and advancing it through the trachea and left main bronchus (as shown). Use the blue line on the catheter as a guide. Then apply intermittent suction by depressing the thumb control valve.

• Pull the catheter back slightly and turn it to the left by rotating it to the 11 o'clock position and advancing it into the patient's right lung. Again, apply intermittent suction by depressing the thumb control valve.

• Keeping a grip on the T-piece, gently withdraw the catheter completely so that the extended length of the catheter is in the sleeve and the black mark on the catheter is visible at the back of the T-piece.

• When you've completed suctioning, flush the catheter through the irrigation port by starting the suction; then slowly instill the flushing solution while maintaining suction. To prevent inadvertent suctioning, lift and turn the thumbpiece 180 degrees to the lock position on the suction control valve.

tion exercises. If possible, help the patient perform active exercises.

• Provide meticulous skin care and reposition the patient every 2 hours. To prevent skin breakdown, also reposition the endotracheal tube from side to side every 24 hours.

• Provide an alternative means of communication for the patient on mechanical ventilation.

Patient teaching

• Provide emotional support to the patient and family members. Try to answer questions as fully as possible to help allay their fears or concerns.

• Explain the disorder to the patient and family members. Tell them what signs and symptoms may occur, and review the required treatment.

• Orient the patient and family members to the hospital environment.

curs with time. Until then, patients often have dyspnea at rest or on exertion, restrictive or obstructive defect on pulmonary function tests, and chest X-ray abnormalities. (See *Ensuring continued care for the patient with ARDS*.)

EVALUATION

To evaluate the patient's response to your care, gather your reassessment data and compare this information with the patient outcomes specified in your plan of care.

Teaching and counseling
Begin by determining the effectiveness of your teaching. Consider the following questions:
• Does the patient understand the disorder, its possible complications, and its treatment?
• Does he know the signs and symptoms to report to the doctor?
• Does he show evidence of reduced anxiety?

Physical condition
Consider the following questions:
• Are the patient's airways clear?
• Have coughing, suctioning, and postural drainage and percussion cleared the airway, as evidenced by clear, thin mucus and mobilized secretions? Does lung auscultation substantiate your findings?
• Is he receiving adequate nutrition?
• Is the patient able to sustain spontaneous ventilation? Does he exhibit a normal respiratory rate and feeling of comfort? Are pain, dyspnea, and fatigue absent?
• Is his fluid balance stable?
• Is his weight within an acceptable range?
• Does he demonstrate a heart rate within established parameters and is he free of arrhythmias?
• Is he maintaining systolic blood pressure above 90 mm Hg, MAP above

• Tell the recuperating patient that recovery will take some time and that he will feel weak for a while. Urge him to share his concerns with the staff.
• Reassure your patient that most ARDS patients regain a satisfactory level of pulmonary functioning. However, some may need continued follow-up with the pulmonary specialist and a pulmonary rehabilitation program. Reduction of fibrosis usually oc-

80 mm Hg, urine output more than 30 ml/hour, and S$\overline{v}$O$_2$ between 60% and 80%?
• Does he exhibit warm, dry skin?
• Are his PAWP, CVP, and PAP readings normal?
• Are cardiac output, cardiac index, and systemic vascular resistance maintained within specified ranges?
• Does he exhibit any signs of infection?

Upper airway obstruction

Upper airway obstruction refers to any interruption in the airflow to the lungs through the nose, mouth, or throat. The obstruction can be partial or complete and may be life-threatening.

Causes
Causes of upper airway obstruction include tumors, vocal cord paralysis, edema of the epiglottis and larynx (resulting from tonsillitis, for example), infection of the nasopharynx and oropharynx, thickened secretions, tongue occlusion, foreign body aspiration, Ludwig's angina, palatal paresis, and thyroid enlargement. (See *Key points about upper airway obstruction.*) Other causes of upper airway obstruction include laryngeal and tracheal trauma (such as tracheal stricture or tracheomalacia) and anaphylaxis.

ASSESSMENT

The patient's signs and symptoms will vary with the cause, location, and severity of the upper airway obstruction. Regardless of the cause, quick and accurate assessment is urgent. If the condition is not treated promptly, complete airway obstruction can bring on hypoxia and lead to loss of consciousness, cardiopulmonary collapse, and possible death within minutes. Follow

FactFinder
Key points about upper airway obstruction

• *Dangers:* Complete airway obstruction causes anoxia. If left untreated, it can lead to brain damage and death in 4 to 6 minutes.
• *Causes:* The most common cause of complete airway obstruction in a conscious patient is foreign body aspiration. An adult is most likely to aspirate food. An infant or a child may aspirate food or some other object.
• *Risk factors:* Risk factors for choking include drug and alcohol use, diseases affecting motor coordination (such as Parkinson's disease), absence of or poorly fitting dentures, and conditions that affect mental functioning (such as cerebrovascular accident).

your hospital's protocol for emergency interventions.

Physical examination
The patient may show increasing or sudden anxiety and distress. If he's conscious, ask him to speak. This will help you determine whether his airway is partly or fully blocked.

If the patient can't speak, his airway is completely occluded. He may place his hands on his neck, a common sign of airway obstruction. He may gag, salivate, and sweat profusely. No air will flow from his nose and mouth, and you won't hear any breath sounds. You will see intercostal retractions and abdominal muscle movements. The patient may quickly become cyanotic and lose consciousness.

If the patient can speak, his airway is only partially occluded. Accompanying signs may include dyspnea, inspiratory stridor, wheezing, and dry, paroxysmal coughing (which means air

Signs and symptoms of upper airway obstruction

Complete obstruction
In the conscious patient, look for:
• anxiety
• gagging and cyanosis
• salivation
• lack of air movement or phonation.
In the unconscious patient, look for:
• intercostal retractions
• accessory muscle use
• lack of air movement.

Partial obstruction
In the conscious patient, look for:
• inspiratory stridor (crowing)
• altered speech
• coughing (air movement present).
In the unconscious patient, look for:
• snoring respirations (air movement present).

movement is present), and tachycardia. You may also note decreased breath sounds. Snoring respirations may be heard in the unconscious (or sleeping) patient. Cyanosis and accessory muscle use may be evident depending on the severity of the obstruction. (See *Signs and symptoms of upper airway obstruction.*)

Diagnostic test results
Depending on the degree of obstruction, diagnostic tests may include:
• radiographic studies, such as X-rays, computed tomography scans of the neck, and bronchography, which can help identify the nature and location of a partial obstruction
• laryngoscopy and bronchoscopy, which can help pinpoint the nature, size, and location of an obstruction
• arterial blood gas (ABG) analysis, which will reveal decreased partial pressure of oxygen and increased par-

tial pressure of carbon dioxide. ABG analysis will also show respiratory and metabolic acidosis, which occur with severe partial or complete airway obstruction.

Timesaving tip: Pulse oximetry quickly defines the degree of oxygen saturation, which is an indicator of patient status and response to treatment.

NURSING DIAGNOSIS

Common nursing diagnoses for a patient with upper airway obstruction include:
• Inability to sustain spontaneous ventilation, related to complete airway obstruction
• Impaired gas exchange, related to impaired ventilation due to obstruction
• Anxiety related to acute respiratory distress and fear of impending death.

PLANNING

Because upper airway obstructions can be fatal, focus your immediate care on helping your patient to breathe and on relieving his anxiety.

Based on the nursing diagnosis *inability to sustain spontaneous ventilation*, develop appropriate patient outcomes. For example, your patient will:
• breathe spontaneously after the obstruction is removed or resolved
• maintain baseline respiratory rate
• attain baseline ABG levels
• maintain baseline breathing pattern
• be free of dyspnea.

Based on the nursing diagnosis *impaired gas exchange*, develop appropriate patient outcomes. For example, your patient will:
• attain baseline ABG levels
• maintain baseline breath sounds
• express a feeling of comfort in maintaining air exchange
• achieve an acceptable baseline respiratory rate.

Based on the nursing diagnosis *anxiety*, develop appropriate patient outcomes. For example, your patient will:
• state that he feels less anxious
• express knowledge of ways to prevent repeated obstruction.

IMPLEMENTATION

Your nursing care will depend on the cause and severity of the patient's upper airway obstruction. In addition to a quick and accurate response, he will need your support and reassurance. (See *Medical care in upper airway obstruction*.)

Nursing interventions
• If you suspect aspiration of a foreign body and the patient can cough forcefully — indicating adequate air exchange — do not interfere with his attempts to expel the foreign body. Call for assistance, but stay with the patient at all times because air exchange may stop.
• If a patient stops eating and suddenly clutches his throat and can't speak or cough, suspect complete airway obstruction due to aspiration of a foreign body. Intervene immediately by using the antichoking techniques recommended by the American Heart Association (AHA). In an adult, these maneuvers may include abdominal thrust, chest thrust, and finger-sweeps.
• As a last resort, a doctor, specially trained nurse, or other trained medical personnel *only* should perform a cricothyrotomy or percutaneous transtracheal catheter ventilation.

 Timesaving tip: The tongue is the most common cause of airway obstruction. Therefore, if a patient suddenly loses consciousness, you may be able to restore a patent airway by performing the head-tilt, chin-lift maneuver. Avoid hyperextending the patient's neck, which can cause cervical

Treatments
Medical care in upper airway obstruction

Treatment for upper airway obstruction depends on the location, cause, and severity of the condition. Your interventions may include:
• using a chin-lift or jaw-thrust maneuver
• performing finger-sweeps and abdominal and chest thrusts to clear a foreign body
• suctioning secretions
• providing an artificial airway
• administering prescribed drugs
• assisting with emergency surgery.

spine injury. (See *Performing the head-tilt, chin-lift maneuver,* page 96).
• Insert a nasopharyngeal or oropharyngeal airway if necessary.
• If obstruction is caused by secretions, suctioning may restore patency.
• If obstruction is related to edema associated with an infection, allergic reaction, or other inflammation, administer prescribed medications, such as antibiotics, epinephrine, or corticosteroids.
• Assist the doctor in performing an emergency tracheotomy, if necessary.
• Briefly and calmly explain all procedures to the patient to help alleviate anxiety. Stay with the patient and provide reassurance as needed to the patient and family members.
• Assess the patient's respiratory status throughout all procedures. Notify the doctor promptly at the first signs of clinical deterioration.
• If airway obstruction is related to fixed lesions such as tumors, surgery or endoscopic removal may be necessary to restore the airway. Explain preoperative and postoperative care to your patient.

Performing the head-tilt, chin-lift maneuver

If a patient loses consciousness because his tongue is obstructing his airway, perform the head-tilt, chin-lift maneuver to restore a patent airway. Follow these steps.
• Place the patient in the supine position.
• Put your hand on the patient's forehead and apply pressure that is firm enough to tilt the patient's head back.
• Place the fingertips of your other hand under the bony part of his lower jaw and lift the patient's chin. At the same time, keep his mouth partially open.
Avoid placing your fingertips on the soft tissue under the patient's chin; this may inadvertently obstruct the airway you're trying to open.
If you know or suspect that the patient has a neck injury, use the jaw-thrust maneuver instead of the head-tilt, chin-lift maneuver.

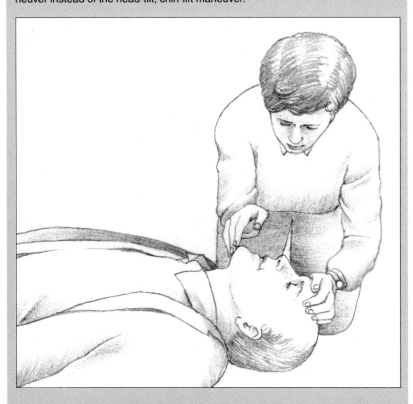

Discharge TimeSaver

Ensuring continued care for the patient with upper airway obstruction

Review the following teaching topics, referrals, and follow-up appointments to make sure that your patient is adequately prepared for discharge.

Teaching topics

Make sure that the following topics have been covered and that your patient's learning has been evaluated:
□ an explanation of upper airway obstruction and its causes and possible complications
□ explanation of techniques to avoid choking, if needed
□ medications, such as those to guard against further allergic reactions, as indicated
□ signs and symptoms to report to the doctor.

Referrals

Make sure that the patient has been provided with necessary referrals to:
□ allergist
□ medical identification bracelet supplier, if needed
□ insect-sting emergency kit supplier, if necessary
□ American Heart Association or American Red Cross for instruction on basic life-support techniques.

Follow-up appointments

Make sure that the necessary follow-up appointments have been scheduled and that the patient has been notified:
□ doctor or clinic.

• Attempt to relieve your patient's anxiety, and don't hesitate to touch him to provide reassurance.

Patient teaching

• If the upper airway obstruction was caused by aspiration of a foreign body, teach your patient how to avoid choking. Instruct him to cut food into small pieces, chew slowly and thoroughly, and avoid laughing and talking when chewing or swallowing. Also warn him to avoid excessive alcohol use before and during meals, which can dull reactions and cause careless chewing and swallowing.

• Caution the patient to keep small objects away from toddlers and not to allow children to run, walk, talk, or play while they are chewing or swallowing.

• If the upper airway obstruction was caused by an allergic reaction, explain to the patient how he can protect himself in the future. This knowledge will help alleviate the patient's anxiety. Provide the patient with information on getting a medical identification bracelet, and instruct him to wear the bracelet at all times. Teach the patient how to avoid allergens and provide referral to an allergist for treatment. Also teach him how to use an insect-sting emergency kit.

• Encourage your patient and his family members to learn basic life-support techniques from the AHA or the American Red Cross. (See *Ensuring continued care for the patient with upper airway obstruction.*)

EVALUATION

When evaluating your patient's response to nursing care, gather reassessment data and compare this information with the patient outcomes specified in your plan of care.

Teaching and counseling

Evaluate the effectiveness of your teaching. Listen for statements from the patient indicating:

• knowledge of measures to prevent choking, including prevention measures for young children, if applicable
• understanding of how to guard against allergic reactions, how to order a medical identification bracelet, and how to use an insect-sting emergency kit, if necessary.

Physical condition

Make sure that the cause of the obstruction has been eliminated or resolved. Consider the following questions:

• Is the patient breathing spontaneously, with normal breath sounds?
• Are there any signs of dyspnea?
• Has the patient achieved a stable and acceptable baseline respiratory rate?
• Are his breathing pattern and ABG levels at baseline?

Acute respiratory failure in COPD

Acute respiratory failure occurs when the lungs can't adequately maintain arterial oxygenation or eliminate carbon dioxide. If the condition is left unchecked and untreated, it leads to tissue hypoxia, organ failure, and respiratory and cardiac arrest. Patients with chronic obstructive pulmonary disease (COPD) are at especially high risk for acute respiratory failure. (See *Detecting acute respiratory failure in COPD*.)

Causes

Acute respiratory failure may develop in COPD patients from any condition that increases the work of breathing and decreases the respiratory drive. (See *Causes of acute respiratory failure,* page 100.)

ASSESSMENT

Your assessment should include consideration of the patient's health history, physical examination findings, and diagnostic test results.

Timesaving tip: Signs and symptoms will alert you to the need for prompt diagnosis and treatment, but they aren't usually reliable in diagnosing acute respiratory failure in COPD or in evaluating the degree of hypoxemia or hypercapnia. Arterial blood gas (ABG) analysis is necessary for an accurate assessment.

Health history

The patient with acute respiratory failure in COPD will be anxious and have difficulty breathing. In most instances, you won't have time to conduct an in-depth patient interview because acute respiratory failure is life-threatening. You'll probably have to rely on family members or the patient's medical records to help you determine the precipitating incident.

Physical examination

On inspection, you will usually note cyanosis of the oral mucosa, lips, and nail beds; nasal flaring; and ashen-colored skin. You may observe the patient using accessory muscles to breathe. He may appear to be restless, anxious, depressed, lethargic, agitated, confused, or comatose.

The patient usually exhibits tachypnea, which signals impending respiratory failure. (Patients with a drug overdose, however, typically have a respiratory rate below 10 breaths/minute.) Respirations may be shallow, deep, or alternate between the two. *When respiratory muscle fatigue occurs, respiratory arrest can occur in seconds or minutes.*

During palpation, you may note cold, clammy skin and asymmetrical chest movement, which suggests pneumothorax. If tactile fremitus (a tremulous vibration of the chest wall) is present, you'll notice that it decreases over an obstructed bronchus or pleural effusion but increases over consolidated lung tissue.

During percussion, especially in patients with COPD, you may note hyperresonance. When acute respiratory failure results from atelectasis or pneumonia, percussion usually produces a dull or flat sound.

Auscultation may reveal diminished breath sounds or egophony (altered transmitted voice sounds and increased vocal resonance that sounds like high-pitched bleating) over an area of consolidation. In patients with pneumothorax, breath sounds may be absent. In some cases of respiratory failure, you may hear breath sounds such as wheezes (in asthma, inflammation, tumor), rhonchi (in bronchitis), and crackles (indicating pulmonary edema).

Tachycardia, with increased cardiac output and mildly elevated blood pressure secondary to adrenal release of catecholamine, may occur early in response to low partial pressure of oxygen in arterial blood (PaO_2). With myocardial hypoxia, arrhythmias may develop. Pulmonary hypertension also occurs.

Diagnostic test results

The following tests may reveal predisposing factors and help identify causes of acute respiratory failure in COPD:

• ABG analysis is the definitive test for diagnosing acute respiratory failure. In patients with COPD, deteriorating ABG values and pH strongly suggest acute respiratory failure, especially when compared with the patient's baseline values. In patients with essentially healthy lung tissue, PaO_2 below 50 mm Hg, partial pressure of carbon dioxide in arterial blood ($PaCO_2$) above 50 mm Hg, and pH below 7.35 usually

---

Detecting acute respiratory failure in COPD

Sometimes, acute respiratory failure is due solely to a failure of arterial oxygenation, or *hypoxemia*. This is generally characterized by partial pressure of oxygen in arterial blood (PaO_2) that's below 50 mm Hg.

Acute respiratory failure may also result from hypoxemia combined with *hypercapnia,* or ventilatory failure. This is generally shown by PaO_2 below 50 mm Hg, partial pressure of arterial carbon dioxide ($PaCO_2$) above 50 mm Hg, and respiratory acidosis (pH below 7.35).

ABG values in COPD patients

Patients with chronic obstructive pulmonary disease (COPD) have a consistently low PaO_2 (hypoxemia) and high $PaCO_2$ (hypercapnia). Their kidneys, however, have time to compensate for the gradual hypercapnia by retaining bicarbonate and buffering the respiratory acidosis. For these patients, then, acute respiratory failure can be shown only by acute deterioration in arterial blood gas (ABG) values with acidemia (an increased hydrogen-ion concentration in the blood) and corresponding clinical deterioration.

---

indicate acute respiratory failure. In patients with COPD, pH is even lower.

• Chest X-rays can help identify underlying pulmonary disease or conditions such as emphysema, atelectasis, lesions, pneumothorax, infiltrates, and effusions. Clear chest X-rays indicate an extrapulmonary source of acute respiratory failure, such as an airway obstruction, neuromuscular disease, or respiratory center depression.

• Electrocardiography (ECG) can demonstrate arrhythmias. Atrial ar-

Causes of acute respiratory failure

Respiratory infection, such as bronchitis or pneumonia, represents the most common cause of acute respiratory failure in patients with chronic obstructive pulmonary disease. Other causes include:
• bronchospasm
• accumulation of secretions from cough suppression
• central nervous system depression resulting from head trauma or injudicious use of sedatives, narcotics, tranquilizers, or oxygen
• cardiovascular disorders, such as myocardial infarction, congestive heart failure, or pulmonary emboli
• airway irritants, including smoke or fumes
• endocrine and metabolic disorders, such as myxedema or metabolic alkalosis
• thoracic abnormalities resulting from chest trauma, pneumothorax, or thoracic or abdominal surgery.

rhythmias are often present. Common ECG patterns point to cor pulmonale and myocardial hypoxia.
• Pulse oximetry reveals a decreasing arterial oxygen saturation (SaO_2) level.
• Blood tests, such as a white blood cell count with differential, can help detect underlying causes. An abnormally low hematocrit and decreased hemoglobin levels signal blood loss, which indicates a decreased oxygen-carrying capacity.
• Pulmonary artery catheterization helps to distinguish between pulmonary and cardiovascular causes of acute respiratory failure. It's also used to monitor hemodynamic pressures and may permit monitoring of mixed venous oxygen saturation, which provides a more accurate assessment of

cellular oxygen delivery and extraction with hemodynamic profiles than ABG levels.
• Additional tests, such as a blood culture, Gram stain, and sputum culture, can identify a pathogen if an infection is present.

NURSING DIAGNOSIS

Common diagnoses for a patient with acute respiratory failure in COPD include:
• Ineffective airway clearance related to excessive secretions or impaired cough
• Anxiety related to acute respiratory distress, fear of impending death, or fear of mechanical ventilation
• Impaired gas exchange related to alveolar hypoventilation and ventilation-perfusion mismatch
• Inability to sustain spontaneous ventilation related to impaired respiratory muscle function secondary to hypoxemia and acidosis
• High risk for infection related to invasive monitoring, therapeutic devices, and debilitation
• Ineffective breathing pattern related to respiratory muscle fatigue or chronic airflow limitations
• Altered tissue perfusion related to hypoxemia.

PLANNING

Because acute respiratory failure in COPD is life-threatening, direct your nursing care toward clearing the patient's airways, easing ventilation, and alleviating his anxiety.

Based on the nursing diagnosis *ineffective airway clearance,* develop appropriate patient outcomes. For example, your patient will:
• produce clear, thin mucus through coughing or suctioning
• be able to mobilize secretions by coughing, suctioning, and postural

drainage and percussion, as evidenced by lung auscultation
• maintain ABG values within specified limits
• have clear or baseline breath sounds
• maintain SaO_2 greater than 95% or near baseline saturation.

Based on the nursing diagnosis *anxiety,* develop appropriate patient outcomes. For example, your patient will:
• state or write down feelings of anxiety
• use available support systems to help him cope
• demonstrate fewer symptoms of anxiety.

Based on the nursing diagnosis *impaired gas exchange,* develop appropriate patient outcomes. For example, your patient will:
• attain baseline PaO_2
• maintain $PaCO_2$ of 35 to 45 mm Hg or baseline for the individual
• maintain baseline breath sounds
• maintain baseline level of consciousness (LOC).

Based on the nursing diagnosis *inability to sustain spontaneous ventilation,* develop appropriate patient outcomes. For example, your patient will:
• maintain a respiratory rate within 5 breaths/minute of baseline
• maintain specified ABG levels
• indicate feelings of comfort and absence of pain, dyspnea, and fatigue
• maintain specified respiratory parameters during and after mechanical ventilation.

Based on the nursing diagnosis *high risk for infection,* develop appropriate patient outcomes. For example, your patient will:
• maintain baseline body temperature
• have clean and dry catheter insertion sites
• demonstrate an absence of pathogen growth as evidenced by fluid cultures
• maintain baseline heart rate
• have clear and odorless respiratory secretions.

Based on the nursing diagnosis *ineffective breathing pattern,* develop appropriate patient outcomes. For example, your patient will:
• maintain a respiratory rate within 5 breaths/minute of baseline
• exhibit baseline ABG values
• demonstrate diaphragmatic pursed-lip breathing
• achieve lung expansion with adequate ventilation.

Based on the nursing diagnosis *altered tissue perfusion,* develop appropriate patient outcomes. For example, your patient will:
• show no signs of arrhythmia
• exhibit strong peripheral pulses
• maintain baseline LOC
• maintain urine output of at least 30 ml/hour or 0.5 ml/kg of body weight/hour
• exhibit baseline vital signs
• maintain baseline ABG levels
• exhibit cardiac output and cardiac index within specified ranges.

IMPLEMENTATION

Nursing care for the patient with acute respiratory failure in COPD involves carefully monitoring the patient and encouraging compliance with treatments. The patient may also need support and reassurance, especially if he is intubated and cannot speak. (See *Medical care of the COPD patient with acute respiratory failure,* page 102.)

Nursing interventions
• Administer oxygen to reverse hypoxemia. Use appropriate concentrations to maintain PaO_2 at a minimum range of 50 to 60 mm Hg. The patient with COPD usually requires low-flow supplemental oxygen because high-flow oxygen may suppress the patient's hypoxic drive to breathe and lead to respiratory arrest. Observe the patient for evidence of a positive response, such as

Treatments

Medical care of the COPD patient with acute respiratory failure

Oxygen represents the primary treatment for acute respiratory failure in chronic obstructive pulmonary disease (COPD). However, you must give oxygen cautiously. For instance, prolonged administration of a high fraction of inspired oxygen (FIO_2) can cause oxygen toxicity. Administration of excessive oxygen to COPD patients can depress the respiratory drive, resulting in apnea.

If significant respiratory acidosis persists, mechanical ventilation with an endotracheal or a tracheostomy tube may be necessary. High-frequency ventilation may be initiated if the patient doesn't respond to conventional mechanical ventilation.

Therapeutic goal
Treatment aims to keep the arterial oxygen saturation level around 95% and

partial pressure of oxygen in arterial blood at 50 to 60 mm Hg, using the lowest possible FIO_2. Oxygen concentrations are kept low by delivering oxygen at 1 to 3 liters/minute through a Venturi mask and nasal prongs.

Other treatments
• Bronchodilation may be used when patients have airflow problems. Theophylline preparations are commonly used, but beta blockers, delivered by nebulization, may also be used.
• Antibiotics may be given to treat an infection.
• Corticosteroids may be used to reduce airway edema and inflammation, but their use in treating COPD patients with acute respiratory failure remains controversial.
• Diuretics may be given if pulmonary edema is present.

improved breathing, color, ABG values, and SaO_2 levels on pulse oximetry.
• Maintain a patent airway. If the patient is intubated and lethargic, reposition him every 1 to 2 hours. Use postural drainage and percussion to help clear secretions.
• Observe the patient closely for respiratory arrest. Auscultate for breath sounds, monitor ABG values, and report any changes immediately. Notify the doctor of any deterioration in SaO_2 levels that are detected by pulse oximetry.
• Monitor vital signs frequently. Report signs of increasing pulse rate, rising or falling respiratory rate, declining blood pressure, or a febrile or hypothermic state.
• Monitor and record serum electrolyte levels carefully. Take steps to correct imbalances. Monitor fluid balance by

recording the patient's intake, output, and daily weight.
• Check the cardiac monitor for arrhythmias, including ectopy or sinus tachycardia.
• Monitor for signs of infection and use strict aseptic technique for all invasive procedures.
• Care for catheter sites according to established protocol, and enforce proper hand-washing technique.
• Perform oral hygiene measures frequently and assess the oral cavity for thrush or viral lesions.
• Apply soft wrist restraints for a confused patient, if necessary, to prevent him from disconnecting the oxygen setup. However, remember that restraints can increase anxiety, fear, agitation and, possibly, the risk of falling.
• Give emotional support to the patient and family members. Allow them to

openly express fears and anxieties. Give brief explanations. Help the patient to use positive coping mechanisms and methods of relaxation.

• Position the patient for comfort and optimal gas exchange. Place the call button within his reach.

• Maintain the patient in a normothermic state to reduce his body's demand for oxygen.

• Plan patient activities that maximize his energy level, allow for needed rest, and achieve adequate oxygen delivery.

Mechanical ventilation

If the patient requires mechanical ventilation, perform the following nursing interventions:

• Check ventilator settings, cuff pressures, and ABG values often to ensure the correct fraction of inspired oxygen (FIO_2) settings, which are determined by ABG levels.

• Draw blood samples for ABG analysis every 20 to 30 minutes after each change in the FIO_2 setting.

• Suction the trachea, as needed, after oxygenation.

• Note changes in sputum quality, consistency, color, and odor.

• Provide humidification to liquefy secretions.

• Perform postural drainage and percussion to mobilize and promote expulsion of secretions. (See *Positioning patients for postural drainage,* pages 104 to 106).

• Watch for complications of mechanical ventilation, such as reduced cardiac output, pneumothorax or other barotrauma, increased pulmonary vascular resistance, diminished urine output, increased intracranial pressure, and GI bleeding.

• Routinely assess endotracheal (ET) tube position and patency. Make sure the ET tube is placed properly and taped securely.

• Check for accidental intubation of the esophagus or the mainstem bronchus (which may occur during ET tube insertion).

• Be alert for tracheal or laryngeal perforation, aspiration, broken teeth, epistaxis, vagal reflexes (such as bradycardia), arrhythmias, and hypertension.

• Watch for complications after endotracheal intubation, such as tube displacement, herniation of the tube's cuff, respiratory infection, or tracheal malacia (softness or sponginess), or stenosis.

• Prevent infection by using sterile technique while suctioning, by changing ventilator tubing every 24 hours, and by enforcing strict hand-washing technique.

• Prevent tracheal erosion, which can result from an overinflated artificial airway cuff that compresses the tracheal wall's vasculature.

• Use the minimal-leak technique and a cuffed tube with high residual volume (low-pressure cuff), a foam cuff, or a pressure-regulating valve on the cuff.

• Measure cuff pressure every 8 hours.

• Implement measures to prevent nasal tissue necrosis. Position and maintain the nasotracheal tube midline within the nostrils and provide meticulous care.

• Periodically reposition the tape securing the tube to prevent skin breakdown.

• Avoid excessive movement of any tube, and check that the ventilator tubing has adequate support.

• Monitor the patient for signs and symptoms of stress ulcers (such as blood in gastric secretions, nausea, vomiting, or epigastric tenderness), which are common in intubated patients.

• Inspect gastric secretions for blood, especially if the patient has a nasogastric tube or reports epigastric tenderness, nausea, or vomiting.

(Text continues on page 107.)

Positioning patients for postural drainage

The following illustrations show you the various postural drainage positions and the areas of the lungs affected by each.

Lower lobes: Posterior basal segments
Elevate the foot of the bed 30 degrees. Have the patient lie prone with his head lowered. Position pillows under his chest and abdomen. Percuss his lower ribs on both sides of his spine.

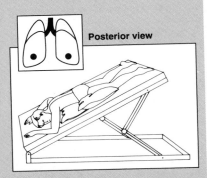

Posterior view

Lower lobes: Lateral basal segments
Elevate the foot of the bed 30 degrees. Instruct the patient to lie on his abdomen with his head lowered and his upper leg flexed over a pillow for support. Then have him rotate a quarter turn upward. Percuss his lower ribs on the uppermost portion of his lateral chest wall.

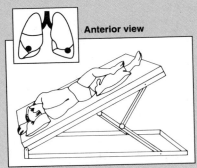

Anterior view

Lower lobes: Anterior basal segments
Elevate the foot of the bed 30 degrees. Instruct the patient to lie on his side with his head lowered. Position pillows under head and between legs. Percuss with a slightly cupped hand over his lower ribs just beneath the axilla. If an acutely ill patient has trouble breathing in this position, adjust the bed to an angle he can tolerate. Then begin percussion.

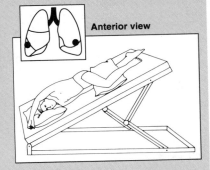

Anterior view

Positioning patients for postural drainage *(continued)*

Lower lobes: Superior segments
With the bed flat, have the patient lie on his abdomen. Place two pillows under his hips. Percuss on both sides of his spine at the lower tip of his scapulae.

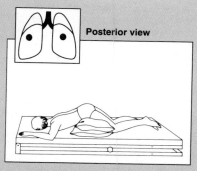

Posterior view

Right middle lobe: Medial and lateral segments
Elevate the foot of the bed 15 degrees. Have the patient lie on his left side with his head down and his knees flexed. Then have him rotate a quarter turn backward. Place a pillow beneath him. Percuss with your hand moderately cupped over the right nipple. For a woman, cup your hand so that its heel is under the armpit and your fingers extend forward beneath the breast.

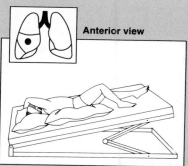

Anterior view

Left upper lobe: Superior and inferior segments, lingular portion
Elevate the foot of the bed 15 degrees. Have the patient lie on his right side with his head down and knees flexed. Then have him rotate a quarter turn backward. Place a pillow behind him, from shoulders to hips. Percuss with your hand moderately cupped over his left nipple. For a woman, cup your hand so that its heel is beneath the armpit and your fingers extend forward beneath the breast.

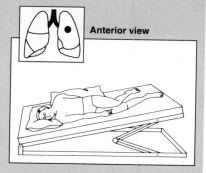

Anterior view

(continued)

Positioning patients for postural drainage *(continued)*

Upper lobes: Anterior segments
Make sure the bed is flat. Have the patient lie on his back with a pillow folded under his knees. Then have him rotate slightly away from the side being drained. Percuss between his clavicle and nipple.

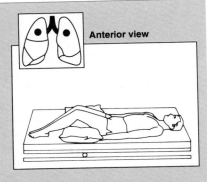

Anterior view

Upper lobes: Apical segments
Keep the bed flat. Have the patient lean back at a 30-degree angle against you and a pillow. Percuss with a cupped hand between his clavicles and the top of each scapula.

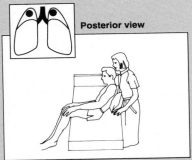

Posterior view

Upper lobes: Posterior segments
Keep the bed flat. Have the patient lean over a pillow at a 30-degree angle. Percuss and clap his upper back on each side.

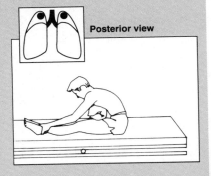

Posterior view

Discharge TimeSaver

Ensuring continued care for the COPD patient with acute respiratory failure

Review the following teaching topics, referrals, and follow-up appointments to make sure that your patient is adequately prepared for discharge.

Teaching topics
Make sure that the following topics have been covered and that your patient's learning has been evaluated:
☐ an explanation of acute respiratory failure in chronic obstructive pulmonary disease (COPD) and its causes, symptoms, and possible complications
☐ activity restrictions, as needed
☐ medications, as indicated
☐ signs and symptoms (including respiratory infections) to report to the doctor.

Referrals
Make sure that the patient has been provided with necessary referrals to:
☐ smoking cessation program or support group, if necessary
☐ home health care agency
☐ pulmonary rehabilitation program, if necessary
☐ medical equipment supplier, if needed.

Follow-up appointments
Make sure that the necessary follow-up appointments have been scheduled and that the patient has been notified:
☐ doctor or clinic
☐ diagnostic tests for reevaluation.

• Monitor hemoglobin and hematocrit levels, and check all stools for occult blood. Administer antacids or histamine-receptor antagonists, as directed.
• Help the patient to communicate using a pen and tablet, a word chart, or an alphabet board.

Patient teaching
Most patients with acute respiratory failure receive intensive care. Orient the patient and family members to the procedures, sounds, and sights of the unit to help minimize their anxiety.
• Teach the patient about the effects of smoking and provide referrals to a smoking cessation program, if appropriate.
• Describe all tests and procedures to the patient and family members. For example, discuss the reasons for suctioning, postural drainage and percussion, blood tests and, if used, soft wrist restraints.
• If the patient is intubated or has a tracheostomy, explain why he can't speak.

Provide referral to a speech therapist, if needed.
• Inform the patient about the signs of respiratory infection and instruct him to report any such signs immediately.
• Instruct the patient and family members in proper home care techniques, such as those for postural drainage and percussion, tracheostomy care, or drug administration. (See *Ensuring continued care for the COPD patient with acute respiratory failure.*)

EVALUATION

To evaluate the patient's response to your care, gather reassessment data and compare this information with the patient outcomes specified in your plan of care.

Teaching and counseling
Assess the effectiveness of your teaching by considering the following questions:

• Is the patient's activity level appropriate, and does he pace activities to preserve energy and promote oxygenation?
• Has the patient's anxiety been alleviated, and is he able to identify ways to cope with symptoms of anxiety?
• Is he able to identify signs and symptoms of infection that should be reported to the doctor?
• Is he free of all signs of infection?
• Does he know how to perform home health care techniques, such as postural drainage and percussion and tracheostomy care?

Physical condition

Evaluate the patient's physical condition by answering the following questions:
• Can the patient sustain spontaneous ventilation on his own, and are his airways now open and clear?
• Has his respiratory rate returned to baseline?
• Are his PaO_2, $PaCO_2$, and pH within specified ranges?
• Is he maintaining satisfactory systemic tissue perfusion, as indicated by vital signs, pulse oximetry, urine output, LOC, peripheral pulses, and skin temperature?
• Has he achieved a stable heart rate and rhythm?

Respiratory acidosis

In this acid-base disturbance, the patient develops increased carbon dioxide in the blood (hypercapnia) and decreased pH. The condition may be *acute*, resulting from sudden failure in alveolar ventilation, or *chronic*, stemming from long-term pulmonary disease. (See *What happens in respiratory acidosis.*)

The prognosis depends on the severity of the underlying disturbance and on the patient's clinical condition. Possible complications of acute or chronic respiratory acidosis include shock and cardiac arrest.

Causes

Any patient with reduced alveolar ventilation may be at risk for respiratory acidosis. (See *Causes of respiratory acidosis,* page 110.)

ASSESSMENT

Because a number of factors may predispose a patient to respiratory acidosis, your assessment should include a health history, a medication history, a physical examination, and consideration of diagnostic test results.

Health history

When taking the patient's health history, you usually find clues to a predisposing condition. Initially, the patient may report headaches and dyspnea. Nausea and vomiting may occur. The patient or his family members may have noticed a reduced attention span or other changes in his mental status.

Medication history

Find out if the patient is taking any drugs that depress the sensitivity of the respiratory center. Drugs that produce such a response include narcotics, hypnotics, and sedatives.

Physical examination

When you examine the patient, you may see that he's dyspneic and diaphoretic or, conversely, he may display slowed respirations. His skin may appear pale to cyanotic. Palpation may disclose bounding pulses. Auscultation may reveal rapid, shallow respirations; tachycardia; and possibly hypertension (in acute respiratory acidosis) or hypotension (in chronic respiratory acidosis).

What happens in respiratory acidosis

Respiratory acidosis is characterized by reduced alveolar ventilation and manifested by hypercapnia (partial pressure of arterial carbon dioxide [$PaCO_2$] above 45 mm Hg). The flowchart below shows what happens in respiratory acidosis.

Pulmonary ventilation diminishes

When pulmonary ventilation decreases, retained carbon dioxide (CO_2) in the red blood cells combines with water (H_2O) to form excessive amounts of carbonic acid (H_2CO_3). The H_2CO_3 dissociates to release free hydrogen (H^+) and bicarbonate ions (HCO_3^-).

Look for increased $PaCO_2$ (over 45 mm Hg) and reduced blood pH (below 7.35).

Oxygen saturation drops

As pH falls and 2,3-diphosphoglycerate (2,3-DPG) increases in red blood cells, 2,3-DPG alters hemoglobin (Hb) so it releases oxygen (O_2). This reduced Hb, which is strongly basic, picks up H^+ and CO_2, eliminating some free H^+ and excess CO_2.

Look for decreased arterial oxygen saturation (SaO_2) and shift of Hb dissociation curve to the right.

Respiratory rate rises

Whenever $PaCO_2$ increases, CO_2 levels increase in all tissues and fluids, including the medulla and the cerebrospinal fluid. CO_2 reacts with H_2O to form H_2CO_3, which dissociates into H^+ and HCO_3^-. Increased $PaCO_2$ and H^+ have a potent stimulatory effect on the medulla, increasing respirations and eliminating CO_2 from the lungs.

Look for rapid, shallow respirations and decreasing $PaCO_2$.

Blood flow increases to the brain

CO_2 and H^+ also dilate cerebral blood vessels and increase blood flow to the brain, causing cerebral edema and depressed central nervous system activity.

Look for headache, confusion, lethargy, and nausea and vomiting.

Kidneys compensate

As respiratory mechanisms fail, increasing $PaCO_2$ stimulates the kidneys to retain HCO_3^- and sodium ions and to excrete H^+. As a result, more sodium bicarbonate is available to buffer free H^+. Ammonium ions are also excreted to remove H^+.

Look for increased acid and ammonium content in the urine, increasing serum pH and HCO_3^-, and shallow, depressed respirations.

Acid-base balance fails

As H^+ concentration overwhelms compensatory mechanisms, H^+ ions move into the cells and potassium ions move out. Without sufficient O_2, anaerobic metabolism produces lactic acid. Electrolyte imbalance and acidosis critically depress brain and cardiac function.

Look for increased $PaCO_2$, decreased PaO_2 and pH, hyperkalemia, arrhythmias, tremors, decreased level of consciousness, and coma.

FactFinder
Causes of respiratory acidosis

Respiratory acidosis can result from:
• drugs, such as narcotics, anesthetics, hypnotics, and sedatives, which depress the sensitivity of the respiratory center
• central nervous system trauma, such as medullary injury, which may impair the ventilatory drive
• neuromuscular diseases, such as Guillain-Barré syndrome, myasthenia gravis, and poliomyelitis, in which respiratory muscles fail to respond properly to respiratory drive, reducing alveolar ventilation.

Respiratory acidosis can also result from these conditions:
• airway obstruction or parenchymal lung disease that interferes with alveolar ventilation
• chronic obstructive pulmonary disease
• asthma
• severe adult respiratory distress syndrome
• chronic bronchitis
• pneumothorax
• extensive pneumonia
• pulmonary edema.

Ophthalmoscopic examination may disclose papilledema, a swelling of the optic disk. A neurologic examination may disclose a level of consciousness (LOC) ranging from restlessness, confusion, and apprehension to somnolence. During the examination, you may note depressed reflexes, possibly with a fine or flapping hand tremor (asterixis).

Diagnostic test results
Arterial blood gas (ABG) analysis will confirm respiratory acidosis when partial pressure of carbon dioxide in arterial blood is above 45 mm Hg. The patient's pH is typically below the normal range of 7.35 to 7.45. Levels of bicarbonate are normal in acute respiratory acidosis but elevated in chronic respiratory acidosis.

NURSING DIAGNOSIS
Common nursing diagnoses for a patient with respiratory acidosis include:
• Fear related to a possible need for mechanical ventilation or to thoughts of impending death
• Impaired gas exchange related to alveolar hypoventilation
• Ineffective breathing pattern related to altered respirations
• Altered thought processes related to cerebral depression.

PLANNING
Based on the nursing diagnosis *fear,* develop appropriate patient outcomes. For example, your patient will:
• identify and express his fear
• use available support systems to help him cope with fear
• exhibit evidence that fear is reduced or absent.

Based on the nursing diagnosis *impaired gas exchange,* develop appropriate patient outcomes. For example, your patient will:
• regain and maintain normal ABG values
• exhibit absence of signs or symptoms of profound central nervous system (CNS) and cardiovascular deterioration
• demonstrate compliance with prescribed treatments for underlying causes of respiratory acidosis.

Based on the nursing diagnosis *ineffective breathing pattern,* develop appropriate patient outcomes. For example, your patient will:
• reestablish a respiratory rate that is within defined limits

- express a feeling of comfort while breathing
- exhibit normal breath sounds on auscultation.

Based on the nursing diagnosis *altered thought processes,* develop appropriate patient outcomes. For example, your patient will:

- remain free of injury
- express awareness of a need for assistance
- remain oriented to person, place, and time
- be able to follow simple commands
- maintain baseline LOC.

IMPLEMENTATION

Treatment seeks to control the patient's condition and avoid complications. You will need to teach the patient about respiratory acidosis and provide emotional support to both the patient and his family members. (See *Medical care of the patient with respiratory acidosis*, page 112.)

Nursing interventions

- Be prepared to treat an underlying cause such as an airway obstruction.
- Watch for changes in the patient's respiratory, CNS, and cardiovascular functions, and report them immediately.
- Report variations in ABG levels and electrolyte status.
- Maintain adequate hydration by administering I.V. fluids.
- Administer oxygen, as ordered, if the partial pressure of arterial oxygen drops. (In patients with chronic obstructive pulmonary disease [COPD], administer oxygen at low concentrations only; too much oxygen can depress the respiratory drive, resulting in apnea.)
- Give aerosolized or I.V. bronchodilators, as prescribed. Monitor and record the patient's response to these medications.

- Anticipate using mechanical ventilation if hypoventilation cannot be corrected immediately. Monitor the ventilator settings continually.
- Maintain a patent airway and provide adequate humidification during mechanical ventilation.
- Perform tracheal suctioning regularly and postural drainage and percussion as ordered.
- Closely monitor a patient with COPD and chronic carbon dioxide retention for signs of developing respiratory acidosis.
- Closely monitor all patients who receive narcotics and sedatives for signs of developing respiratory acidosis.
- Maintain a safe environment if the patient's LOC changes. Avoid physical restraints, if possible, but if restraints are necessary, follow your hospital's protocol.
- Frequently orient your patient to person, place, and time.
- Reduce environmental stimuli and give short, simple explanations to the patient during care procedures.
- Reassure the patient as much as possible, depending on his LOC. Help ease the family's fears and concerns by keeping them informed about the patient's status. Support the family's attempts to interact with the patient.

Patient teaching

- Alert the patient and family members to possible adverse effects of prescribed medications, especially sedatives, that should be reported to the doctor.
- Inform the patient and family members about the signs and symptoms of respiratory acidosis that should be reported to the doctor.
- Teach the patient and family members about the safe use of oxygen, if it will be used after his discharge. If the patient will receive home oxygen therapy for COPD, stress the importance

Treatments

Medical care of the patient with respiratory acidosis

The goal of treating respiratory acidosis is to correct the source of alveolar hypoventilation. If alveolar ventilation is significantly reduced, the patient may need mechanical ventilation until the underlying condition can be addressed.
 Treatment includes:
• bronchodilators, oxygen, and antibiotics in chronic obstructive pulmonary disease
• drug therapy for conditions such as myasthenia gravis

• removal of foreign bodies from the airway in cases of obstruction
• antibiotics for pneumonia
• dialysis to eliminate toxic drugs.
 Dangerously low pH levels (less than 7.15) can cause profound central nervous system and cardiovascular deterioration. I.V. sodium bicarbonate may be administered in this case. In chronic lung disease, however, elevated carbon dioxide levels may persist despite treatment.

of maintaining his dose at the prescribed flow rate.
• Teach deep-breathing exercises.
• Demonstrate the proper use of assistive-adaptive devices (such as a bedside spirometer), if necessary, and supervise the patient and family members as they repeat the demonstration. (See *Ensuring continued care for the patient with respiratory acidosis.*)

EVALUATION

When evaluating your patient's response to nursing care, gather reassessment data and compare this information with the patient outcomes specified in your plan of care.

Teaching and counseling
Determine the effectiveness of teaching and counseling. Consider the following questions:
• Does the patient understand what precipitated his condition?
• Is he complying with treatment to address the underlying cause?
• Do the patient and family members recognize the signs and symptoms of

adverse drug reactions and other conditions that should be reported to the doctor?
• Does the patient exhibit signs of reduced feelings of fear?
• Does he display coping skills, such as using support systems?

Physical condition
Continue your assessment by documenting your patient's physiologic status. Consider these questions:
• Is the patient's respiratory rate within established parameters?
• Is he comfortable while breathing, and has he learned deep-breathing exercises?
• Are the patient's ABG levels within specified limits?
• Is he free of signs of CNS or cardiovascular deterioration? Has he achieved a stable cardiovascular status?
• Have his thought processes returned to baseline? Is he oriented to his surroundings and able to follow simple directions?

Discharge TimeSaver
Ensuring continued care for the patient with respiratory acidosis

Review the following teaching topics, referrals, and follow-up appointments to make sure that your patient is adequately prepared for discharge.

Teaching topics
Make sure that the following topics have been covered and that your patient's learning has been evaluated:
□ an explanation of respiratory acidosis and its causes, symptoms, and possible complications
□ deep-breathing exercises
□ use of home oxygen therapy, if indicated, including safety measures
□ activity restrictions, as needed
□ medications and possible adverse effects
□ signs and symptoms to report to the doctor.

Referrals
Make sure that the patient has been provided with necessary referrals to:
□ social services
□ home health care agency
□ medical equipment supplier
□ pulmonary rehabilitation program.

Follow-up appointments
Make sure that the necessary follow-up appointments have been scheduled and that the patient has been notified:
□ doctor or clinic
□ additional diagnostic tests.

Respiratory alkalosis

Respiratory alkalosis is marked by a decrease in carbon dioxide (CO_2) in the blood (hypocapnia) and an elevated blood pH. The condition may be either acute or chronic. Hypocapnia occurs when the pulmonary ventilation rate exceeds normal limits, causing the lungs to eliminate more CO_2 than the body produces at the cellular level. Blood pH increases because of a decrease in hydrogen ions.

In extreme cases of respiratory alkalosis, the patient may experience cardiac arrhythmias that do not respond to conventional treatment.

Causes
Respiratory alkalosis is commonly caused by either active or passive alveolar hyperventilation, which can be precipitated by pulmonary or non-

pulmonary conditions. (See *Causes of respiratory alkalosis,* page 114.)

ASSESSMENT

Your assessment should include consideration of the patient's health history, physical examination findings, and diagnostic test results.

Health history
Your patient's health history may reveal a predisposing factor associated with respiratory alkalosis. The patient may report light-headedness or numbness and tingling in his arms and legs (paresthesia). He may also report muscle cramping and twitching.

Physical examination
During an initial inspection, your patient may seem anxious, and you will note visibly deep, rapid breathing. Auscultation may reveal tachycardia. In acute respiratory alkalosis, tetany (or

FactFinder

Causes of respiratory alkalosis

Respiratory alkalosis can result from:
• congestive heart failure
• injury to the respiratory control center
• extreme anxiety
• fever
• excessive ventilation (during mechanical ventilation)
• pulmonary embolism
• salicylate intoxication (early stages)
• compensation for metabolic acidosis.

severe cramping) may be apparent with visible twitching and flexion of the wrists and ankles.

Diagnostic test results
Arterial blood gas (ABG) analysis can confirm respiratory alkalosis and rule out compensation for metabolic acidosis. Respiratory alkalosis is confirmed when:
• partial pressure of arterial carbon dioxide ($PaCO_2$) is below 35 mm Hg
• blood pH increases (above 7.45) as $PaCO_2$ declines
• bicarbonate (HCO_3^-) level remains normal (22 to 26 mEq/liter)

Chronic respiratory alkalosis is confirmed when:
• $PaCO_2$ is below 35 mm Hg
• blood pH approaches normal (7.35 to 7.45) as $PaCO_2$ declines
• HCO_3^- level falls below 22 mEq/liter.

In addition, serum electrolyte studies may help detect metabolic acid-base disorders.

NURSING DIAGNOSIS

Common nursing diagnoses for a patient with respiratory alkalosis include:

• Anxiety related to the underlying cause
• Ineffective breathing pattern related to deep, rapid breathing.

PLANNING

Based on the nursing diagnosis *anxiety*, develop appropriate patient outcomes. For example, your patient will:
• identify and express feelings of anxiety
• perform stress reduction techniques to prevent or minimize anxiety symptoms
• demonstrate that physical symptoms of anxiety have decreased.

Based on the nursing diagnosis *ineffective breathing pattern*, develop appropriate patient outcomes. For example, your patient will:
• reestablish baseline respiratory rate and pattern
• express feelings of comfort while breathing
• exhibit normal breath sounds on auscultation.

IMPLEMENTATION

Treatment seeks to control the condition and prevent complications. You'll also need to teach the patient about respiratory alkalosis and its treatment. (See *Medical care of the patient with respiratory alkalosis.*)

Nursing interventions
• Watch for and report changes in neurologic, neuromuscular, and cardiovascular functioning. Note twitching and cardiac arrhythmias, which may be associated with alkalemia and electrolyte imbalances.
• Monitor ABG and serum electrolyte levels closely. Report any change immediately.
• Stay with the patient during periods of extreme stress and anxiety. Offer re-

Treatments

Medical care of the patient with respiratory alkalosis

Treatment of respiratory alkalosis aims to eradicate the underlying condition. It may entail:
• removal of ingested toxins
• management of fever, sepsis, or diseases of the central nervous system
• use of sedatives and tranquilizers if respiratory alkalosis is caused by anxiety.

In severe respiratory alkalosis, the patient may need to breathe into a paper bag, which helps relieve acute anxiety and increase carbon dioxide levels.

Preventing hyperventilation
To prevent hyperventilation in patients on mechanical ventilation, monitor arterial blood gas levels and adjust the *dead-space* or minute ventilation volume.

---

assurance, as needed, and maintain a calm, quiet environment.
• If the patient is coping with anxiety-induced respiratory alkalosis, help him identify factors that cause anxiety. Help him develop coping mechanisms and encourage activities that promote relaxation.

Patient teaching
• Explain all care procedures to the patient and answer his questions.
• Teach the patient to use anxiety-reducing techniques, such as guided imagery, meditation, or yoga.
• Instruct the patient on how to counter hyperventilation with a controlled breathing pattern. (See *Ensuring continued care for the patient with respiratory alkalosis,* page 116.)

EVALUATION

When evaluating your patient's response to nursing care, gather reassessment data and compare this information with the patient outcomes specified in your plan of care.

Teaching and counseling
Talk to the patient and family members to determine the effectiveness of teaching and counseling. Consider the following questions:
• Does the patient understand what precipitated his condition?
• Is he complying with prescribed treatments to address the underlying cause?
• Can he identify feelings of anxiety and does he demonstrate effective anxiety-reducing techniques, such as guided imagery, meditation, or yoga?
• Has he learned how to counter hyperventilation with a controlled breathing pattern?

Physical condition
Evaluate your patient's physiologic status by considering the following questions:
• Has the underlying cause of respiratory alkalosis been addressed?
• Are the patient's respiratory rate and rhythm within established limits?
• Does he exhibit normal breath sounds, and does he express feelings of comfort while breathing?
• Are his ABG levels within specified parameters?
• Have his neurologic and cardiac functions returned to baseline, with no signs of seizures or arrhythmias?

Discharge TimeSaver
Ensuring continued care for the patient with respiratory alkalosis

Review the following teaching topics, referrals, and follow-up appointments to make sure that your patient is adequately prepared for discharge.

Teaching topics
Make sure that the following topics have been covered and that your patient's learning has been evaluated:
☐ an explanation of respiratory alkalosis and its causes, symptoms, and possible complications
☐ anxiety-reduction techniques
☐ activity restrictions, as needed
☐ medications and their possible adverse effects
☐ signs and symptoms to report to the doctor.

Referrals
Make sure that the patient has been provided with necessary referrals to:
☐ home health care agency
☐ social services
☐ support groups.

Follow-up appointments
Make sure that the necessary follow-up appointments have been scheduled and that the patient has been notified:
☐ doctor or clinic
☐ diagnostic tests for reevaluation.

Atelectasis

In this disorder, alveolar clusters (lobules) or lung segments fail to expand completely, producing partial or complete lung collapse. This prevents the exchange of carbon dioxide and oxygen in some parts of the lung. Unoxygenated blood may pass unchanged through regions of collapsed tissue, thereby producing hypoxia. (See *Looking at atelectatic alveoli.*)

Lung collapse may be acute or chronic. Prognosis depends on how promptly the airway obstruction is removed, the hypoxia relieved, and the collapsed lung reexpanded. Complications of atelectasis include pneumothorax, hypoxemia, and acute respiratory failure. Static (or nonmoving) secretions resulting from atelectasis may cause pneumonia.

Causes
Atelectasis occurs in many patients undergoing upper abdominal or thoracic surgery. It may result from hypoventilation, which commonly leads to collapsed alveoli and mucus retention. The problem may also be caused by lung tissue compression. (See *Causes of atelectasis,* page 118, and *Understanding atelectasis resulting from compression,* page 119.)

ASSESSMENT

You'll find that clinical effects vary depending on the cause of the lung collapse, the degree of hypoxia, and the underlying cause. Your assessment should include a patient health history, a physical examination, and consideration of diagnostic test results.

Health history
If atelectasis affects a small area of the lung, the patient's symptoms may be minimal and transient. With massive collapse, however, the patient may re-

port severe dyspnea and pleuritic chest pain.

Physical examination

Inspection of your patient may disclose decreased chest wall movement, cyanosis, diaphoresis, substernal or intercostal retractions, use of accessory muscles for breathing, and anxiety.

Palpation may reveal decreased fremitus and mediastinal shift to the affected side. Percussion may disclose dullness or flatness over the lung fields.

During auscultation, you may hear crackles at the end of inspiration and decreased (or absent) breath sounds with major lung involvement. You may also detect tachycardia.

Diagnostic test results

The following tests can help establish the diagnosis and reveal predisposing factors:

• Chest X-rays are the primary diagnostic tool, although extensive areas of "microatelectasis" may exist without abnormalities appearing on the films. In widespread atelectasis, X-ray findings define characteristic horizontal lines in the lower lung zones. In segmental or lobar collapse, the films reveal characteristic dense shadows that are commonly associated with hyperinflation of neighboring lung zones.
• Bronchoscopy can rule out the presence of an obstructing neoplasm or foreign body.
• Arterial blood gas (ABG) analysis may detect respiratory acidosis and hypoxemia.
• Pulse oximetry may show a deteriorating arterial oxygen saturation level.

Looking at atelectatic alveoli

Normally, the alveoli exchange oxygen and carbon dioxide. In atelectasis, the alveoli fail to expand completely, preventing gas exchange.

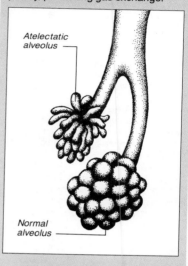

Atelectatic alveolus

Normal alveolus

• High risk for infection related to retained pulmonary secretions
• Impaired gas exchange related to decreased availability of lung tissue for gas exchange
• Ineffective breathing pattern related to decreased chest wall movement
• Fear related to possible suffocation and dying
• Knowledge deficit related to atelectasis and its treatment.

NURSING DIAGNOSIS

Common nursing diagnoses for a patient with atelectasis include:
• Ineffective airway clearance related to bronchial obstruction

PLANNING

Based on the nursing diagnosis *ineffective airway clearance*, develop appropriate patient outcomes. For example, your patient will:

FactFinder

Causes of atelectasis

- Obstruction by mucus plugs, which may occur in patients with chronic obstructive pulmonary disease, bronchiectasis, and cystic fibrosis and in patients who smoke heavily. (Smoking increases mucus production and damages cilia.)
- Occlusion caused by aspiration of foreign bodies, bronchogenic carcinoma, or inflammatory lung disease
- Idiopathic respiratory distress syndrome of newborn
- Oxygen toxicity
- Pulmonary edema
- Adult respiratory distress syndrome
- Prolonged immobility, which promotes ventilation of one lung area over another
- Mechanical ventilation that doesn't supply intermittent deep breaths
- Central nervous system depression that suppresses periodic sighing, possibly resulting from a drug overdose
- External compression or pain, which inhibits full lung expansion. This can result from tumors, upper abdominal surgical incisions, rib fractures, pleuritic chest pain, tight chest dressings, and obesity (which elevates the diaphragm and reduces tidal volume).

- maintain an open airway
- exhibit diminished adventitious breath sounds or none at all
- report symptoms that indicate a need for medical intervention.

Based on the nursing diagnosis *high risk for infection,* develop appropriate patient outcomes. For example, your patient will:
- maintain normal body temperature and baseline white blood cell count
- perform bronchial hygiene measures correctly

- not exhibit signs and symptoms of pulmonary infection.

Based on the nursing diagnosis *impaired gas exchange,* develop appropriate patient outcomes. For example, your patient will:
- not exhibit signs of hypoxia, such as restlessness and dyspnea
- maintain baseline level of consciousness (LOC)
- maintain baseline ABG levels and show baseline pulse oximetry readings.

Based on the nursing diagnosis *ineffective breathing pattern,* develop appropriate patient outcomes. For example, your patient will:
- reestablish baseline respiratory rate and pattern
- achieve maximum lung expansion with adequate ventilation.

Based on the nursing diagnosis *fear,* develop appropriate patient outcomes. For example, your patient will:
- express fears related to atelectasis
- report reduced feelings of fear
- ask questions about treatment progress and make decisions about care.

Based on the nursing diagnosis *knowledge deficit,* develop appropriate patient outcomes. For example, your patient will:
- express a willingness to learn about atelectasis and how to control it
- communicate an understanding of atelectasis and its risks, and of how to manage the disorder and prevent complications
- identify appropriate actions to be taken if airway obstruction recurs.

IMPLEMENTATION

Your nursing responsibilities will include carefully monitoring the patient and urging him to comply with treatment. Provide emotional support, as needed, especially if he is in pain or frightened by his limited breathing capacity. (See *Medical care of the patient with atelectasis,* page 120.)

Understanding atelectasis resulting from compression

Atelectasis may result from compression of lung tissue from a source outside the alveoli, such as a tumor within the lung.

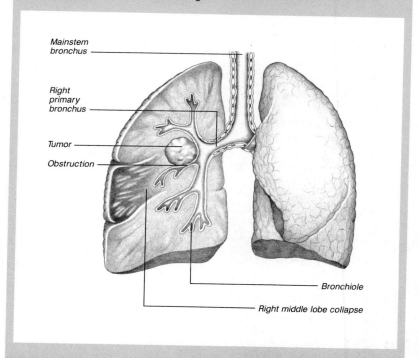

Mainstem bronchus

Right primary bronchus

Tumor

Obstruction

Bronchiole

Right middle lobe collapse

Nursing interventions
• Encourage the patient recovering from surgery (or other patients at high risk for atelectasis) to perform coughing and deep-breathing exercises every 1 to 2 hours. To minimize pain during these exercises, hold a pillow tightly over the patient's incisional area. Teach the patient how to do this for himself.

• Gently reposition him frequently and help him walk as soon as possible.

• Administer analgesics, as prescribed, to control pain.

• Maintain tidal volume at 10 to 15 cc/kg of the patient's body weight if the patient is receiving mechanical ventilation. This will ensure adequate lung expansion. Use the sigh mechanism on the ventilator, if appropriate, to intermittently increase tidal volume at the rate of 3 or 4 sighs/hour.

• Provide an incentive spirometer to encourage deep breathing.

Medical care of the patient with atelectasis

The treatment for atelectasis seeks to remove the underlying cause of the disorder.

Removal of secretions
Suctioning, coughing and deep-breathing exercises, postural drainage and percussion, or bronchoscopy may help to facilitate removal of secretions.

Drug therapy
Humidity and bronchodilator medications may be used concurrently to improve mucociliary clearing and to dilate airways. Medications may be administered by nebulizer or by a face mask that establishes continuous positive-airway pressure.

Mechanical ventilation
Positive end-expiratory pressure may be used to maintain open alveoli if the patient is intubated. Alternatively, intermittent positive-pressure breathing may be used.

Other treatments
If the patient has atelectasis secondary to obstructing neoplasm, surgery or radiation therapy may be required. To minimize the risk of atelectasis after thoracic and abdominal surgery, analgesics are given to facilitate deep breathing.

• Mobilize secretions by humidifying inspired air, and encourage the patient to drink adequate amounts of fluid. Use postural drainage and chest percussion to remove secretions.
• Provide suction, as needed, for an intubated or uncooperative patient.
• Administer prescribed sedatives cautiously and monitor the patient closely for possible depressed respirations and cough reflex. These medications also suppress sighs.
• Assess breath sounds and respiratory status frequently. Report any changes immediately.
• Monitor the patient's pulse oximetry readings and ABG values for evidence of hypoxia.

Patient teaching
• Teach the patient how to use the incentive spirometer and urge him to use it every 1 to 2 hours. Make sure he understands the importance of performing the exercise regularly to maintain alveolar inflation. Instruct the patient to exhale normally and then inhale as slowly and as deeply as possible. If the patient has difficulty with this step, tell him to suck as he would through a straw, but to do so more slowly. Ask the patient to retain the entire volume of air he inhaled for 3 seconds or, if he's using a device with a light indicator, until the light turns off.
• Show the patient and family members how to perform postural drainage and percussion. Explain that postural drainage seeks to empty peripheral pulmonary secretions into the major bronchi or trachea. First, the patient should assume a position that will allow gravity to drain his lungs of mucus. Teach the patient different positions that will enable him to drain specific areas of the lungs; he should maintain each position for 10 minutes. To perform chest percussion, teach family members to cup their hands to create an air pocket and use their cupped hands to clap the patient's chest or back. Tell them the hand should clap the chest with a hollow sound, like a horse galloping.

After postural drainage and percussion, instruct the patient to cough to remove loosened secretions. First, tell him to inhale deeply through his nose and then exhale in three short huffs. Then have him inhale deeply again and

Discharge TimeSaver

Ensuring continued care for the patient with atelectasis

Review the following teaching topics, referrals, and follow-up appointments to make sure that your patient is adequately prepared for discharge.

Teaching topics
Make sure that the following topics have been covered and that your patient's learning has been evaluated:
☐ an explanation of atelectasis and its causes, symptoms, and possible complications
☐ use of an incentive spirometer, if indicated
☐ postural drainage and percussion, if indicated
☐ activity restrictions, as needed
☐ prescribed medications, including possible adverse effects
☐ signs and symptoms to report to the doctor.

Referrals
Make sure that the patient has been provided with necessary referrals to:
☐ home health care agency
☐ social services
☐ smoking cessation program, if necessary
☐ weight loss program, if necessary.

Follow-up appointments
Make sure that the necessary follow-up appointments have been scheduled and that the patient has been notified:
☐ doctor or clinic
☐ diagnostic tests for reevaluation.

cough through a slightly open mouth. Tell him to perform three consecutive coughs. An effective cough sounds deep, low, and hollow; an ineffective one, high-pitched.

• Inform the patient of symptoms to report to the doctor: an upper respiratory infection, influenza, difficulty breathing, a persistent cough, and an elevated temperature.

• Encourage the patient to stop smoking and to lose weight, if necessary. Refer him to appropriate support groups for help.

• Demonstrate comfort measures that promote relaxation to help the patient conserve energy. Advise him to alternate periods of rest and activity to save energy and to prevent fatigue. Inform the patient's family members about the importance of these measures. (See *Ensuring continued care for the patient with atelectasis.*)

EVALUATION

To evaluate your patient's response to nursing care, gather reassessment data and compare this information with the patient outcomes specified in your plan of care.

Teaching and counseling
Determine the effectiveness of teaching and counseling by considering the following questions:

• Does the patient appear willing to learn about atelectasis and how to control it?

• Does he communicate an understanding of atelectasis and its risks?

• Does he communicate an understanding of how to manage the disorder and prevent complications?

• Can he identify appropriate actions to be taken if airway obstruction recurs?

• Can he demonstrate effective use of the incentive spirometer?
• Can the patient and family members correctly perform bronchial hygiene measures?
• Can they correctly perform postural drainage and percussion measures?
• Can they correctly perform deep-breathing and coughing exercises?
• Can the patient identify symptoms to report to the doctor?
• Is he able to demonstrate comfort measures that promote relaxation?
• Has he expressed fears related to atelectasis?
• Does he report feeling less fearful?
• Does he ask questions about treatment progress?
• Is he able to participate in decisions about care?

Physical condition

Evaluate the patient's physiologic status by considering the following questions:
• Are the patient's breath sounds clear?
• Does he exhibit any signs and symptoms of pulmonary infection?
• Does he maintain baseline respiratory rate and pattern?
• Are his body temperature and white blood cell count within established parameters?
• Is his chest expansion normal?
• Does he show any signs of hypoxia, such as restlessness or dyspnea?
• Are his mentation and LOC at baseline?
• Is he maintaining baseline ABG levels?

CHAPTER 5

Caring for patients with obstructive pulmonary disease

Asthma

Asthma is marked by inflammation of the tracheobronchial tree and excessive responsiveness of its lining to various stimuli. Smooth-muscle contraction and hypertrophy, inflammation and edema of the bronchial wall, and increased mucus production cause narrowing of the airways. This narrowing causes an asthma attack. (See *How asthma narrows the bronchial airways.*)

An asthma attack may begin dramatically, with the simultaneous onset of severe, multiple symptoms. Alternatively, it may develop insidiously, with gradually worsening respiratory distress. Effects may range from mild to severe. The attack may resolve spontaneously or require treatment.

Status asthmaticus refers to an acute worsening of bronchial asthma marked by ongoing bronchospasm, edema, and the formation of mucus plugs. Unless quickly reversed, status asthmaticus can lead to respiratory acidosis and acute respiratory failure that results in death.

Causes

Extrinsic asthma is triggered by specific allergens, such as grasses, pollens, molds, animal dander, or dust. *Intrinsic* asthma is triggered by nonallergenic factors, such as exercise, emotional stress, chilling of the airways, respiratory infections, or cigarette smoke. Many patients have a mixed disorder, which can't be attributed exclusively to intrinsic or extrinsic causes. (See *Asthma triggers*, page 126.)

Asthma is often classified according to its precipitating factors, such as exercise-induced asthma, aspirin-induced asthma, asthmatic bronchitis (chronic bronchitis with bronchospasm), and triad asthma (intrinsic asthma, aspirin sensitivity, and nasal polyposis).

Hereditary factors are thought to play a role in asthma. About one-third of asthma patients have at least one close relative with the disorder. (See *Key points about asthma,* page 127.)

ASSESSMENT

Your assessment should include a careful consideration of the patient's health history, physical examination findings, and diagnostic test results.

Health history

Typically, the patient reports exposure to a particular allergen followed by sudden onset of dyspnea, wheezing, and tightness in the chest accompanied by a cough that produces fresh, clear or yellow sputum. The cough can range from barely noticeable to intense and persistent. In 50% of asthma patients, symptoms may occur 4 to 8 hours after exposure (late phase reaction).

Ask the patient about his lifestyle, particularly about smoking and exposure to allergens in the home, at work, or from hobbies. Ask about precipitating factors, such as exercise, upper respiratory infection, or exposure to cold air. Also inquire about sleep disturbances and a family history of asthma.

Consider the following questions to determine the severity of the patient's asthma:
• Has the patient ever been intubated or received oral corticosteroids?
• How often does he use an inhaler?
• How often do exacerbations occur?
• How frequently does the patient miss school or work because of his symptoms?
• How many times has he been hospitalized or taken to the emergency department because of an asthma attack?
• Do symptoms occur at night?

Physical examination

During an asthma attack, your patient may be visibly dyspneic and able to

How asthma narrows the bronchial airways

When certain triggers come in contact with the respiratory passageways of an asthma patient, the smooth muscles that spiral around these passageways contract and constrict the bronchial tubes, thereby inhibiting airflow. Swelling of the membranous lining of these tubes and increased mucus production may further narrow the lumina. Airflow into and especially out of the lungs is blocked to varying degrees. The lungs' ability to provide oxygen and remove carbon dioxide is impaired, leading to ventilation-perfusion mismatch and altered arterial blood gas levels.

Smooth-muscle contraction

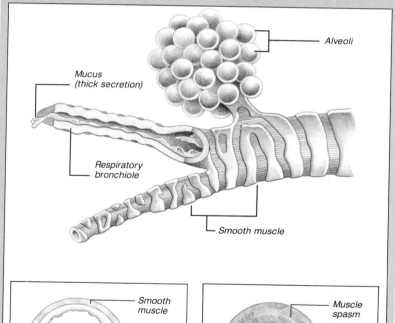

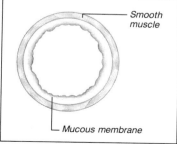

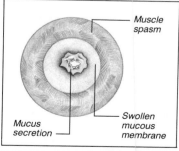

Asthma triggers

Asthma can be caused by an allergic response to an antigen (extrinsic or allergic asthma) or by an abnormal response to a nonspecific, nonallergenic factor (intrinsic asthma). However, many patients with asthma don't fit neatly into either category. They may have a mixed disorder, having elements of both extrinsic and intrinsic asthma.

Extrinsic asthma
The triggers of extrinsic asthma include the following:
- certain foods, such as eggs, shellfish, or chocolate
- molds, especially Alternaria and Cladosporium genera
- pollens of trees, grasses, and weeds
- air pollutants
- dust and dust mites
- animal feather or dander.

Intrinsic asthma
The triggers of intrinsic asthma include the following:
- upper respiratory tract infection
- sinusitis
- gastroesophageal reflux
- psychological stress
- exercise
- cold or hot air, very dry air, or high humidity
- cigarette smoke
- aspirin, other nonsteroidal anti-inflammatory drugs, beta blockers, and other drugs
- cold drinks
- food additives containing sulfites
- variations in menstrual cycle
- fumes—for example, from automobiles, cooking, and wood smoke
- strong perfumes
- personal care products, such as sprays, cosmetics, and powders.

speak only a few words before pausing to catch his breath. You may see him using accessory respiratory muscles to breathe. He may be agitated, restless, anxious, sweating profusely or lack concentration. He may experience syncope or near syncope. You may observe an increased anteroposterior thoracic diameter.

Percussion may reveal hyperresonance, whereas palpation may disclose vocal fremitus. Auscultation may reveal tachycardia, tachypnea, mild systolic hypertension, harsh breathing with inspiratory and expiratory wheezes, prolonged expiratory phase, and diminished or absent breath sounds.

Hypoxemia and acidemia may produce cyanosis, confusion, and lethargy, indicating the onset of life-threatening status asthmaticus and respiratory failure.

Diagnostic test results
The bronchial provocation test is the most specific test for diagnosing asthma. A known bronchoconstricting agent (methacholine, histamine, or cold air) is inhaled in increasing amounts with expiratory flow rates being measured between each inhalation. An asthmatic patient will have decreased flow rates, while someone with normal lungs will show no change in flow rates. The test shouldn't be given to known asthma patients or to patients with already low flow rates.

The following tests can help confirm the diagnosis:
- Pulmonary function tests determine the degree of airway obstruction and the patient's responsiveness to bronchodilator therapy. In asthma patients, they will reveal decreased flow rates and forced expiratory volume in 1 second (FEV_1), low-normal or decreased vital capacity, and increased total lung and residual capacities. Despite abnormal findings during attacks, pulmo-

nary function may be normal between them.

In mild asthma, signs of small airway disease are usually noted: a rise in residual volume and a decline in forced expiratory flow between 25% and 75% of vital capacity. In moderate to severe asthma, the large airways are affected, showing a decline in FEV_1 and forced vital capacity, while diffusing capacity remains normal.

Peak flow studies usually correlate with FEV_1 and can be used to detect early signs of an acute exacerbation and to evaluate the effectiveness of treatment. Peak flow studies are usually done during an acute attack or when the patient is hospitalized and may be continued at home with a simple monitoring device.

• Serum immunoglobulin E levels may rise because of an allergic reaction.

• Complete blood count with differential reveals increased eosinophil count.

• Chest X-rays can help diagnose asthma or monitor its progress. During an asthma attack, X-rays may show hyperinflation with areas of focal atelectasis or pneumonia. Chest X-rays of an asymptomatic patient are normal.

• Arterial blood gas (ABG) analysis can detect hypoxemia, hypercapnia, and acidosis and can be used to guide treatment. During an asthma attack, the patient typically has diminished levels of partial pressure of oxygen in arterial blood (PaO_2) and partial pressure of carbon dioxide in arterial blood ($PaCO_2$). However, in severe asthma, $PaCO_2$ may be normal or increased, indicating severe bronchial obstruction. Initiating treatment tends to improve airflow.

• Skin tests may identify specific allergens. Test results are read in 1 to 2 days to detect an early reaction and then again after 4 or 5 days to reveal a late reaction. (See *Determining asthma's severity*, page 128.)

FactFinder

Key points about asthma

• *Incidence:* Asthma is the most common chronic disease in industrialized nations. Although asthma can strike at any age, about half of all patients are under age 10, with almost twice as many boys affected as girls.

• *Prognosis:* Up to 50% of persons with asthma remain free of symptoms, or nearly so, for life, particularly if disease onset was before age 16. Adult-onset asthma usually improves or disappears as the patient grows older.

• *Chief diagnostic methods:* Bronchial provocation test, pulmonary function tests, peak flow studies

• *Treatment:* Avoidance or removal of precipitating factors

• *Leading complication:* Respiratory failure following status asthmaticus

• *Other complications:* Chronic bronchitis, emphysema, pulmonary hypertension, and cor pulmonale

NURSING DIAGNOSIS

Common nursing diagnoses for a patient with asthma include:

• Impaired gas exchange related to ventilation-perfusion mismatch caused by bronchoconstriction

• Ineffective airway clearance related to increased secretion of thick mucus

• Ineffective breathing pattern related to limited airflow

• Anxiety related to dyspnea associated with an asthma attack

• Knowledge deficit related to asthma treatment and prevention of an attack.

PLANNING

Based on the nursing diagnosis *impaired gas exchange,* develop appropri-

Determining asthma's severity

Assessment	Mild asthma	Moderate asthma	Severe asthma
Signs and symptoms during acute phase	• Cough • Mild dyspnea on exertion • Weakness • Adequate air exchange • Intermittent, brief (less than 1 hour) wheezing, cough, or dyspnea once or twice a week • Asymptomatic between exacerbations	• Respiratory distress at rest • Hyperpnea • Marked coughing and wheezing • Air exchange normal or below normal • Exacerbations that may last several days	• Marked respiratory distress • Marked wheezes or absent breath sounds • Pulsus paradoxus greater than 10 mm • Chest wall contractions • Continuous symptoms • Frequent exacerbations
Diagnostic test results	• Forced expiratory volume in 1 second (FEV_1) or peak flow 80% of normal values • pH normal or increased • Partial pressure of oxygen in arterial blood (PaO_2) normal or decreased • Partial pressure of carbon dioxide in arterial blood ($PaCO_2$) normal or decreased • Chest X-ray normal	• FEV_1 or peak flow 60% to 80% of normal values; may vary 20% to 30% with symptoms • pH generally elevated • PaO_2 reduced • $PaCO_2$ generally decreased • Chest X-ray that shows hyperinflation	• FEV_1 or peak flow less than 60% of normal values; may normally vary 20% to 30% and up to 50% with exacerbations • pH normal or reduced • PaO_2 decreased • $PaCO_2$ normal or increased • Chest X-ray that may show hyperinflation
Other assessment findings	• One attack per week (or none) • Positive response to bronchodilator therapy within 24 hours • No signs of asthma between episodes • No sleep interruption • No hyperventilation • Minimal evidence of airway obstruction • No or minimal increase in lung volume	• More than one attack per week • Coughing and wheezing between episodes • Diminished exercise tolerance • Possible sleep interruption • Increased lung volumes	• Frequent severe attacks • Daily wheezing • Poor exercise tolerance • Frequent sleep interruption • Bronchodilator therapy doesn't completely reverse airway obstruction • Markedly increased lung volumes

ate patient outcomes. For example, your patient will:
• demonstrate peak flows of 80% to 100% of predicted values for his age, sex, height, and weight or return to 80% to 100% of his highest values
• maintain $PaCO_2$ at established levels (usually between 35 and 45 mm Hg)
• display normal level of consciousness
• maintain arterial oxygen saturation (SaO_2) between 95% and 100%, or at baseline
• exhibit clear breath sounds on auscultation
• recover from an asthma attack with no residual lung damage.

Based on the nursing diagnosis *ineffective airway clearance,* develop appropriate patient outcomes. For example, your patient will:
• expectorate mucus when breathing deeply and coughing
• exhibit clear breath sounds on auscultation
• demonstrate ABG values within acceptable range.

Based on the nursing diagnosis *ineffective breathing pattern,* develop appropriate patient outcomes. For example, your patient will:
• perform diaphragmatic and pursed-lip breathing during an asthma attack
• demonstrate a stable breathing pattern when carrying out activities of daily living
• exhibit a normal respiratory rate
• report that he feels rested
• report that he feels comfortable when breathing
• demonstrate effective coughing.

Based on the nursing diagnosis *anxiety,* develop appropriate patient outcomes. For example, your patient will:
• perform relaxation techniques and breathing exercises
• use support systems to assist with emotional coping
• demonstrate abated signs of anxiety and report feeling less anxious.

Based on the nursing diagnosis *knowledge deficit,* develop appropriate patient outcomes. For example, your patient will:
• develop educational goals leading to the management of his asthma
• identify asthma triggers and state a plan for eliminating or reducing them
• demonstrate effective coughing and breathing techniques
• demonstrate effective relaxation techniques
• express a knowledge of the action, dosage, and adverse effects of all prescribed medications
• demonstrate the use of a metered-dose inhaler, peak flow meter, or a nebulizer
• describe the warning signs of respiratory infection and ways to prevent it.

IMPLEMENTATION

Focus your nursing care on assisting the patient during an asthma attack, monitoring drug therapy, and teaching him about asthma. (See *Medical care of the patient with asthma,* page 130.)

Nursing interventions
Your interventions can be divided into acute and long-term care.

Acute care
• In an acute asthma attack, find out if the patient has a nebulizer and if he has used it; he should have an albuterol or metaproterenol inhaler available at all times. Instruct him to take no more than two or three puffs every 4 hours. If he needs the nebulizer before 4 hours pass, let him use it and call the doctor for further instructions. Keep in mind that excessive nebulizer use can gradually weaken the patient's response and mask underlying inflammation. Rarely, extended overuse can lead to cardiac arrest and death.
• Reassure your patient during an asthma attack and stay with him. Place him

Treatments

Medical care of the patient with asthma

Immediate treatment for asthma aims to decrease bronchoconstriction, reduce the edema of the bronchial airways, and increase pulmonary ventilation. Treatment after an acute episode includes avoiding or removing precipitating factors, such as environmental allergens or irritants.

If asthma results from a particular antigen, it may be treated by desensitizing the patient through a series of injections of limited amounts of the antigen. The aim is to curb the patient's immune response to the antigen.

Drug therapy
This usually includes bronchodilators (theophyllines and beta-adrenergic agents), corticosteroids, cromolyn (mast-cell stabilizer) and, occasionally, anticholinergic bronchodilators. If asthma results from an infection, antibiotics are prescribed. Drug therapy proves most effective when begun soon after the onset of signs and symptoms.
• Bronchodilators decrease bronchoconstriction. Commonly used bronchodilators include the methylxanthines, such as theophylline and aminophylline, and the beta$_2$-adrenergic agonists, such as albuterol and terbutaline.
• Corticosteroids are prescribed for their anti-inflammatory and immunosuppressive effects, which decrease inflammation and edema of the airways. Commonly used corticosteroids include hydrocortisone sodium succinate, prednisone, methylprednisolone, and beclomethasone dipropionate.
• Cromolyn and nedocromil help to prevent the release of the chemical mediators, such as histamine and leukotrines, that cause bronchoconstriction.
• Anticholinergics, such as ipratropium bromide, block acetylcholine, another chemical mediator.

Management of asthma attacks
For the most part, asthma treatment must be tailored to each patient, depending on the severity of the episode. However, the following treatments are generally used:
• *Chronic mild asthma.* A beta-adrenergic bronchodilator by metered-dose inhaler or cromolyn is used before exercise, exposure to an allergen, or other stimuli to prevent symptoms. A beta$_2$-adrenergic agonist is used every 3 to 4 hours if symptoms occur.
• *Chronic moderate asthma.* Initially, an inhaled beta-adrenergic bronchodilator and an inhaled corticosteroid or cromolyn are prescribed. If symptoms persist, inhaled corticosteroids may be increased or sustained-release theophylline may be added. Short courses of oral corticosteroids may also be used.
• *Chronic severe asthma.* Initially, around-the-clock oral bronchodilator therapy with a long-acting theophylline or a beta-adrenergic drug may be required, supplemented with an inhaled beta-adrenergic agent and an inhaled corticosteroid. An oral corticosteroid, such as prednisone, may be added in cases of acute exacerbations.
• *Acute asthma attack.* Acute attacks that don't respond to self-treatment may require a visit to the emergency department or hospitalization. Treatment may include large doses of beta-adrenergic agents by inhalation or nebulization, oral or I.V. corticosteroids, I.V. aminophylline, and S.C. epinephrine. If severe, I.V. fluid therapy and low-flow oxygen therapy by nasal cannula or mask may also be needed. Patients not responding to this treatment who continue to have significant airway obstruction and increasing respiratory difficulty are at risk for status asthmaticus and may require mechanical ventilation.

Treatments

Medical care of the patient with asthma *(continued)*

Management of status asthmaticus
Treatment for this medical emergency consists of aggressive drug therapy (with the same drugs used to treat an acute asthma attack), I.V. fluids, and oxygen. If the patient becomes extremely fatigued (as evidenced by rising partial pressure of carbon dioxide in arterial blood), endotracheal intubation and mechanical ventilation may be necessary. Monitor arterial blood gas levels and pH frequently. Perform postural drainage and chest percussion, if tolerated, to remove bronchial secretions and mucus plugs.

in high Fowler's position and encourage pursed-lip and diaphragmatic breathing. Help him to relax as much as possible.

• Monitor the patient's vital signs. Keep in mind that developing or increasing tachypnea may indicate worsening asthma, and that tachycardia may indicate worsening disease or drug toxicity. Blood pressure readings may reveal pulsus paradoxus, indicating severe asthma. Hypertension may indicate asthma-related hypoxemia.

• Administer prescribed humidified oxygen by nasal cannula at 2 liters/minute to ease breathing and to increase SaO_2. Later, adjust oxygen according to the patient's vital signs and ABG levels.

• Anticipate intubation and mechanical ventilation if the patient fails to maintain adequate oxygenation because of the increased work of breathing and fatigue, respiratory arrest, progressive hypercapnia with respiratory acidosis, or progressive hypoxemia with mental deterioration.

• Give prescribed drugs and I.V. fluids, including aerosolized $beta_2$-adrenergic agonists. If prescribed, give a loading dose of I.V. aminophylline. Follow with I.V. drip, as prescribed. When possible, use an infusion pump. Don't infuse I.V. aminophylline faster than 25 mg/minute. Simultaneously, give an I.V. loading dose of a prescribed corticosteroid.

• Monitor serum theophylline levels to ensure they're in the therapeutic range. Observe your patient for signs of theophylline toxicity, such as vomiting, diarrhea, and headache, as well as for signs of subtherapeutic dosage, such as respiratory distress and increased wheezing.

• Observe the frequency and severity of your patient's cough, and note whether it's productive. Then, auscultate his lungs, noting adventitious or absent sounds. If his cough isn't productive and rhonchi are present, explain effective coughing techniques. If the patient can tolerate postural drainage and chest percussion, perform these procedures to clear secretions. Suction an intubated patient as needed.

• Treat dehydration with I.V. fluids until the patient can tolerate oral fluids, which will help loosen secretions.

• If conservative treatment fails to improve the airway obstruction, anticipate bronchoscopy or bronchial lavage when the area of collapse is a lobe or larger.

Long-term care
• Monitor the patient's respiratory status to detect baseline changes, to assess response to treatment, and to prevent or detect complications.

- Auscultate the lungs frequently, noting the degree of wheezing and quality of air movement.
- Review ABG levels, pulmonary function test results, and SaO_2 readings.
- If the patient is taking systemic corticosteroids, observe for complications, such as elevated blood glucose levels, osteoporosis, friable skin and bruising, and psychosis (if high dosages are used).
- If cushingoid effects result from long-term use of corticosteroids, they may be minimized by alternate-day dosage or use of inhaled corticosteroids, such as beclomethasone, flunisolide, or triamcinolone acetonide.
- If the patient is taking corticosteroids by inhaler, watch for signs of candidal infection in the mouth and pharynx. Using an extender device and rinsing the mouth afterward can prevent such infection.
- Observe the patient's anxiety level. Keep in mind that measures which reduce hypoxemia and breathlessness should help relieve anxiety. Encourage the patient to express his fears and concerns about his illness. Answer his questions honestly and offer reassurance. Provide relaxation measures, such as massage and soothing music.
- Keep the room temperature comfortable and use an air conditioner in hot, humid weather. A fan creates air movement that helps to lessen dyspnea.
- Monitor the patient's compliance with drug therapy and the avoidance of asthma-triggering factors.
- Control exercise-induced asthma by instructing the patient to use a bronchodilator or cromolyn 30 minutes before exercise. Also instruct him to use pursed-lip breathing while exercising.

Patient teaching
Include the following in your teaching program:

- Explain what asthma is and what happens during an attack. Inform the patient of complications that can occur if treatment isn't followed.
- Discuss factors that commonly bring on an asthma attack. Encourage the patient to keep a diary helping him to identify asthma-triggering factors.
- Teach the patient and his family to avoid known allergens and irritants. Refer him to a smoking cessation program, if warranted.
- Describe prescribed drugs, including their names, dosages, actions, adverse effects, and special instructions.
- Teach the patient how to use a metered-dose inhaler. (See *Using a metered-dose inhaler.*)
- If he has difficulty using an inhaler, he may need an extender device. These devices use valves or a reservoir bag to delay medication delivery to patients. They fit most oral inhalers. The addition of an extender device optimizes drug delivery and lowers the risk of candidal infection with orally inhaled corticosteroids.
- If the patient has moderate to severe asthma, explain how to use a peak flow meter to measure the degree of airway obstruction. Tell him to keep a record of peak flow readings and to bring it to medical appointments. Explain the importance of calling the doctor at once if the peak flow drops suddenly. (A drop can signal severe respiratory problems.)
- Tell the patient to notify the doctor of an asthma attack if he develops a fever over 100° F (37.8° C), chest pain, shortness of breath without coughing or exercising, or uncontrollable coughing. (See *Controlling an asthma attack,* page 134.) If he has a severe, uncontrollable asthma attack, he should get medical help immediately.
- Show the patient how to clean any special equipment.
- Teach him diaphragmatic and pursed-lip breathing. Explain effective

Teaching TimeSaver

Using a metered-dose inhaler

Using an inhaler correctly requires a certain degree of psychomotor coordination. So try to break down the instructions for its use into steps. Doing so will save you time and help you improve compliance.

You should instruct your patient to do the following:

• Use pursed-lip breathing to slow down his rate of breathing.

• Shake the inhaler for 5 to 10 seconds. The canister should be above the mouthpiece.

• At the end of a normal breath, put the inhaler in or just in front of his open mouth.

• With his head tilted back slightly, he should begin to inhale slowly and deeply (for 5 to 6 seconds) as he presses the canister down once (one press equals one dose).

• Hold the mist in his lungs for 5 to 10 seconds to allow the medication to settle on the airways. He should purse his lips and exhale slowly.

• If the doctor has prescribed a second dose, the patient should wait 2 minutes and repeat all the steps.

• If he's using an inhaled bronchodilator and an inhaled corticosteroid, he should use the bronchodilator first.

• Rinse or gargle after using an inhaled corticosteroid. This will decrease the risk of developing a yeast infection in his mouth.

• Take the mouthpiece off the canister and rinse it once a day.

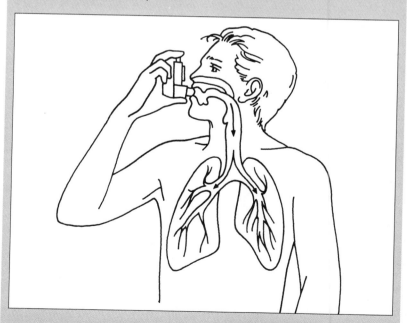

Teaching TimeSaver

Controlling an asthma attack

If you have limited time to teach your asthma patient, focus first on how he can control asthma attacks. Explain how to recognize warning signs and respond to them. Point out that early warning signs are more likely to occur at night because the airways are smallest between 3 a.m. and 5 a.m.

Recognizing warning signs
Emphasize that the patient must heed these warning signs:
• chest tightness
• coughing
• awareness of his breathing
• wheezing
• restlessness, irritability, and fatigue.

Responding to warning signs
Once the patient recognizes warning signs, he should take the following steps:
• Take his prescribed medication, as directed, to keep the attack from getting worse.
• Try to relax as the medication takes effect. Anxiety and fear worsen the shortness of breath. To help relax, he should sit upright in a chair; rest his arms on his knees, arms of a chair, or a table; close his eyes; and breathe slowly and evenly. Then he should concentrate on tightening and relaxing the muscles of the body.
• Tighten his face muscles and count one-1,000, two-1,000, and so forth. He shouldn't hold his breath.
• Then relax these muscles and repeat with the muscles of his arms and hands, and then with his legs and feet. Finally, he should let his body go limp.
• Regain control of breathing by using pursed-lip breathing. He should avoid gasping and continue pursed-lip breathing until he no longer feels breathless.
• If the attack triggers a coughing spell, he should use the following coughing technique (or a similar one) to bring up mucus and help clear the airways: Lean forward slightly, keeping both feet on the floor, and inhale deeply and exhale. Then inhale deeply again and hold that breath for one or two seconds. Cough twice into a tissue: first to loosen mucus, and then to bring it up.

Stress to the patient that if the attack worsens despite these steps, he should call his doctor immediately.

---

coughing techniques and, if necessary, how to perform postural drainage and chest percussion to clear mucus from the lungs.
• Encourage him to exercise according to guidelines established by the doctor or respiratory therapist. Many patients don't exercise for fear that it will worsen their asthma. In fact, exercise helps control asthma. Also, teach energy conservation techniques.
• Explain how to perform relaxation techniques and encourage the patient to practice them as needed.

• Urge him to drink plenty of fluids (at least 3 quarts [3 liters] daily) to help loosen secretions and maintain hydration.
• Encourage him to maintain a balanced diet to help prevent respiratory infection and fatigue. (See *Ensuring continued care for the patient with asthma.*)

EVALUATION

When evaluating the patient's response to your nursing care, gather reassess-

Ensuring continued care for the patient with asthma

Review the following teaching topics, referrals, and follow-up appointments to ensure that your patient is adequately prepared for discharge.

Teaching topics

Make sure that the following topics have been covered and that your patient's learning has been evaluated:

☐ explanation of the disorder, including its process and potential complications

☐ triggers of asthma attacks and how to avoid them

☐ importance of rinsing mouth after using inhaled corticosteroids

☐ warning signs and symptoms and when to see the doctor or go to the emergency department

☐ exercise and activity guidelines

☐ breathing and coughing techniques

☐ correct use and cleaning of equipment, including metered-dose inhaler, extender device, and peak flow meter.

Referrals

Make sure that the patient has been provided with necessary referrals to:

☐ social services for financial consultation regarding equipment and medications

☐ dietary consultation to discuss allergies (if applicable)

☐ smoking cessation program and importance of avoiding secondhand smoke

☐ sources of information and support, including the American Lung Association, National Allergy & Asthma Network, and National Asthma Education Program.

Follow-up appointments

Make sure that the necessary follow-up appointments have been scheduled and that the patient has been notified:

☐ doctor

☐ allergist

☐ diagnostic tests for reevaluation.

---

ment data and compare this information with the patient outcomes specified in your plan of care.

Teaching and counseling

Begin by determining the effectiveness of your teaching and counseling. Consider the following questions:

• Does the patient understand asthma and what happens during an attack?

• Does he know the factors that trigger his asthma and the importance of avoiding them?

• Does he know the warning signs of respiratory infection and how to prevent it?

• Is he knowledgeable about his prescribed drugs, including their names, dosages, actions, adverse effects, and special instructions?

• Does he understand how to use a peak flow meter and metered-dose inhalers?

• Does he know when to call the doctor?

Physical condition

A physical examination and diagnostic tests will provide additional information. If treatment has been successful, you should note the following outcomes:

• Breath sounds are clear on auscultation.

• Respiratory rate and pattern are at acceptable baseline values.

• ABG, pulmonary function, and (SaO_2) levels are within an acceptable range.
• Peak flow readings are 80% to 100% of predicted values or 80% to 100% of the patient's highest values.
• The patient maintains a normal activity level.
• Asthma attacks are prevented or reduced in frequency.
• The patient hasn't missed time from work or school because of asthma.
• He exhibits no asthma symptoms or only minor ones.
• He can sleep through the night without asthma symptoms.
• He experiences few or no adverse effects from medication.

Chronic bronchitis

Marked by excessive production of tracheobronchial mucus, chronic bronchitis is characterized by daily coughing lasting at least 3 months of the year for 2 consecutive years. Its severity varies widely, depending on the individual response of the lungs, the amount of cigarette smoke or other pollutants inhaled by the patient, and the duration of the inhalation. A respiratory tract infection typically worsens the cough and related symptoms.

Chronic bronchitis results in pathologic changes in the lungs:
• hypertrophy and hyperplasia of the bronchial mucous glands
• increased goblet cells
• ciliary damage
• squamous metaplasia of the columnar epithelium
• chronic leukocytic and lymphocytic infiltration of bronchial walls.

Additional effects may include widespread inflammation, airway narrowing, and mucus within the airways that can be obstructing. Because oxygen can't reach the alveolocapillary membrane, a severe ventilation-perfusion mismatch with hypoxemia and hypercapnia may develop. (See *Understanding chronic bronchitis*.)

In later stages, chronic bronchitis may lead to polycythemia, cyanosis, pulmonary hypertension, cor pulmonale, or acute respiratory failure. (See *Key points about chronic bronchitis*, page 138.)

Causes

Cigarette smoking represents the most common cause of chronic bronchitis. Upper respiratory tract infection and inhaled atmospheric pollutants, such as sulfur dioxide, nitrogen oxides, and ozone, exacerbate symptoms and cause the disorder to progress. Some patients may have a genetic predisposition to the disorder.

ASSESSMENT

Knowledge of the patient's health history aids diagnosis of chronic bronchitis. Typically, the patient is a long-time cigarette smoker who experiences frequent upper respiratory tract infections. Your assessment should include a careful consideration of physical examination findings and diagnostic test results.

Health history

The patient's chief complaint is a productive cough. He may reveal that the cough was initially prevalent during the winter but gradually became a year-round problem with increasingly severe episodes. Dyspnea, usually a later complaint, typically worsens and requires an increasingly long time to subside. Very often the patient does not seek help until dyspnea becomes a frequent problem.

Physical examination

Inspection usually reveals a cough that produces copious gray, white, or yel-

Understanding chronic bronchitis

In chronic bronchitis, irritants inhaled over a prolonged period inflame the tracheobronchial tree, leading to increased mucus production and a narrowed or blocked airway.

As inflammation continues, the mucus-producing goblet cells undergo hypertrophy, as do the ciliated epithelial cells that line the upper respiratory tract. Hypersecretion from the goblet cells blocks the free movement of the cilia, which normally sweep dust, irritants, and mucus from the airways.

As a result, the airways become blocked and mucus and debris accumulate in the respiratory tract.

Cross section of normal bronchial tube

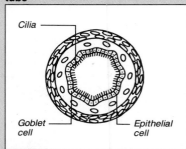

Inflamed bronchiole

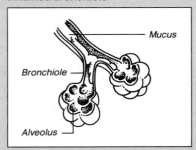

Narrowed bronchial tube in chronic bronchitis

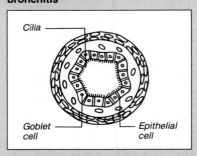

low sputum. If bronchitis is advanced, the patient's skin may appear reddish blue (from cyanosis and polycythemia), and he may have gained a substantial amount of weight from edema brought on by right ventricular failure. The patient with chronic bronchitis who exhibits cyanosis, polycythemia, and edema is commonly referred to as a "blue bloater." He may use accessory respiratory muscles for breathing and be tachypneic. However, he usually

doesn't have a barrel chest (increased anteroposterior diameter).

Palpation may disclose pedal edema, hepatic congestion, and neck vein distention, if severe pulmonary hypertension is present.

Auscultation may reveal diminished breath sounds, wheezing, prolonged expiratory time, and rhonchi. Heart sounds may be distant and an S_3 may be present, indicating right ventricular failure. (See *What to look for in chronic bronchitis,* page 139.)

FactFinder

Key points about chronic bronchitis

- *Incidence:* Children of parents who smoke are at a higher risk for upper respiratory tract infections that can lead to chronic bronchitis. Most patients with moderate to severe bronchitis also have some degree of emphysema.
- *Prognosis:* If the patient stops smoking and avoids exposure to irritants, symptoms may improve significantly at first and some reversal in airway obstruction may be noted.
- *Chief diagnostic methods:* Pulmonary function studies and patient history
- *Treatment:* The best therapy is smoking cessation and the avoidance of air pollutants. Other treatments alleviate symptoms.
- *Leading complication:* Respiratory tract infection
- *Other complications:* Right ventricular hypertrophy, cor pulmonale, and acute respiratory failure

Diagnostic test results

The following tests aid diagnosis of chronic bronchitis:
- Pulmonary function tests demonstrate increased residual volume, reduced vital capacity and forced expiratory flow, and normal static compliance and diffusing capacity. Both inspiratory and expiratory flow rates are decreased.
- Arterial blood gas (ABG) analysis reveals a diminished partial pressure of oxygen in arterial blood (PaO_2) and a normal or elevated partial pressure of carbon dioxide in arterial blood ($PaCO_2$).
- Sputum culture may reveal increased microorganisms and neutrophils.
- Electrocardiography may detect atrial arrhythmias; peaked P waves in leads II, III, and aV_F; and, occasionally, right ventricular hypertrophy.
- Complete blood count (CBC) may show elevated hemoglobin (in polycythemia) and increased red blood cell (RBC) production.
- Chest X-rays may be useful to exclude other causes of productive cough, such as lung cancer and tuberculosis.

NURSING DIAGNOSIS

Common nursing diagnoses for a patient with chronic bronchitis include:
- Ineffective breathing pattern related to chronic airflow obstruction
- Ineffective airway clearance related to increased tracheobronchial secretions or bronchoconstriction
- Impaired gas exchange related to ventilation-perfusion mismatch increasing difficulty of breathing
- Fluid volume excess related to edema from right ventricular failure
- High risk for infection related to ineffective airway clearance and decreased pulmonary function
- Altered nutrition: Less than body requirements related to dyspnea and fatigue.

PLANNING

Focus your nursing care on teaching the patient controlled breathing and coughing techniques, as well as emphasizing the importance of smoking cessation and maintaining normal weight.

Based on the nursing diagnosis *ineffective breathing pattern,* develop appropriate patient outcomes. For example, your patient will:
- demonstrate controlled breathing techniques (including pursed-lip and diaphragmatic breathing) regularly, with activity, and during acute episodes

• exhibit a respiratory rate that returns to baseline

• demonstrate ways to decrease dyspnea.

Based on the nursing diagnosis *ineffective airway clearance,* develop appropriate patient outcomes. For example, your patient will:

• demonstrate effective postural drainage, percussion, and coughing techniques

• exhibit diminished cough and sputum production

• have diminished or no rhonchi and wheezes

• describe the plan to decrease or eliminate dyspnea

• exhibit ABG levels within a normal range.

Based on the nursing diagnosis *impaired gas exchange,* develop appropriate patient outcomes. For example, your patient will:

• carry out activities of daily living without weakness or fatigue

• maintain adequate ventilation

• exhibit optimal PaO$_2$ and PaCO$_2$ levels.

Based on the nursing diagnosis *fluid volume excess,* develop appropriate patient outcomes. For example, your patient will:

• achieve a weight that is normal for his height and age or that is at baseline

• exhibit decreased pedal edema or jugular vein distention

• comply with treatment plan including oxygen therapy, sodium restriction, and diuretic therapy.

Based on the nursing diagnosis *high risk for infection,* develop appropriate patient outcomes. For example, your patient will:

• verbalize signs and symptoms of infection and plan of action

• exhibit a normal temperature

• remain free of all signs and symptoms of infection

• exhibit a cough productive of clear, mucoid secretions.

Assessment TimeSaver

What to look for in chronic bronchitis

• *Onset of signs and symptoms:* Ages 40 to 50
• *Appearance:* Stocky body build with no history of weight loss; use of accessory muscles to breathe (late stage)
• *Chief complaint:* Productive cough
• *Clinical course:* Variable
• *Arterial blood gas levels:* Decreased partial pressure of oxygen in arterial blood and normal or increased partial pressure of carbon dioxide in arterial blood
• *Additional findings:* Frequent episodes of right ventricular failure with dependent edema (late stage)

Based on the nursing diagnosis *altered nutrition: less than body requirements,* develop appropriate patient outcomes. For example, your patient will:

• develop and maintain a low-salt, balanced diet plan that meets his nutritional needs

• identify activities that increase fatigue

• take measures to conserve energy and prevent or minimize fatigue.

IMPLEMENTATION

Treatment for chronic bronchitis includes smoking cessation, drug therapy, and measures to prevent fatigue and decrease dyspnea. (See *Medical care of the patient with chronic bronchitis,* page 140.)

Nursing interventions

Answer the patient's questions, and encourage him and his family to express their concerns about the illness. Include the patient and his family in deci-

Medical care of the patient with chronic bronchitis

The most effective treatment for chronic bronchitis is cessation of smoking and avoidance of air pollutants as much as possible. In the early stage of the disorder, when obstruction is limited to the small airways, it may be reversed once its causative factors are eliminated. In later stages, however, chronic bronchitis is irreversible.

Drug therapy
The following drugs may be prescribed as part of the treatment plan:
- Antibiotics can be used to treat recurring bacterial infections.
- Bronchodilators may relieve bronchospasm and facilitate mucus clearance. Ipratropium, an anticholinergic, and theophylline, a methylxanthine, are the bronchodilators of choice.
- Corticosteroids may be prescribed to relieve inflammation.
- A mucolytic or an expectorant may be prescribed to facilitate expectoration.

- Diuretics may be used to treat edema.

Other treatments
The following measures may also be necessary:
- Low-flow oxygen helps to treat hypoxemia.
- Ultrasonic or mechanical nebulizer treatments may help to loosen and mobilize secretions.
- A sodium-restricted diet may be ordered to treat edema.
- Adequate fluid intake may help to liquefy secretions and prevent dehydration.
- Postural drainage, chest percussion, coughing, and possibly vibration may be needed to mobilize secretions.
- Pulmonary rehabilitation, including exercise, may help the patient to become desensitized to dyspnea and to increase overall conditioning.

---

sions regarding care. Refer them to support services as appropriate.
- Administer prescribed medications and note the patient's response to them. Inform the patient that it may take about 4 weeks to notice the effects of inhaled corticosteroids. Provide mouth care or encourage the patient to rinse his mouth after respiratory therapy.
- Provide low-flow oxygen therapy as necessary to maintain adequate oxygenation. Monitor ABG and oximetry readings.
- Assess for respiratory changes. Evaluate sputum quality and quantity, restlessness, increased tachypnea, altered breath sounds, and ABG values. Report significant changes to the doctor immediately.

- Monitor the patient's fluid status by weighing him three times weekly, and assess for edema.
- Watch for signs and symptoms of respiratory infection such as fever; increased cough; purulent, copious sputum; and increased fatigue and dyspnea. Administer prescribed antibiotics.
- Unless contraindicated, make sure that the patient receives adequate fluids (at least 3 quarts [3 liters] a day) to loosen secretions.
- Encourage the patient to cough effectively to clear secretions. If prescribed, perform postural drainage, chest percussion and, in some instances, vibration for involved lobes.
- If appropriate, offer small, frequent meals to conserve the patient's energy

and prevent fatigue. Large meals can worsen abdominal distention, thereby diminishing chest excursion.

• Encourage daily activity, and provide diversional activities, when appropriate. To conserve the patient's energy and prevent fatigue, help him to alternate periods of rest and activity.

• Schedule respiratory therapy at least 1 hour before or after meals.

Patient teaching

Include the following in your teaching program:

• Explain chronic bronchitis, its relationship to cigarette smoke and other types of air pollutants, and its serious complications.

• Teach pursed-lip and diaphragmatic breathing and energy conservation techniques to the patient experiencing dyspnea. Instruct him to use pursed-lip breathing during all activities and to keep breathing as slow and deep as possible at all times.

• Review all medications, including their purpose, dosage, and adverse effects. If appropriate, teach the patient how to use a metered-dose inhaler and extender device. Stress the importance of blood work to monitor drug levels (especially theophylline) and potassium, if he is taking diuretics. Advise him to immediately report any adverse reactions to the doctor.

• Advise the patient to avoid crowds and people with known infections and to obtain influenza and pneumococcal immunizations.

• Describe the warning signs and symptoms that should be reported to the doctor.

• If the patient is receiving oxygen therapy at home, explain the treatment rationale. Show him how to operate the equipment safely. Refer him to a medical equipment supplier.

• Teach the patient and his family how to perform postural drainage and chest percussion. Instruct the patient to maintain each position for 10 minutes before a caregiver performs percussion and the patient coughs. Also teach the patient coughing and deep-breathing techniques to promote good ventilation and to remove secretions.

• Encourage the patient to drink plenty of fluids, unless contraindicated, to prevent dehydration and help loosen secretions.

• Instruct the edematous patient about prescribed measures that may include a sodium-restricted diet and diuretic therapy.

• If the patient smokes, assess his level of knowledge about how smoking affects pulmonary functioning and instruct him, as needed. Also assess his motivation to stop smoking. Provide positive reinforcement for smoking cessation efforts, and supply him with smoking cessation resources or counseling, as needed.

• Urge the patient to avoid exposure to inhaled irritants, such as automobile exhaust fumes, aerosol sprays, industrial pollutants, and secondhand cigarette smoke.

• If the patient takes theophylline, warn him that smoking cigarettes or marijuana significantly increases plasma clearance of theophylline. Also, if the patient quits smoking, he should notify the doctor because he may experience the onset of adverse effects of higher blood levels of theophylline.

• Tell the patient not to take any over-the-counter medications unless approved by the doctor. (See *Ensuring continued care for the patient with chronic bronchitis,* page 142.)

EVALUATION

When evaluating the patient's response to your nursing care, gather reassessment data and compare this information with the patient outcomes specified in your plan of care.

Discharge TimeSaver
Ensuring continued care for the patient with chronic bronchitis

Review the following teaching topics, referrals, and follow-up appointments to ensure that your patient with chronic bronchitis is adequately prepared for discharge.

Teaching topics
Make sure that patient teaching has been provided on the following topics and that your patient's learning has been evaluated:
☐ an explanation of the disorder, including its causes, symptoms, and complications
☐ smoking as a major risk factor
☐ prescribed medications, including possible adverse effects
☐ energy conservation techniques
☐ postural drainage, chest percussion, coughing, and breathing techniques, as needed
☐ importance of monitoring weight at least three times a week
☐ warning signs and symptoms to report to the doctor (weight gain of more than 5 lb [2.3 kg] in 2 days, increased coughing, fatigue, change in sputum, and signs and symptoms of hypoxemia and right ventricular failure)
☐ treatment of dyspnea.

Referrals
Make sure that your patient has been provided with these necessary referrals:
☐ social services (financial consultation regarding equipment and medications)
☐ home oxygen equipment supplier
☐ smoking cessation program
☐ pulmonary rehabilitation program
☐ other sources of information and support.

Follow-up appointments
Make sure that the necessary follow-up appointments have been scheduled and that your patient has been notified:
☐ doctor
☐ pulmonary rehabilitation
☐ diagnostic tests for reevaluation.

Teaching and counseling
Begin by determining the effectiveness of your teaching and counseling. Note statements by the patient indicating he:
• understands the relationship of chronic bronchitis to cigarette smoke and inhalation of other pollutants
• understands the need to avoid crowds and people with infections
• knows the warning signs that must be reported to the doctor
• knows his medication's purpose, dosage, and reportable adverse effects.

Physical condition
If interventions are successful, your evaluation should indicate the following:

• absence or reduction in rhonchi and wheezes
• ABG values within normal range for your patient
• normal temperature
• decreased dyspnea
• diminished coughing and sputum production
• absence or decrease in edema, jugular vein distention, and hepatic congestion
• minimal fatigue.

Emphysema

In emphysema, recurrent obstruction of airflow results from the excessive inflation and destruction of lung tissue beyond the terminal bronchioles. (See *What happens in emphysema,* page 144.)

Emphysema is one of three major types of chronic obstructive pulmonary disease (the other two are asthma and chronic bronchitis), which frequently overlap as they progress. For instance, many emphysema patients also have chronic bronchitis; and many emphysema and chronic bronchitis patients have some aspects of asthma as well. (See *Key points about emphysema,* page 145.)

Causes
Cigarette smoking is the leading cause of emphysema. However, in 1% to 2% of patients, deficiency of alpha$_1$-antitrypsin, an enzyme that breaks down trypsin, causes the disorder. If trypsin accumulates, it can destroy lung tissue.

ASSESSMENT

Your assessment should include a thorough health history, physical examination, and a review of diagnostic test findings.

Health history
Typically, the patient with emphysema is a cigarette smoker who is age 50 or older. He usually reports dyspnea that occurs when performing daily activities. Dyspnea occurs with progressively lower levels of activity and, eventually, during rest. The patient may report anorexia with resultant weight loss and a general feeling of malaise. Rarely, he may complain of a chronic nonproductive cough.

Physical examination
The patient may be barrel-chested, breathe through pursed lips, and use accessory muscles to breathe. You may notice a markedly increased expiratory effort and tachypnea. However, the patient isn't usually hypoxic or cyanotic. Typically, he appears underweight for his height.

Palpation performed while the patient sits and leans forward in a tripod position (to increase chest excursion) may reveal decreased tactile fremitus and chest expansion. Percussion may reveal hyperresonance. On auscultation, you may hear decreased breath sounds, crackles and wheezing during inspiration, a prolonged expiratory phase with grunting respirations, and distant heart sounds. Edema isn't present early in the disease, but may occur later due to cor pulmonale. The patient may have resting tachycardia. (See *What to look for in emphysema,* page 146.)

Diagnostic test results
The following tests may confirm a diagnosis of emphysema:
• Pulmonary function tests (PFTs) typically indicate increased residual volume and total lung capacity, reduced diffusing capacity, and decreased expiratory flow, especially forced expiratory volume in 1 second. Inspiratory flow is normal.
• Arterial blood gas (ABG) analysis may show a normal partial pressure of arterial oxygen or a mild to moderate decrease. Partial pressure of arterial carbon dioxide (PaCO$_2$) is normal until late in the disease.
• Electrocardiography may reveal tall, symmetrical P waves in leads II, III, and aV$_F$; a vertical QRS axis; and signs of right ventricular hypertrophy late in the disease.
• In advanced disease, chest X-rays may show a flattened diaphragm, reduced vascular markings at the lung

What happens in emphysema

Emphysema is characterized by destruction of the alveolar walls and the creation of large air spaces distal to the terminal bronchioles. Its pathophysiology isn't fully understood, but research indicates that destructive enzymes attack the lung's connective tissue and alveolar walls.

During inspiration, alveoli can't recoil normally after expanding. During expiration, bronchioles collapse causing increased airway resistance and air entrapment within the lungs. Gradually, the lungs become larger and press down on the diaphragm, causing the diaphragm to flatten and lose its ability to contract adequately. The patient begins to use accessory muscles to increase chest diameter during inspiration.

Healthy lung

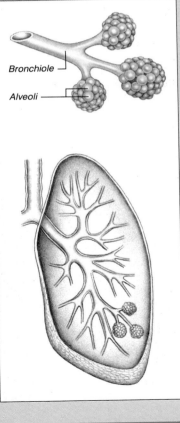

Bronchiole

Alveoli

Emphysematous lung

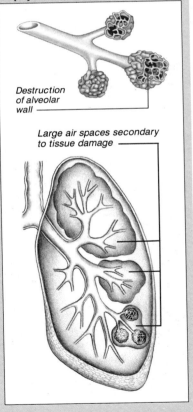

Destruction of alveolar wall

Large air spaces secondary to tissue damage

periphery, overaeration of the lungs, a vertical heart, increased anteroposterior thoracic diameter, and large retrosternal air space.
• Liver function tests may reveal cor pulmonale.
• The red blood cell count usually demonstrates an increased hemoglobin level late in the disease process when the patient has persistent severe hypoxemia.
• Serum electrolyte studies may indicate reduced sodium, potassium, calcium, magnesium, and phosphorus levels. Diminished levels may cause reduced respiratory muscle strength and endurance.
• Albumin and total protein levels may be measured to evaluate nutritional status.

NURSING DIAGNOSIS

Common nursing diagnoses for a patient with emphysema include:
• Activity intolerance related to dyspnea, fear, and anxiety
• Altered nutrition: Less than body requirements related to shortness of breath, low energy levels, and depression
• Ineffective breathing pattern related to chronic airflow limitations and respiratory muscle weakness
• Impaired gas exchange related to loss of lung tissue caused by destruction of alveolar walls
• High risk for infection related to the effects of poor nutrition and altered immunity on lungs
• Knowledge deficit related to emphysema and its treatment
• Ineffective individual coping related to the lifestyle effects of an obstructive respiratory disorder
• Anxiety related to breathlessness, fear of death, or decreased functional status.

FactFinder
Key points about emphysema

• *Incidence:* Emphysema is the most common cause of death from respiratory disease in North America.
• *Cause:* Smoking represents the most common cause of emphysema. Other causes may include environmental pollution, heredity, and recurrent infections.
• *Prognosis:* No cure exists for emphysema. Airway obstruction is persistent and irreversible.
• *Chief diagnostic methods:* Pulmonary function tests and chest X-rays
• *Treatment:* Therapy focuses on alleviating symptoms and preventing complications.
• *Leading complications:* Recurrent respiratory tract infections, primary pulmonary hypertension, acute pulmonary embolism, and respiratory failure
• *Other complications:* Peptic ulcer disease affects 20% to 25% of emphysema patients. Also, alveolar blebs and bullae may rupture, causing spontaneous pneumothorax or pneumomediastinum.

PLANNING

Based on the nursing diagnosis *activity intolerance,* develop appropriate patient outcomes. For example, your patient will:
• identify controllable factors that cause fatigue
• demonstrate skill in conserving energy while carrying out daily activities to tolerance level
• use a bronchodilator, if prescribed, carrying out an activity to prevent shortness of breath
• seek assistance when needed to complete an activity

Assessment TimeSaver

What to look for in emphysema

- *Onset of signs and symptoms:* Ages 50 to 75
- *Appearance:* Cachectic, with history of major weight loss, reflecting chronic shortness of breath and increased work of breathing; use of accessory muscles to breathe
- *Chief complaint:* Shortness of breath
- *Clinical course:* Progressive deterioration
- *Arterial blood gas levels:* Slightly decreased partial pressure of arterial oxygen and normal partial pressure of arterial carbon dioxide
- *Additional findings:* Normal skin color, absence of edema, possible barrel-chested appearance.

• pace activities to decrease shortness of breath.

Based on the nursing diagnosis *altered nutrition (less than body requirements),* develop appropriate patient outcomes. For example, your patient will:
• maintain his weight within an acceptable range for his sex, age, and height
• maintain a normal serum albumin level
• eat small, frequent meals.

Based on the nursing diagnosis *ineffective breathing pattern,* develop appropriate patient outcomes. For example, your patient will:
• demonstrate pursed-lip and diaphragmatic breathing techniques.

Based on the nursing diagnosis *impaired gas exchange,* develop appropriate patient outcomes. For example, your patient will:
• maintain ABG levels within an acceptable range.

Based on the nursing diagnosis *high risk for infection,* develop appropriate patient outcomes. For example, your patient will:
• avoid crowds and people with known infections
• obtain influenza and pneumococcal immunizations
• identify signs and symptoms of respiratory infection and notify the doctor immediately if they develop.

Based on the nursing diagnosis *knowledge deficit,* develop appropriate patient outcomes. For example, your patient will:
• verbalize understanding of self-care requirements for emphysema
• describe factors that influence compliance with the health care regimen
• adhere to prescribed treatment measures, as agreed upon
• use available support resources as needed.

Based on the nursing diagnosis *ineffective individual coping,* develop appropriate patient outcomes. For example, your patient will:
• describe resources available to help him cope with his disorder.

Based on the nursing diagnosis *anxiety,* develop appropriate patient outcomes. For example, your patient will:
• seek help, as necessary, to prevent episodes of anxiety
• demonstrate ability to control his anxiety with breathing and relaxation techniques
• list symptoms of anxiety or depression to report to the doctor.

IMPLEMENTATION

Because emphysema has no cure, treatment seeks only to alleviate the patient's symptoms. Therefore, nursing interventions are extremely important. (See *Medical care of the patient with emphysema.*)

Nursing interventions

- Encourage the patient to use deep, slow, pursed-lip breathing to control episodes of shortness of breath.
- Encourage the patient to express his fears and concerns about his illness. Answer his questions as honestly as possible. Include the patient and his family in decisions related to his care. Remain with the patient during periods of extreme stress and anxiety. Encourage the patient and his family to join a support group and refer them to other appropriate support services, such as the local chapter of the American Lung Association.
- Monitor the patient's respiratory function regularly. Auscultate breath sounds, noting improvement or deterioration. Obtain ABG levels and PFTs as ordered. Be alert to the development of complications such as pneumothorax, infection, and cor pulmonale.
- If prescribed, perform postural drainage and chest percussion several times daily.
- If hypoxemia is evident, administer oxygen, as prescribed, at low flow rates. Remember that the condition of the patient with late-stage emphysema may deteriorate further in response to a high fraction of inspired oxygen. Deterioration would be evidenced by a decreased level of consciousness, shallow breathing, and an increased $PaCO_2$ above the patient's baseline.
- Assess the patient's nutritional status. If needed, provide the patient with a high-caloric, high-fat, protein-rich diet to promote health and healing. Provide small, frequent meals to conserve energy and prevent fatigue. Consult a dietitian to find ways to increase the patient's caloric intake with nutrient-dense foods. Avoid foods that cause gas with resulting abdominal distention. The patient may require nutritional supplements.
- Schedule respiratory treatments at least 1 hour before or after meals. Pro-

Treatments

Medical care of the patient with emphysema

Emphysema management usually includes drug therapy, oxygen therapy, and additional measures as required.

Drug therapy

Bronchodilators (inhalers and nebulizers), such as albuterol, pirbuterol, and I.V. or oral theophylline, are used to treat reversible bronchospasm, which may occur in emphysema. Corticosteroids are used during acute exacerbation to decrease inflammation of the throat and lungs. Antibiotics are used during acute flare-ups and to treat respiratory tract infection.

Oxygen therapy

The doctor may prescribe oxygen at low flow rates to correct hypoxemia. Oxygen may be delivered continuously, only at night, or during exercise. Some patients may desire transtracheal catheterization to receive oxygen at home.

Additional measures

Although excessive mucus production does not usually accompany pure emphysema, for patients who also have chronic bronchitis, additional measures may include ensuring adequate hydration and performing postural drainage and chest percussion to mobilize secretions. Immunizations may be prescribed to prevent influenza and pneumococcal pneumonia. Anxiolytics or antidepressants may be prescribed to decrease anxiety or to treat depression.

vide mouth care after bronchodilator therapy.
- Make sure that the patient receives adequate fluids (at least 3 quarts [3 liters] a day) to loosen secretions.

Teaching TimeSaver

Avoiding bronchial irritants

If you have limited time to teach your patient, focus first on two key topics: smoking cessation and avoidance of other bronchial irritants.

Quitting smoking
• Tell your patient about the dangers of smoking and the benefits of quitting. Provide him with literature about these topics and about ways to quit smoking.
• Encourage him to set a date for quitting his habit.
• If he's not smoking while hospitalized, provide lots of encouragement. Suggest some diversional activities and supply him with gum or hard candy, if allowed. Also, encourage liberal fluid intake.
• If the patient continues to smoke, understand that he needs more than teaching to get over his addiction. He needs effective coping strategies and help in changing his self-image. Recommend counseling or a smoking cessation program while he's in the hospital. Your local chapter of the American Lung Association, American Heart Association, or American Cancer Society can usually provide a list of resources. In addition, many hospitals have their own programs.
• Family members who aren't ready to quit smoking should be encouraged to smoke in a separate, well-ventilated room and to use smokeless ashtrays or air filters.

Avoiding other irritants
Provide the patient with a list of potential bronchial irritants other than cigarette smoke. These may include cold air, strong winds, high humidity, air pollution, cooking fumes, perfumes (including perfumed deodorants, hair sprays, lotions, and powders). Exercise can induce bronchospasm in some patients.
Emotional stress can act as a bronchial irritant. Suspect stress-induced bronchial irritation if the emphysema patient has emotional problems or is repeatedly hospitalized. Such a patient may benefit from stress management programs or counseling. Make the patient aware of the significance of stress as an exacerbating factor in his illness.

• Encourage daily activity and provide diversionary activities as appropriate. To conserve energy and prevent fatigue, help the patient to pace his activity and alternate periods of rest and activity. Also help him develop realistic expectations for his activity.
• Because of the potential for infection, advise the patient to avoid crowds and people with known infections and to obtain influenza and pneumococcal immunizations. Identify signs and symptoms of respiratory infection and tell the patient to notify the doctor promptly if they occur.

• Administer prescribed medications and record the patient's response.
• Monitor the patient's compliance with the recommended treatment program.

Patient teaching
• Explain emphysema, its physiologic effects, and its complications.
• If the patient smokes, encourage him to stop. Provide him with information on smoking cessation resources or counseling.
• Urge the patient to avoid exposure to respiratory irritants, such as automobile exhaust fumes, aerosol sprays, in-

dustrial pollutants, and secondhand cigarette smoke. (See *Avoiding bronchial irritants.*)

• For the patient receiving home oxygen therapy, explain the rationale, the need for weaning, and the safe use of the equipment. Emphasize that the oxygen flow rate should never be increased above the prescribed level.

• Help the patient to identify factors that cause stress or fatigue. Teach relaxation and energy conservation techniques.

• Review the patient's medications and explain the rationale for their use, their dosages, and their possible adverse effects. Advise him to report any adverse reactions to the doctor immediately.

Timesaving tip: The best time to explain each medication is when you administer it, but don't try to explain all of the patient's medications at once. Talk about one medication the first day, then another the next day. Explain their action in simple terms. State, for instance, that bronchodilators open the breathing passages and antibiotics fight infection. Later, ask the patient to explain the purpose of each medication.

• Instruct the patient to avoid over-the-counter medications, unless prescribed by the doctor, because of possible drug interactions. This is particularly important for patients on theophylline. If appropriate, show the patient how to use an inhaler and extender device correctly.

Timesaving tip: Because the patient with emphysema may need to take several medications each day, devise a schedule listing the types and number of medications to take with each meal and at bedtime. The patient may also benefit from a system to help him remember, such as using a partitioned box or marked envelopes. Refer the patient to a home health care agency that will help him establish a system tailored to his individual needs.

• Encourage the patient to eat high-calorie, high-fat, protein-rich foods. Urge him to drink plenty of fluids to prevent dehydration and to help loosen secretions.

Timesaving tip: To help the patient with emphysema get the nutrition he needs, advise him to rest for 30 minutes before eating. Encourage him to rest periodically while preparing meals (cooking can be as tiring as eating) and suggest using a microwave oven. Tell him to avoid exercise and breathing treatments for at least 1 hour before and after eating.

• Teach the patient controlled coughing and effective breathing techniques. (See *Overcoming shortness of breath,* page 150.)

• Urge the patient to remain as active as possible. Tell him that inactivity leads to depression and further deconditioning.

• If appropriate, describe signs and symptoms of peptic ulcer disease. Instruct the patient to check his stools every day and to notify the doctor if he sees blood or experiences persistent nausea, vomiting, heartburn, indigestion, constipation, or diarrhea.

• Inform the patient about the signs and symptoms of ruptured alveolar blebs and bullae. Explain the seriousness of a possible spontaneous pneumothorax. Urge him to notify the doctor if he feels sudden, sharp pleuritic pain that worsens with chest movement, breathing, or coughing.

• Inform the patient about pulmonary rehabilitation programs in his area. (See *Ensuring continued care for the patient with emphysema,* page 151.)

EVALUATION

When evaluating the patient's response to your nursing care, gather reassessment data and compare this information with the patient outcomes specified in your plan of care.

Overcoming shortness of breath

Shortness of breath limits the activity of the emphysema patient and causes anxiety and depression. Although the patient can't expect to remain as active as he once was, he can learn to cope with his shortness of breath and remain as active as possible. To help him, focus on teaching him pursed-lip breathing, diaphragmatic breathing, and positioning techniques, which will help him gain control of his breathing.

Encourage the patient to practice breathing techniques four times a day (with 6 to 10 repetitions each time) until they become familiar.

Pursed-lip breathing
Instruct the patient to inhale slowly through the nose while counting: one-1,000, two-1,000, three-1,000. Then the patient should exhale slowly through pursed lips, producing a soft whistling, and count to six-1,000. Exhalation must take longer than inhalation. Alternatively, tell the patient to breathe in to a count of 2 and breathe out to a count of 4. Encourage him to use pursed-lip breathing whenever he feels short of breath.

Instruct him to use pursed-lip breathing during activities by inhaling first, then exhaling during exertion. For example, when climbing stairs, he should inhale while standing still and exhale while stepping up.

Explain that exhaling through pursed lips:

- slows down breathing
- helps remove stale air trapped in the lungs
- increases the level of oxygen
- promotes relaxation.

Diaphragmatic breathing
Instruct the patient to sit or lie down with one hand placed lightly on the abdomen, the other hand on the chest. Then have him breathe slowly through the nose, using his abdominal muscles. The hand on his abdomen should rise during inspiration and fall during expiration. The hand on his chest should remain almost still.

Positioning techniques
Instruct the patient to use the following positioning techniques to help expand his lungs and gain control of breathing when he's short of breath:
- Sit, leaning forward slightly, with his elbows on the knees.
- Stand facing a wall. Then lean forward, resting his hands and forearms against the wall at shoulder height.
- Stand with one foot forward, and then lean back against the wall.

Additional techniques
Teach the patient guided imagery and progressive relaxation techniques to help him relax. Tell him that using a fan can help shortness of breath by circulating air.

Teaching and counseling
Begin by evaluating your patient's response to teaching and counseling. Consider the following questions:
- Does he understand emphysema and its effects and complications?
- Does he know the purposes of his medications, the correct dosages, and the importance of reporting any adverse reactions to the doctor?
- Can he demonstrate controlled coughing, pursed-lip and diaphragmatic breathing, postural drainage, and chest percussion techniques?
- Does he comply with the recommended treatment?

Review the following teaching topics, referrals, and follow-up appointments to make sure that your patient is adequately prepared for discharge.

Teaching topics
Make sure that the following topics have been covered and that your patient's learning has been evaluated:
☐ explanation of emphysema, including its causes, symptoms, and potential complications
☐ smoking as a major risk factor
☐ prevention of upper respiratory tract infection
☐ drug therapy, including inhalers or nebulizers, antibiotics, and corticosteroids
☐ signs and symptoms to report to the doctor
☐ energy conservation techniques and activity guidelines
☐ breathing and controlled coughing techniques
☐ relaxation techniques
☐ safe use of home oxygen.

Referrals
Make sure that the patient has been provided with necessary referrals to:
☐ social services for consultation regarding equipment, medications, and home health care visits
☐ medical equipment supplier for home oxygen
☐ smoking cessation program
☐ dietitian
☐ pulmonary rehabilitation program
☐ other sources of information and support.

Follow-up appointments
Make sure that the necessary follow-up appointments have been scheduled and that the patient has been notified:
☐ doctor.

• Does he understand the importance of avoiding respiratory irritants, such as automobile exhaust fumes, aerosol sprays, secondhand cigarette smoke, and industrial pollutants?
• Does he understand the signs and symptoms that suggest ruptured alveolar blebs and bullae and the necessity of contacting the doctor if he experiences them?
• Is he able to control his anxiety?
• Has he sought help for anxiety and depression?
• Does he know what signs and symptoms of anxiety and depression to report to the doctor?

Physical condition
A physical examination and diagnostic tests will help evaluate the effectiveness of care. Consider the following questions:
• Are the patient's ABG levels within an acceptable range or at baseline?
• Does he maintain body weight within a target range?
• Are nutritional indices, such as the serum albumin level, within acceptable ranges?

Bronchiectasis

Bronchiectasis is marked by chronic abnormal dilation of the bronchi and destruction of the bronchial walls. This destruction may be confined to one lung segment or lobe or occur throughout the tracheobronchial tree. Fre-

FactFinder

Key points about bronchiectasis

• *Incidence:* Bronchiectasis affects males and females of all ages. The incidence has decreased dramatically over the past 20 years because of the availability of immunizations for childhood diseases and antibiotics to treat acute respiratory tract infection.
• *Prognosis:* Bronchiectasis is not curable but, with adequate treatment, can be controlled.
• *Chief diagnostic method:* Bronchography or computed tomography scan
• *Treatment:* Control of infection with antibiotics and postural drainage, chest percussion, and coughing techniques
• *Leading complications:* Pneumonia and atelactasis
• *Other complications:* Advanced bronchiectasis can produce chronic malnutrition, right ventricular failure, primary pulmonary hypertension, acute pulmonary embolism, cor pulmonale, and respiratory failure.

quently bilateral, it usually involves the basilar segments of the lower lobes.

In bronchiectasis, sputum stagnates in the dilated bronchi and leads to secondary infection characterized by inflammation and leukocytic accumulations. Additional debris collects and occludes the bronchi. Increasing pressure from the retained secretions induces mucosal injury. (See *Key points about bronchiectasis.*)

Causes and types

Bronchiectasis results from conditions associated with repeated damage to bronchial walls and abnormal mucociliary clearance, which causes a breakdown of supporting tissue adja-

cent to the airways. (See *Causes of bronchiectasis.*)

Bronchiectasis is classified by the three different configurations of the bronchial dilation: cylindrical, fusiform (or varicose), and saccular. (See *Looking at types of bronchiectasis,* page 154.)

ASSESSMENT

The health history may suggest the presence of bronchiectasis, which then can be confirmed by a computed tomography (CT) scan or bronchography.

Health history

The health history commonly includes frequent bouts of pneumonia or a history of coughing up blood or blood-tinged sputum. Typically, the patient has a chronic cough that produces copious, foul-smelling, mucopurulent secretions (up to several cups daily). He may also report fever, dyspnea, wheezing, weight loss, and malaise.

Physical examination

In mild bronchiectasis, the patient may be asymptomatic. If he has a complicating condition, such as pneumonia or atelectasis, percussion may reveal dullness over lung fields. Auscultation may reveal coarse crackles during inspiration over involved lobes or segments, occasional wheezes, and diminished breath sounds. Inspection of sputum may show a frothy top layer, a middle layer of clear mucosa, and a heavy, thick, purulent bottom layer. Rarely, in advanced disease, the patient may have clubbed fingers and toes and cyanotic nail beds.

Diagnostic test results

The following test results may confirm the diagnosis of bronchiectasis:
• Chest X-rays show peribronchial thickening, atelectatic areas, scattered

cystic changes, and air bronchograms that suggest bronchiectasis.
• CT scans can determine the location and extent of the disease.
• Bronchography will provide a more accurate definition of bronchiectatic lesions and their extent than will a CT scan. This procedure is essential for considering and selecting surgical resection.
• Bronchoscopy may identify the source of secretions or the bleeding site in hemoptysis.
• A sputum culture and a gram stain identify the predominant pathogens.
• A complete blood count and white blood cell differential reveal possible anemia and leukocytosis.
• Pulmonary function tests (PFTs) help evaluate disease severity, therapeutic effectiveness, and the patient's suitability for surgery. If the disease is severe, PFTs may reveal decreased vital capacity and decreased expiratory flow.
• Arterial blood gas (ABG) analysis may show hypoxemia, but most ABG abnormalities will depend on the severity of the disease and complications.

Additional tests that may be ordered include a urinalysis and electrocardiography. If cystic fibrosis is suspected as the underlying cause of bronchiectasis, a sweat test may be ordered.

FactFinder

Causes of bronchiectasis

Some of the known or suspected causes of bronchiectasis include:
• cystic fibrosis
• immune disorders (such as agammaglobulinemia)
• recurrent, inadequately treated respiratory tract infections (from *Mycobacterium tuberculosis*, *Klebsiella* and *Staphylococcus* species, fungi, viruses, and other bacteria)
• complications of measles, pneumonia, pertussis, or influenza
• allergic bronchopulmonary aspergillosis
• bronchial obstruction by a foreign body, a tumor, or stenosis, with recurrent infection
• inhalation of corrosive gas or repeated aspiration of gastric juices
• congenital anomalies (rare), such as bronchomalacia, congenital bronchiectasis, and Kartagener's syndrome (bronchiectasis, sinusitis, and dextrocardia), and rare disorders, such as immotile cilia syndrome
• immunodeficiency states, such as immunoglobulin E and immunoglobulin M deficiencies in the blood or immunosuppression produced by drugs.

NURSING DIAGNOSIS

Suggested nursing diagnoses for a patient with bronchiectasis include:
• Impaired gas exchange related to damage to the bronchial walls
• Ineffective airway clearance related to excessive pulmonary secretions
• Altered nutrition: Less than body requirements related to chronic malnutrition.

PLANNING

Based on the nursing diagnosis *impaired gas exchange,* develop appropriate patient outcomes. For example, your patient will:
• demonstrate breath sounds that reveal a decrease in congestion, crackles, and wheezes
• demonstrate ABG levels within a normal range or at an acceptable baseline.

Based on the nursing diagnosis *ineffective airway clearance,* develop ap-

Looking at types of bronchiectasis

There are three types of bronchiectasis: cylindrical, fusiform (or varicose), and saccular. In cylindrical bronchiectasis, bronchioles are usually symmetrically dilated. In fusiform bronchiectasis, bronchioles are deformed. In saccular bronchiectasis, large bronchi become enlarged and balloon-like.

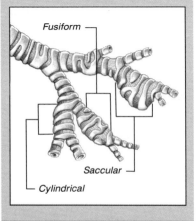

Fusiform

Saccular

Cylindrical

propriate patient outcomes. For example, your patient will:
• perform bronchial hygiene skillfully and regularly
• demonstrate skill in conserving energy when attempting to clear airways
• demonstrate effective coughing technique
• produce decreased amount and consistency of mucus when coughing
• demonstrate breath sounds that reveal less congestion
• take antibiotics, if prescribed.

Based on the nursing diagnosis *altered nutrition: less than body requirements,* develop appropriate patient outcomes. For example, your patient will:

• consume a balanced diet that contains sufficient calories to regain lost weight and to maintain normal weight
• minimize fatigue during the day so that he will have strength to eat at mealtimes.

IMPLEMENTATION

Treatment for bronchiectasis usually includes drug therapy, supportive care to clear secretions, prompt treatment of infections, interventions to make the patient more comfortable and, in some instances, surgery. (See *Medical care of the patient with bronchiectasis.*)

Nursing interventions
• Administer prescribed antibiotics and record the patient's response to the medications.
• Perform postural drainage, chest percussion, and coughing exercises for involved lobes several times a day, especially in the early morning and before bedtime.
• Administer oxygen as ordered.
• Make sure that the patient receives adequate hydration to help thin secretions and promote easier removal.
• Give frequent mouth care to remove foul-smelling sputum. Provide the patient with tissues and a waxed bag in which to discard the contaminated tissues.
• Provide supportive care and help the patient adjust to the lifestyle changes brought on by irreversible lung damage.
• Monitor the patient's respiratory rate and pattern and ABG levels regularly.
• Monitor the patient's breath sounds and sputum production for changes that might indicate a respiratory infection or worsening of his condition.
• Watch for developing complications, such as right ventricular failure, primary pulmonary hypertension, and acute pulmonary embolism.

Treatments

Medical care of the patient with bronchiectasis

Removal of the affected lung portion provides the only cure for bronchiectasis. However, surgery is reserved for severe, localized bronchiectasis.

Drug therapy
Oral or I.V. antibiotics are administered for at least 14 days, or until sputum production decreases.

Supportive treatment
• Postural drainage, chest percussion, and coughing techniques remove secretions if the patient has thick, tenacious sputum.
• Bronchodilators may be administered if the patient has bronchospasm.
• Bronchoscopy may be used to remove secretions.
• Bronchial artery embolization may be used for hemoptysis. Segmental resection or lobectomy may be indicated for severe hemoptysis.
• Oxygen may be administered to treat hypoxemia.

• Provide a warm, quiet, comfortable environment.
• Help the patient to alternate rest and activity periods.
• Provide well-balanced, high-calorie meals. Small, frequent meals can help prevent fatigue.
• If surgery is to be performed to remove an affected lung portion, prepare the patient accordingly.

Postoperative care
• Encourage deep breathing and position changes to ensure maximal oxygenation.
• Provide chest-tube care.
• Monitor the patient's vital signs, respiratory status, and incision for signs of postoperative complications such as wound infection or atelectasis.

Patient teaching
Include the following in your patient-teaching program:
• Show the patient and his family how to perform postural drainage and percussion. Teach the patient coughing and deep-breathing techniques to promote good ventilation and assist in secretion removal. Teach pursed-lip breathing and cough control to decrease dyspnea. Instruct him to maintain each postural drainage position for 10 minutes. Then direct the caregiver in performing percussion and instructing the patient to cough.
• If appropriate, advise the patient to stop smoking because it stimulates secretions and irritates the airways. Refer the patient to a smoking cessation group.
• Instruct the patient to avoid air pollutants and people with known upper respiratory tract infections.
• Teach the patient to identify signs of infection, such as fever, increased cough and sputum production, and fatigue, and to seek prompt medical attention.
• Instruct the patient to take medications (especially antibiotics) exactly as prescribed. Make sure that he knows the adverse effects associated with his medications and instruct him to notify the doctor if any occur.
• Teach the patient to dispose of all secretions properly to avoid spreading the infection to others. Advise him to wash his hands thoroughly after discarding contaminated tissues.

Ensuring continued care for the patient with bronchiectasis

Review the following teaching topics, referrals, and follow-up appointments to make sure that your patient is adequately prepared for discharge.

Teaching topics
Make sure that the following topics have been covered and that your patient's learning has been evaluated:
☐ explanation of bronchiectasis, including its causes, symptoms, and potential complications, especially hemoptysis
☐ postural drainage and chest percussion
☐ breathing and coughing techniques
☐ warning signs and symptoms, including change in sputum color, consistency, and odor
☐ prevention and recognition of upper respiratory tract infection
☐ smoking as a major risk factor
☐ prescribed medications, including their possible adverse effects
☐ energy conservation techniques and activity guidelines
☐ explanation of surgery, including preoperative, postoperative, and home care.

Referrals
Make sure that your patient has been provided with necessary referrals to:
☐ social services for consultation regarding equipment, medications, and home health care visits
☐ medical equipment supplier (for home oxygen use)
☐ smoking cessation program
☐ occupational therapist for energy conservation techniques
☐ dietitian
☐ other sources of information and support.

Follow-up appointments
Make sure that the necessary follow-up appointments have been scheduled and that the patient has been notified:
☐ doctor
☐ surgeon, if needed
☐ diagnostic tests for reevaluation.

• Advise the patient to pace his activities.
• Encourage the patient to follow a balanced, high-protein diet with small, frequent meals. Explain that whole milk products may increase the viscosity of secretions, so nonfat or low-fat dairy products are preferable.
• Encourage the patient to drink plenty of fluids to thin secretions and to aid expectoration.
• If the patient needs surgery, provide complete preoperative and postoperative instructions. Forewarn the patient if he is to have an I.V. line and chest tubes inserted. Explain the reason for these procedures. (See *Ensuring contin-* *ued care for the patient with bronchiectasis.*)

EVALUATION

When evaluating a patient's response to your nursing care, gather assessment data and compare this information with the patient outcomes specified in your plan of care.

Teaching and counseling

Begin by evaluating the effectiveness of your teaching and counseling. Consider the following questions:
• Can the patient perform coughing and deep-breathing techniques?

• Does he perform bronchial hygiene techniques skillfully and regularly?

• Can he demonstrate how to conserve energy when attempting to clear his airways?

• Does he follow a balanced diet and consume enough calories to regain lost weight and maintain a normal weight?

• Does he take measures to minimize fatigue during the day so that he will have strength to eat at mealtimes?

• Does he understand the importance of avoiding crowds and people with upper respiratory tract infections?

• Does he understand the purposes of his medications and the importance of contacting the doctor if he experiences any adverse reactions?

Physical condition
A physical examination and diagnostic tests will help evaluate the effectiveness of care. Consider the following questions:

• Are the patient's breath sounds less congested with reduced rhonchi, crackles, and wheezes?

• Does his cough produce thin mucus?

• Are his ABG values within a normal range or at baseline?

Cystic fibrosis

A chronic, progressive disease, cystic fibrosis affects the exocrine (mucus-secreting) glands, resulting in extremely thick, tenacious secretions that obstruct ducts in the lungs, pancreas, and other parts of the body.

Progressive pulmonary infection represents the most important clinical problem in patients with cystic fibrosis. Accumulation of secretions in the bronchioles and alveoli may cause severe atelectasis, and recurrent infections and inflammation leading to bronchiectasis.

When thickened secretions obstruct the pancreatic ducts, they cause a deficiency of the enzymes trypsin, amylase, and lipase, which interferes with the digestion of food and the absorption of fat-soluble vitamins (A, D, E, and K). In the pancreas, fibrotic tissue, multiple cysts, thick mucus, and fat replace the acini (small, saclike swellings normally found in this gland), resulting in pancreatic insufficiency. (See *Complications of cystic fibrosis,* page 158.)

Causes
Cystic fibrosis results from a genetic mutation that appears to interfere with chloride channel transport across the cell membrane. This mutation is passed from parents to children as an autosomal recessive trait. The onset and progression of the disease may vary. (See *Key points about cystic fibrosis, page* 159.)

ASSESSMENT

Clinical findings in cystic fibrosis primarily involve the respiratory and GI systems. During your assessment, you should also investigate for a family history of cystic fibrosis.

Health history
If the patient is a child, parents or family members may report that he has failed to gain sufficient weight or to grow adequately, despite a healthy or often excessive appetite. They may describe the child's stools as frequent, bulky, foul-smelling, and pale, and oil droplets may be seen in the toilet or his diaper. Kissing the child may reveal that his sweat tastes unusually salty.

Common respiratory complaints include a productive cough (which may awaken the patient at night or occur upon awakening in the morning and when engaging in physical activity) and frequent upper respiratory tract infections. As the disease progresses, the

FactFinder

Complications of cystic fibrosis

Cystic fibrosis produces widespread complications that affect the lungs, pancreas, biliary tract, reproductive system, and sweat glands.

Pulmonary complications
- Nasal polyps and sinusitis
- Hemoptysis
- Atelectasis
- Bronchiectasis
- Emphysema
- Pneumothorax
- Cor pulmonale

Pancreatic complications
- Malabsorption
- Nutritional deficiencies
- Insufficient insulin production, abnormal glucose tolerance, glycosuria (secondary to pancreatic insufficiency)
- Diabetes mellitus
- Pancreatitis
- Clotting problems

Biliary complications
- Prolonged neonatal jaundice (secondary to biliary obstruction and fibrosis)

- Portal hypertension
- Cirrhosis
- Esophageal varices, episodes of hematemesis, hepatomegaly (brought on by portal hypertension and cirrhosis)
- Cholecystitis

Other GI complications
- Distal intestinal obstruction
- Gastroesophageal reflux
- Rectal prolapse

Reproductive complications
- Azoospermia
- Secondary amenorrhea
- Increased viscosity of cervical mucus, leading to decreased fertility

Complications of sweat gland dysfunction
- Hypochloremia
- Hyponatremia
- Cardiac arrhythmias, shock (from hypochloremia and hyponatremia; may occur during hot weather when the patient sweats profusely)

patient or his family may report dyspnea and activity intolerance.

Physical examination
Inspection of a child with cystic fibrosis may reveal a barrel chest and clubbing of the fingers and toes.

Timesaving tip: Pay special attention to finger clubbing in a patient with cystic fibrosis. It may be the first sign of respiratory compromise. Cyanotic mucous membranes may be another early indicator of respiratory compromise.

The patient may cough up tenacious, yellow or green sputum. Palpation may show a distended abdomen. On auscultation, you may hear crackles or rhonchi.

Approximately 10% of neonates with cystic fibrosis may have meconium ileus — obstruction of the intestine secondary to failure to excrete meconium, the dark green mucilaginous material found in the intestine at birth. In such a neonate, you may observe signs of intestinal obstruction, such as abdominal distention, vomiting, constipation, and dehydration. A child with cystic fibrosis may be smaller than normal for his age. If an adult, he may show signs of stunted growth because of malnutrition.

Diagnostic test results

The Cystic Fibrosis Foundation's standard for definitive diagnosis consists of:

• two clearly positive sweat tests using a pilocarpine solution (a sweat inducer) and one of the following: an obstructive pulmonary disease, confirmed pancreatic insufficiency or failure to thrive, and a positive family history of cystic fibrosis (See *Understanding the sweat test*, page 160.)

• chest X-rays indicating early signs of obstructive lung disease

• stool specimen analysis indicating the absence of trypsin, suggesting pancreatic insufficiency.

The following test results may support the diagnosis:

• Deoxyribonucleic acid (DNA) testing can locate the presence of the Delta 508 deletion. About 70% of cystic fibrosis patients have this deletion, although the disease can also cause more than 100 other mutations.

• If pulmonary exacerbation exists, pulmonary function tests (PFTs) reveal decreased vital capacity, elevated residual volume due to air entrapments, and decreased forced expiratory volume in 1 second.

• A liver enzyme test may reveal hepatic insufficiency.

• A sputum culture reveals organisms that cystic fibrosis patients typically and chronically colonize, such as *Staphylococcus* and *Pseudomonas*.

• A serum albumin level helps assess nutritional status.

• Electrolyte analysis assesses dehydration and glucose levels.

FactFinder

Key points about cystic fibrosis

• *Incidence:* Cystic fibrosis occurs most commonly in people of northern European ancestry, affecting about 1 in 2,000 live births. About 5% of the Caucasian population carries the recessive gene for transmitting the disorder. The disorder occurs less commonly in Blacks, Native Americans, and Asians. Boys and girls are equally affected.

• *Genetic transmission:* The disorder is transmitted as an autosomal recessive trait. When both parents carry this gene, each of their offspring has a 25% chance of inheriting the disorder, a 50% chance of being a genetic carrier, and a 25% chance of being both free of the disorder and a noncarrier.

• *Prognosis:* Cystic fibrosis is incurable. But as medical research progresses, it has allowed patients to live longer lives. Although the disorder's progression varies widely, the average life expectancy of affected patients in North America is slightly less than 30 years.

ficiency and resulting malabsorption of nutrients that increases the metabolic requirements of patient

• Ineffective airway clearance related to the viscosity of respiratory secretions

• Ineffective individual coping related to chronic health impairment and its complex treatment regimen.

NURSING DIAGNOSIS

Common nursing diagnoses for a patient with cystic fibrosis include:

• Altered nutrition: Less than body requirements related to pancreatic insuf-

PLANNING

Focus your nursing care on helping the patient manage his condition independently.

Understanding the sweat test

The sweat test plays a key role in diagnosing cystic fibrosis.

Implementation
Two electrodes covered with pads are attached to the patient's forearm (or the right leg of an infant). One pad is saturated with saline solution and the other with pilocarpine solution (a sweat inducer). A mild electric current is administered to produce sweat, and the electrodes are removed. A dry gauze pad or filter paper is then applied to the damp area for 30 to 40 minutes, removed, and analyzed for electrolyte concentration.

Implications
Normal sodium values in sweat range from 10 to 30 mEq/liter. Normal chloride values range from 10 to 35 mEq/liter. Although sodium and chloride concentrations normally rise with age, concentrations of 50 to 60 mEq/liter strongly suggest cystic fibrosis and call for repeated testing. Concentrations greater than 60 mEq/liter, with typical clinical features, confirm the diagnosis of cystic fibrosis.

Based on the nursing diagnosis *altered nutrition: less than body requirements,* develop appropriate patient outcomes. For example, your patient (or his caregiver) will:

• express an understanding of the need for a well-balanced, high-calorie, high-protein diet
• demonstrate skill in selecting appropriate foods
• identify ways to increase salt intake and use pancreatic enzyme replacements correctly

• describe daily stools and make appropriate changes in enzyme supplements, if necessary
• maintain an acceptable weight
• grow at an acceptable rate
• notify a member of the health care team if his weight decreases.

Based on the nursing diagnosis *ineffective airway clearance,* develop appropriate patient outcomes. For example, your patient (or his caregiver) will:

• express an understanding of the need for prescribed medications, adequate hydration, and bronchial hygienic measures
• demonstrate skill in performing postural drainage, chest percussion, vibration, deep breathing, coughing exercises, and in using nebulizers
• maintain or achieve baseline PFT results after treatment for pulmonary exacerbation
• demonstrate reduced crackles and rhonchi during auscultation
• describe daily amount, color, and consistency of secretions.

Based on the nursing diagnosis *ineffective individual coping,* develop appropriate patient outcomes. For example, your patient (or his caregiver) will:

• seek support from available resources, including his family, his friends, a support group, and the health care team
• consult with social worker as needed
• establish short- and long-term career and personal goals.

IMPLEMENTATION

Treatment for cystic fibrosis includes drug therapy and measures to help the patient lead as normal a life as possible. (See *Medical care of the patient with cystic fibrosis.*)

Treatments

Medical care of the patient with cystic fibrosis

Treatment for cystic fibrosis seeks to improve the patient's quality of life and includes drug therapy, exercise, dietary guidelines, and supportive measures.

Drug therapy

Antibiotics may be prescribed to prevent or treat acute respiratory infection. Aerosol bronchodilators (methylxanthines and sympathomimetics) reverse or control wheezing and airway spasm. Inhalable and intranasal corticosteroids reduce the frequency and severity of airway spasm and dyspnea, as do mast-cell stabilizers, such as cromolyn.

Oral pancreatic enzymes may be taken before each meal and snack to treat pancreatic enzyme deficiency. Enzyme replacements improve absorption and digestion. Histamine-2 blockers may be added to enhance absorption of enzymes.

Exercise

The doctor will probably prescribe exercise to improve breathing, posture, and chest mobility and enhance overall fitness. Exercise improves the function and efficiency of respiratory muscles, enhances cardiopulmonary function and activity tolerance, and can dislodge mucus from the lungs.

Diet

Because a patient with cystic fibrosis does not absorb food completely, a high-calorie diet, rich in fat, protein, and carbohydrates, is crucial because chronic lung infection increases the need for calories. The patient should eat salty foods to replace high levels of sodium lost in sweat, and should drink enough fluids to maintain good hydration. Although pancreatic supplements are usually needed for digestion, fats are an important way to increase calories in the diet.

Supportive treatment

Aerosolized medication can be delivered by an air compressor, metered-dose inhaler, or both. Aerosol therapy may be followed by postural drainage, percussion, vibration, and coughing. Together these treatments open the airways and thin the mucus so that it can be expelled from the lungs. If hypoxemia occurs, home oxygen therapy may also be ordered.

Experimental drugs

Researchers are developing new drugs to treat the lungs, the site mainly affected by cystic fibrosis. Experimental drugs such as DNase, Pulmozyne, and amiloride thin the thick mucus in the airways so that it can be expectorated. These drugs may halt the progression of lung disease, but cannot be considered cures for cystic fibrosis since they are unable to repair already damaged lung tissue, and are not targeted for other affected systems yet.

Since the discovery of the basic genetic defect in cystic fibrosis, researchers have been exploring the safety and feasibility of gene therapy for treatment of lung disease. Researchers hope to develop a nasal or oral aerosol, containing corrected genetic material delivered via retroviruses, which can be sprayed into the lung.

Nursing interventions

• Continue to monitor the patient's respiratory and nutritional status, and evaluate individual and family coping mechanisms. Seek consultations as needed.

• Give medications as prescribed.

• Perform prescribed postural drainage and chest percussion several times a day.

• Administer prescribed oxygen therapy if hypoxemia occurs. Check arterial oxygen saturation levels using pulse oximetry while the patient is awake and asleep.

• Provide a well-balanced, high-calorie, high-protein diet. Include plenty of fats, which are often used to increase caloric intake without increasing the quantity of food. Give prescribed pancreatic enzymes to help combat the effects of fat malabsorption. Vitamins A, D, and E are often prescribed to prevent deficiencies, and vitamin K supplements may be prescribed if the patient has cholestatic liver disease.

Timesaving tip: Advise the patient or his family to consult a nutritionist for strategies to maintain or increase his weight.

• Provide exercise and activity periods for the patient to promote health. Encourage him to perform breathing exercises to help improve his ventilation.

• Make sure that the patient receives plenty of liquids and salt to prevent dehydration and hyponatremia, especially in warm weather and during intense activity. *Note:* Athletes with cystic fibrosis especially need to keep up with salt and fluid requirements.

• Provide pediatric patients with play periods, and hospitalized patients with recreational activities, both diversional and therapeutic. Some pediatric hospitals have child life therapists, who provide essential playtime for young patients.

• Provide emotional support to the parents of children with cystic fibrosis.

Because the disease is inherited, the parents may feel enormous guilt. Encourage them to discuss their fears and concerns, and answer their questions as honestly as possible. Refer the patient and his family for professional counseling, if needed.

• Be flexible with care and visiting hours during hospitalization to allow pediatric patients to continue sibling relationships, perform school work, and preserve friendships.

• Include the family in all phases of the patient's care. If the patient is an adolescent, he may want to perform much of his own treatment protocol. Encourage him to do so.

Patient teaching

• Explain to the patient and his family the role of genes in cystic fibrosis. Make sure that they know about tests that can determine if family members carry the cystic fibrosis gene. They may wish to consult a genetic counselor regarding the latest testing information available for mutation identification, carrier testing, and prenatal diagnosis. (See *Genetic transmission in cystic fibrosis.*)

• Assess the need for more information about the complications of the disease and thoroughly explain all treatment measures, if necessary.

• Emphasize the importance of lifelong follow-up care, preferably at a cystic fibrosis center accredited by the Cystic Fibrosis Foundation.

• Teach the patient and his family about all medications. Assess their knowledge regarding routine medications and the rationale for any changes in medications. Describe their possible adverse effects, and urge them to notify the doctor if these effects occur.

• Instruct the patient and his family about aerosol therapy, including intermittent nebulizer treatments before postural drainage and chest percussion.

Teaching TimeSaver

Genetic transmission in cystic fibrosis

Cystic fibrosis is passed on as a recessive trait. If both parents carry the recessive gene for cystic fibrosis, each child has a 25% chance of having the disease. In the diagram below, the large *C* refers to the dominant gene, and the small *c* stands for the recessive gene.

• The child with *CC* has inherited the dominant gene from each parent. She won't have cystic fibrosis and is not at risk for transmitting the disorder to her offspring.

• The child with *Cc* and the one with *cC* have each inherited one dominant and one recessive gene. These children won't have the disease, but they can pass the gene on to their offspring.

• The child with *cc* has inherited the recessive gene from both parents and has cystic fibrosis.

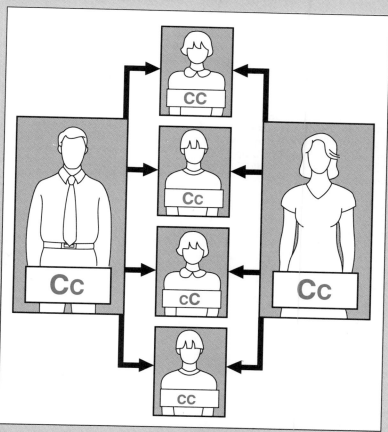

Tell them that these treatments help to loosen secretions and dilate bronchi.

• Stress the importance of pancreatic enzyme replacement therapy to treat malabsorption. Explain that the enzymes should be taken before snacks and meals.

• Discuss the need to observe characteristics of daily stools. The stool pattern indicates the level of malabsorption. If the stool is consistently bulky, foul-smelling, and pale, the patient should consult with the doctor or nutritionist to assess what changes need to be made in enzyme supplements.

• Emphasize the importance of a well-balanced, high-calorie, high-protein diet. Also encourage the patient to eat salty foods to compensate for sodium lost in sweat and to drink plenty of fluids to prevent dehydration.

• Encourage the patient to participate in an exercise program or pulmonary rehabilitation program. Review the importance of building up respiratory muscles and cardiopulmonary function and of improving activity tolerance.

• Stress the importance of keeping all scheduled appointments even when the patient is feeling well.

• Instruct the patient and his family to report to the doctor any signs of exacerbations of chronic pulmonary infection or changes in his condition. They should be aware of chronic, subtle changes such as an increased cough, a decreased appetite, fatigue, weight loss, and shortness of breath, as well as acute symptoms of chest pain, and sputum that increases in amount, thickens, or contains blood.

• Help the patient and his family to cope with the realization that cystic fibrosis can shorten his life. Encourage family members to use the resources available at their cystic fibrosis center, and inform them of any new breakthroughs in research that will give the patient cause for optimism.

• Advise the parents of a child with the disease not to be overly protective. Help them explore ways to enhance the child's quality of life and to foster responsibility and independence in their child from an early age. Stress the importance of good communication so that the child may express his fears and concerns.

Timesaving tip: Counsel parents of a patient with cystic fibrosis to encourage sibling participation in his care. This will help family members cope with the diagnosis, deal with emotions regarding the patient, and expedite his care.

• Counsel the female patient to consult her pulmonologist and to seek genetic counseling before becoming pregnant.

• Counsel the male patient regarding semen analysis. Approximately 98% to 99% of male patients are sterile and should be seen by a urologist to confirm this.

• If the patient is at the end stage of the disease, the option of a lung transplant should be mentioned. If a transplant is not a feasible option, help him and his family to achieve life closure. (See *Ensuring continued care for the patient with cystic fibrosis.*)

EVALUATION

When evaluating the patient's response to your nursing care, gather reassessment data and compare this information with the patient outcomes specified in your plan of care.

Teaching and counseling

Begin by determining the effectiveness of your teaching and counseling. Consider the following questions:

• Are the patient and his family adhering to the recommended regimen? Are there any barriers to the accomplishment of the patient's care in the home?

• How well are the patient and his family coping with the complications

Discharge TimeSaver

Ensuring continued care for the patient with cystic fibrosis

Review the following teaching topics, referrals, and follow-up appointments to make sure that your patient is adequately prepared for discharge.

Teaching topics
Make sure that the following topics have been covered and that your patient's learning has been evaluated:
☐ explanation of cystic fibrosis, including associated signs and symptoms, genetic factors, and recent research
☐ prevention and recognition of complications
☐ medications, including dosages, possible adverse effects, appropriate use of a prescription for higher antibiotic dosage (for patients on long-term antibiotic therapy)
☐ activity guidelines
☐ breathing and coughing techniques
☐ postural drainage and chest percussion
☐ aerosol therapy
☐ warning signs and symptoms
☐ need for follow-up care, preferably at a cystic fibrosis center
☐ sexual and reproductive concerns.

Referrals
Make sure that your patient has been provided with necessary referrals to:
☐ social services for consultation regarding equipment, medications, and home health care visits
☐ respiratory or physical therapist for respiratory treatments and home care
☐ dietitian
☐ genetic counseling
☐ support group
☐ sources of information and support.

Follow-up appointments
Make sure that the necessary follow-up appointments have been scheduled and that the patient has been notified:
☐ pulmonologist
☐ respiratory or physical therapist
☐ nearest cystic fibrosis center
☐ child life therapist or pediatrician.

of daily care? (See *Assessing failure to achieve outcomes in cystic fibrosis therapy,* page 166.)
• Do the patient and family members demonstrate knowledge of breathing exercises, postural drainage, and chest percussion?
• Do they understand the adverse effects of prescribed medications and the importance of contacting the doctor if any occur?
• Do they understand the need for adequate hydration?
• Do they demonstrate skill in administration of medications?
• Do they understand the importance of keeping medical appointments, even when the patient feels well?

• Have they arranged for consultation with a social worker, if necessary?
• Does the patient express an understanding of his dietary needs and demonstrate skill in choosing appropriate foods?
• Has he increased his salt intake and is he using enzyme replacements correctly?
• Does he report the amount, color, and consistency of respiratory secretions?
• Does he report characteristics of stools daily?
• Does he seek help from available support people, such as family, friends, support group members, and members of the health care team?

Evaluation TimeSaver

Assessing failure to achieve outcomes in cystic fibrosis therapy

If your patient fails to respond to nursing interventions, this checklist can help you evaluate the reasons why. Consult with the patient, his family, and members of the health care team to determine the presence or absence of these factors.

Patient factors
☐ Desire to conform with peers (may make patient reluctant to adhere to recommended treatment regimen)
☐ Discouragement at having to be readmitted to hospital despite adherence to treatment regimen
☐ Emotional distress brought on by restrictions of long-term illness
☐ Boredom with repetitious health care regimen

Family factors
☐ Strain on family relationships caused by presence of child with special needs

☐ Lack of adequate support systems
☐ Parental guilt over having transmitted genetic disease to child
☐ Anxiety over progressive nature of disease
☐ Parental tendency to become overly protective of child

Additional factors
☐ Lack of insurance
☐ High cost of medications, home health care, or frequent, extended hospitalizations
☐ Lack of access to health care facilities with resources for treating cystic fibrosis
☐ Complexity of health care regimen
☐ Decreased appetite and lack of desire to eat caused by complex medication regimen required with each meal

• Does he articulate career and educational goals?
• Do parents appear to foster independence?
• Do they encourage the patient to express fears and concerns?
• Are the patient and family members aware of recent research on the causes and treatment of cystic fibrosis?

Physical condition
A physical examination and diagnostic tests will help determine the effectiveness of care. Consider the following questions:
• Does the patient maintain an acceptable weight for his age?
• Is he growing at an acceptable rate?
• Does he maintain baseline PFT levels?

• Does auscultation reveal reduced crackles and rhonchi?
• Are dehydration and hyponatremia absent?
• Does the patient report any signs or symptoms of infection, such as increased cough, decreased appetite, fatigue, weight loss, or shortness of breath?

Caring for patients with pleural disorders

Pleurisy

Also called pleuritis, pleurisy is an inflammation of the visceral and parietal pleurae that line the inside of the thoracic cage and envelop the lungs. This disorder occurs when the pleurae swell and become congested, hampering movement of pleural fluid, thereby increasing friction between the adjacent surfaces of the pleurae. (See *Understanding pleurisy*.)

If pleural membranes are extensively inflamed, permanent adhesions may form and may restrict lung expansion. This inflammation can also stimulate the production of too much pleural fluid while hindering its reabsorption, leading to pleural effusion. In response to chest pain, the pleuritic patient may take only shallow breaths, which could lead to atelectasis. (See *Key points about pleurisy*, page 170.)

Causes
Pleurisy may result from:
- pneumonia
- tuberculosis
- viruses
- systemic lupus erythematosus
- rheumatoid arthritis
- uremia
- Dressler's syndrome
- tumor
- pulmonary infarction
- chest trauma.

ASSESSMENT

Signs and symptoms of pleurisy vary depending on the underlying cause. The patient's health history may suggest the cause.

Health history
The patient may report a sudden, sharp, stabbing pain that worsens on inspiration. This pain results from inflammation or irritation of the sensory nerve endings in the parietal pleurae that rub against one another during respiration. The pain may be so severe that it limits the patient's chest movement on the affected side during breathing. Other symptoms, such as dyspnea, may vary depending on the underlying disorder.

Physical examination
Inspection may reveal shallow tentative breathing or tachypnea. Chest wall motion may be reduced on the affected side.

Auscultation may reveal a characteristic pleural friction rub — a coarse, grating sound heard during late inspiration and early expiration directly over the area of pleural inflammation. Auscultation may also reveal crackles secondary to atelectasis.

Palpation over the affected area of your patient's thorax may reveal coarse vibration and intercostal tenderness.

The patient may also show signs of chills and a fever.

Diagnostic test results
Although diagnosis primarily rests on the patient's health history and physical examination, diagnostic tests help rule out other causes and pinpoint the underlying disorder.
- Electrocardiography rules out coronary artery disease as the source of your patient's pain.
- Chest X-rays can identify pneumonia.

NURSING DIAGNOSIS

Common nursing diagnoses for a patient with pleurisy include:
- Ineffective breathing pattern related to pain on inspiration
- Pain related to inflammation caused by pleurisy.

Understanding pleurisy

Normally, the visceral and parietal pleurae slide easily over each other to reduce friction during breathing. However, in pleurisy, the pleurae become edematous and congested, an exudate collects on pleural surfaces, and cell infiltration occurs. The buildup of fibrinous exudate causes the pleural surfaces to rub together roughly. This causes an audible pleural friction rub. Stretching of the inflamed pleurae causes the pain that's characteristic of pleurisy.

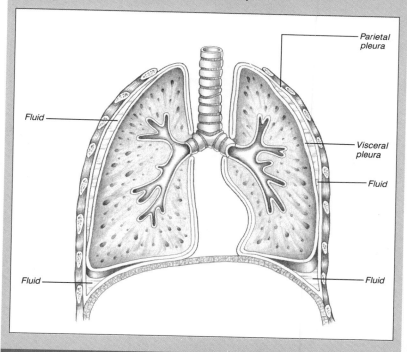

Parietal pleura

Fluid

Visceral pleura

Fluid

Fluid

Fluid

PLANNING

Based on the nursing diagnosis *ineffective breathing pattern,* develop appropriate patient outcomes. For example, your patient will:
• maintain a respiratory rate at rest of 20 breaths/minute or less
• maintain adequate oxygenation as evidenced by an arterial oxygen saturation (SaO_2) level above 95%
• demonstrate full, bilaterally equal breath sounds
• exhibit symmetrical chest wall motion
• exhibit few or no atelectatic crackles during auscultation of breath sounds.

Based on the nursing diagnosis *pain,* develop appropriate patient outcomes. For example, your patient will:
• describe the characteristics of his pain
• list factors that intensify his pain
• identify activities that promote comfort and relaxation
• express feelings of pain relief.

IMPLEMENTATION

Treatment of pleurisy usually focuses on relieving pain and maintaining adequate respiration. (See *Medical care of the patient with pleurisy.*)

Nursing interventions

• Assess your patient for pain every 3 hours. Administer nonsteroidal anti-inflammatory drugs and narcotic analgesics, as prescribed, to relieve pain and thus help your patient breathe deeply. If he has a nonproductive cough, administer prescribed antitussives.
• Encourage him to take deep breaths and to change position frequently in an effort to prevent atelectasis.
• To minimize pain during coughing, apply firm pressure at the site of the pain.
• Have the patient use an incentive spirometer every 1 to 2 hours to improve or maintain oxygenation.
• Place your patient in high Fowler's position to help lung expansion. Having him lie on the affected side may aid in splinting.
• Assess his respiratory status at least every 4 hours to detect early signs of compromise. Report increased dyspnea or reduced breath sounds and monitor for fever.
• Plan your care to allow as much uninterrupted rest as possible.
• If your patient has an associated pleural effusion and requires thoracentesis, remind him to breathe normally and avoid sudden movements, such as coughing or sighing, during the procedure. Monitor his vital signs and watch for syncope. Also look for signs of overly rapid fluid removal, including bradycardia, hypotension, pain, or cardiac arrest. Reassure him throughout the procedure. After thoracentesis, watch for respiratory distress and signs of pneumothorax, including sudden onset of dyspnea and cyanosis.
• Throughout therapy, listen to your patient's fears and concerns, and answer his questions. Remain with him during periods of extreme stress and anxiety. Perform care measures to aid relaxation and encourage him to initiate measures to improve relaxation.

• Whenever possible, include your patient in care decisions, and include the family members in all phases of care.

Patient teaching

• If thoracentesis is required, explain the procedure to your patient. Tell him to expect a stinging sensation from the local anesthetic and a feeling of pressure as the needle is inserted. Instruct him to tell you immediately if he feels uncomfortable or has trouble breathing during the procedure.

• Explain any other procedures to the patient and his family members.

• Encourage the patient to identify actions that will help him relax. Teach him techniques that relieve anxiety and promote relaxation, such as guided imagery, meditation, and yoga.

• If the patient receives a prescription for a narcotic analgesic at discharge, warn him about the dangers of overuse. Explain that the drug suppresses coughing and depresses respirations. Warn him to avoid activities that require alertness while taking a narcotic analgesic. Also, teach him about other possible adverse effects and when to notify the doctor.

• Teach him how to splint the affected area and how to perform deep-breathing exercises.

• Emphasize the need for regular rest periods.

• Teach your patient the signs and symptoms of possible complications, such as worsened dyspnea, fever, increasing fatigue, or any change in the quality or quantity of secretions. Tell him to call the doctor if such signs or symptoms occur.

• Reassure the patient that the pain should subside after several days. (See *Ensuring continued care for the patient with pleurisy,* page 172.)

Treatments

Medical care of the patient with pleurisy

Treatment of pleurisy is usually symptomatic and generally includes anti-inflammatory agents, analgesics, and bed rest. However, other treatments may be required depending on the patient's condition:

• If the patient experiences severe pain, particularly during coughing and deep breathing, an intercostal nerve block may be required.

• If decreased inspiratory effort leads to atelectasis and subsequent hypoxemia, supplementary oxygen may be needed.

• If pleurisy is accompanied by pleural effusion, thoracentesis may be used as both a diagnostic and a therapeutic measure.

EVALUATION

When evaluating the patient's response to nursing care, gather reassessment data and compare this information with the patient outcomes specified in your plan of care.

Teaching and counseling

Begin by determining the effectiveness of your teaching. Consider the following questions:

• Has the patient identified activities that intensify his pain?

• Has he identified activities that promote comfort and relaxation?

• After treatment, does the patient express a feeling of relief from pain?

Physical condition

Consider the following questions:

• Are the patient's breathing patterns within established limits?

• Does his respiratory rate at rest remain at 20 breaths/minute or less?

• Has he achieved adequate oxygenation as evidenced by an SaO₂ level above 95%?
• Is his chest wall motion symmetrical?
• Does he demonstrate full, bilaterally equal breath sounds?
• Does he exhibit few or no atelectatic crackles?

Pleural effusion

Normally, the pleural space contains a small amount of protein-free fluid in dynamic equilibrium. Pleural effusion occurs when inflammation caused by disease increases the permeability of pleural membranes, allowing extracellular fluid to build up in the pleural space. The fluid may contain protein, blood cells (hemothorax), pus and bacteria (empyema), or triglycerides (chylothorax). Complications associated with large pleural effusions include atelectasis, infection, and hypoxia. (See *Looking at pleural effusion*.)

Causes and types
Transudative pleural effusion occurs when excessive hydrostatic pressure or decreased osmotic pressure causes excess fluid with a low protein concentration to pass across intact capillaries into the pleural space. This type of effusion may result from congestive heart failure, hepatic disease with ascites, peritoneal dialysis, hypoalbuminemia, and disorders that increase intravascular volume.

Exudative pleural effusion occurs when capillary permeability increases, allowing protein-rich fluid to leak into the pleural space. This type of effusion may result from tuberculosis, subphrenic abscess, pancreatitis, bacterial or fungal pneumonitis or empyema, influ-

Looking at pleural effusion

The illustration shows the buildup of fluid in the pleural space, the cavity between the visceral and parietal pleurae. This buildup occurs in pleural effusion.

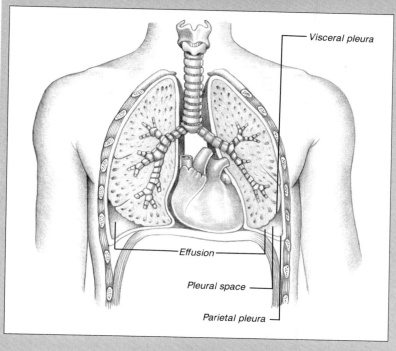

Visceral pleura

Effusion

Pleural space

Parietal pleura

enza, cancer, parapneumonia, pulmonary embolism (with or without infarction), collagen disease (lupus erythematosus and rheumatoid arthritis), myxedema, intra-abdominal abscess, esophageal perforation, and chest trauma.

Empyema, an exudative pleural effusion, usually stems from an infection in the pleural space. The infection may be idiopathic or may be related to pneumonitis, cancer, perforation, penetrat-

ing chest trauma, or esophageal rupture.

ASSESSMENT

Because pleural effusion is associated with many other conditions, your assessment should include a thorough health history. Note the presence of any underlying pulmonary disease.

Health history

The patient with a large pleural effusion may report dyspnea. This may be the only complaint, or he may have a dry, nonproductive cough. If he has pleurisy, he may report pleuritic chest pain. If he has empyema, he may also complain of malaise. Depending on the size of pleural effusion, the patient may report tachycardia, tachypnea, or dyspnea on exertion. Alternatively, the patient may be asymptomatic.

Physical examination

Inspection may reveal tracheal deviation from the affected side. This indicates that the effusion is large enough to shift the mediastinum to the unaffected side.

With a large pleural effusion, palpation may reveal decreased tactile fremitus. Percussion may disclose dullness over the effused area that doesn't change with respiration.

Auscultation may reveal diminished or absent breath sounds over the effusion. Sometimes, you'll hear a pleural friction rub during both inspiration and expiration. (This pleural friction rub is transitory, however, and disappears as fluid accumulates in the pleural space.) You'll also hear bronchial breath sounds, sometimes with your patient's pronunciation of the letter "e" sounding like the letter "a." Bilateral crackles and gallop heart rhythms suggest heart failure, which frequently accompanies pleural effusion.

The patient with empyema will likely have a fever.

Diagnostic test results

A chest X-ray may reveal pleural effusion, but usually only after 200 to 300 ml of fluid have accumulated in the pleural cavity. A computed tomography scan of the chest may be necessary to confirm the diagnosis.

Analysis of fluid aspirated during thoracentesis may show:

- a specific gravity below 1.015 and less than 3 g/dl of protein (in transudative pleural effusion)
- a ratio of protein in the pleural fluid to protein in the serum of at least 0.5, a pleural fluid lactate dehydrogenase (LD) level of at least 200 IU, and a ratio of LD in pleural fluid to LD in serum of at least 0.6 (in exudative pleural effusion)
- leukocytosis and the presence of acute inflammatory white blood cells (WBCs) and microorganisms (in empyema)
- an extremely decreased pleural fluid glucose level (in empyema and rheumatoid arthritis, which may lead to exudative pleural effusion)
- pleural fluid amylase levels that are higher than serum levels (if pleural effusion results from esophageal rupture or pancreatitis).

Aspirated fluid may also be tested for lupus erythematosus cells, antinuclear antibodies, and neoplastic cells. Plus, it may be analyzed for color and consistency; for acid-fast bacillus, fungal, and bacterial cultures; and if chylothorax is suspected.

Additional diagnostic tests

A negative tuberculin skin test helps rule out tuberculosis as a cause. If thoracentesis doesn't provide a definitive diagnosis in exudative pleural effusion, a pleural biopsy may help confirm tuberculosis or cancer. Arterial blood gas (ABG) analysis may reveal decreased partial pressure of arterial oxygen (PaO_2).

NURSING DIAGNOSIS

Common nursing diagnoses for a patient with pleural effusion include:

- High risk for infection related to introduction of thoracentesis needle or chest tube into chest cavity or to fluid accumulation in pleural space

• Ineffective breathing pattern related to restricted movement of chest wall caused by fluid accumulation in the pleural space

• Impaired gas exchange related to alveolar hypoventilation.

PLANNING

Based on the nursing diagnosis *high risk for infection,* develop appropriate patient outcomes. For example, your patient will:

• maintain temperature within normal limits

• maintain a normal WBC count

• maintain skin integrity at insertion site for the chest tube or thoracentesis needle, as evidenced by an absence of purulent drainage, redness, or other signs of infection.

Based on the nursing diagnosis *ineffective breathing pattern,* develop appropriate patient outcomes. For example, your patient will:

• maintain a respiratory rate at rest of 20 breaths/minute or less

• demonstrate full, bilaterally equal breath sounds

• exhibit symmetrical chest wall motion

• demonstrate adequate breath sounds with minimal or absent atelectatic crackles

• report a decrease in episodes of dyspnea.

Based on the nursing diagnosis *impaired gas exchange,* develop appropriate patient outcomes. For example, your patient will:

• demonstrate PaO_2 within established limits

• demonstrate partial pressure of arterial carbon dioxide within established limits.

IMPLEMENTATION

Treatment for pleural effusion focuses on removing excess extracellular fluid from the pleural space through thoracentesis and helping your patient maintain adequate respiration. (See *Medical care of the patient with pleural effusion,* page 176.)

Nursing interventions

• During thoracentesis, remind the patient to breathe normally and to avoid sudden movements, such as coughing or sighing. Monitor his vital signs and watch for syncope. Also be alert for bradycardia, hypotension, pain, and cardiac arrest—indications that fluid is being removed too quickly. Reassure your patient throughout the procedure.

• Allow enough time between premedication and the start of thoracentesis. Postoperative sedatives and analgesics aren't nearly as effective as adequate premedication.

• After thoracentesis, watch for respiratory distress and signs of pneumothorax, including sudden onset of dyspnea and cyanosis.

• Administer oxygen if the patient is hypoxemic.

• Administer prescribed antibiotics to the patient with empyema.

• Use an incentive spirometer to promote deep breathing and encourage the patient to perform deep-breathing exercises with sustained maximal inspiration to promote lung expansion.

• Monitor ABG values and assess for signs and symptoms of tissue hypoxia, such as increased respiratory rate, tachycardia, visual disturbances, cyanosis, and altered levels of consciousness. Also note clinical indications of improvement, such as a decrease in dyspnea, improved chest films, and improved ABG values.

• Reposition your patient every 2 hours. To promote lung expansion, place the patient in high Fowler's position.

• Provide meticulous chest tube care and use aseptic technique for changing dressings around the tube insertion site.

Medical care of the patient with pleural effusion

Depending on the amount of fluid in the pleural space, the patient with symptomatic effusion may require thoracentesis to remove fluid. Effective management also requires identifying and treating the underlying cause: for example, drug therapy for heart failure or radiation therapy for cancer.

Preventing recurrent infections
Chemical pleurodesis — the instillation of a sclerosing agent, such as tetracycline, bleomycin, or nitrogen mustard, through the chest tube to purposely create adhesions between the two pleural surfaces — may prevent recurrent effusions. After instillation of the sclerosing agent, the patient must remain in a single position for an established period of time, and then change positions as directed. This procedure can be painful for the patient.

Treating empyema
The patient with empyema needs one or more chest tubes inserted after thoracentesis. These tubes allow purulent material to drain. He may also need decortication (surgical removal of the thick coating over the lung) or rib resection to allow open drainage and lung expansion. He'll also require parenteral antibiotics and, if he has hypoxia, oxygen administration.

Ensure tube patency by watching for fluctuation in the underwater-seal chamber. Record the amount, color, and consistency of any tube drainage.
• Follow your hospital's policy for milking the chest tube. Keep petroleum gauze at the bedside in case the tube becomes dislodged.
• Don't clamp the chest tube: This may cause tension pneumothorax.
• If your patient has open drainage through a rib resection or intercostal tube, use secretion precautions. Your patient will usually need weeks of such drainage, so make necessary home health care referrals if he'll be discharged with the chest tube in place.
• Monitor for signs of infection, which may include fever, increased WBC count, and purulent chest tube drainage.
• Throughout therapy, listen to your patient's fears and concerns and remain with him during periods of extreme stress and anxiety. Encourage him to identify activities that will help him relax. Perform care measures to help the patient relax and encourage the patient to initiate relaxation measures as well.

Patient teaching
• Explain pleural effusion and its relationship to the underlying disorder.
• Explain all tests and procedures to the patient, including thoracentesis, and answer any questions.
• Explain the importance of deep breathing and show your patient how to use an incentive spirometer.
• Before thoracentesis, tell your patient to expect a stinging sensation from the local anesthetic and a feeling of pressure when the needle is inserted. Instruct him to tell you immediately if he feels uncomfortable or has trouble breathing during the procedure.
• If your patient developed pleural effusion because of pneumonia or influenza, tell him to seek medical attention promptly whenever he gets a chest cold.

Discharge TimeSaver

Ensuring continued care for the patient with pleural effusion

Review the following teaching topics, referrals, and follow-up appointments to ensure that your patient is adequately prepared for discharge.

Teaching topics
Make sure that the following topics have been covered and that your patient's learning has been evaluated:
☐ explanation of pleural effusion and its relationship to the underlying disorder
☐ management of chest tubes after thoracentesis
☐ activity guidelines
☐ drug therapy, including potential adverse effects
☐ need for deep breathing
☐ need for smoking cessation
☐ warning signs and symptoms of atelectasis, infection, and hypoxemia

Referrals
Make sure that the patient has been provided with necessary referrals to:
☐ social services
☐ home health care agency
☐ smoking cessation program.

Follow-up appointments
Make sure that the necessary follow-up appointments have been scheduled and that the patient has been notified:
☐ doctor or clinic
☐ diagnostic tests for reevaluation.

• If the patient is being discharged with the chest tube in place (common in patients with cancer), explain that the tube will be removed only after the problem is resolved. Refer the patient to a home health care agency.

• Teach your patient the signs and symptoms of respiratory complications and tell him to notify his doctor when signs and symptoms occur.

• Explain the medication regimen, including any adverse effects. Emphasize the importance of completing the prescribed drug regimen.

• If your patient smokes, urge him to stop and recommend a smoking cessation program. (See *Ensuring continued care for the patient with pleural effusion.*)

EVALUATION

When evaluating the patient's response to nursing care, gather reassessment data and compare this information

with the patient outcomes specified in your plan of care.

Teaching and counseling
Begin by determining the effectiveness of your teaching. Consider the following questions:

• Does the patient understand the disorder, its possible complications, and its treatment?

• Does he know the signs and symptoms to report to the doctor?

Physical condition
Consider the following questions:

• Are your patient's temperature, WBC count, respiratory rate, and ABG levels within established limits?

• Is the patient's chest wall motion symmetrical?

• Is the insertion site of the chest tube or thoracentesis needle clean and free of redness and purulent drainage?

• Does the patient demonstrate full, bilaterally equal breath sounds with few or no atelectatic crackles?
• Does he report a decrease in episodes of dyspnea?

Pneumothorax

Pneumothorax refers to an accumulation of air or gas between the parietal and visceral pleurae that impairs lung inflation and leads to partial or total lung collapse. The amount of air or gas trapped in the intrapleural space determines the degree of lung collapse.

Causes and types
In *open pneumothorax,* a penetrating chest wound creates a communication (pleurocutaneous fistula) between the outside air and the pleural space that permits air to rush in. An open pneumothorax may be traumatic or iatrogenic.

In *closed pneumothorax,* air enters the pleural space from within the lung without penetrating the chest wall. A closed pneumothorax may be further classified as spontaneous, iatrogenic, or traumatic. Spontaneous pneumothorax occurs without antecedent trauma when air enters the pleural space in the course of pulmonary disease or in an apparently healthy person. Iatrogenic closed pneumothorax may result from mechanical ventilation. Traumatic closed pneumothorax may occur after an injury when the chest wall remains intact; for example, when a fractured rib punctures the lung.

A life-threatening complication, *tension pneumothorax* occurs when a tear in the pleura acts as a one-way valve, permitting air to leak into the pleural space but not to escape. This causes pressure in the pleural space to rise above atmospheric pressure, leading to complete collapse of the lung and forc-ing the mediastinum to shift away from the affected side. (See *Understanding types of pneumothorax,* and *Causes of pneumothorax,* page 180.)

ASSESSMENT

Your assessment should include a thorough health history, a physical examination, and a review of diagnostic test findings. The health history may also reveal a causative factor.

Health history
The patient may report sudden, sharp, pleuritic pain; he may state that chest movement, breathing, and coughing exacerbate the pain. He may also indicate that he has shortness of breath. Additionally, he may report recent chronic respiratory infections or a recent impact to his thorax that was followed by rib pain or lateral chest pain upon inspiration.

Physical examination
Inspection typically reveals asymmetrical chest wall movement with overexpansion and rigidity on the affected side. The patient may exhibit tachypnea and cyanosis. In tension pneumothorax, he may have distended neck veins and pallor and may appear anxious. (Test results may confirm increased central venous pressure.) Palpation may reveal crackling beneath the skin, indicating subcutaneous emphysema (air in tissues), and decreased vocal fremitus. In tension pneumothorax, palpation may disclose tracheal deviation away from the affected side and a weak, rapid pulse. Percussion may demonstrate hyperresonance on the affected side, and auscultation may disclose decreased or absent breath sounds over the collapsed lung.

The patient with tension pneumothorax may be hypotensive and may exhibit a decreased level of consciousness (LOC). Spontaneous pneumotho-

Understanding types of pneumothorax

Review the illustrations below to better understand open, spontaneous, and tension pneumothorax.

Open pneumothorax
In this type of pneumothorax, a penetrating chest wound allows air to enter the pleural space through the chest wall.

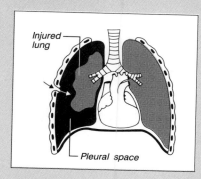

Spontaneous pneumothorax
In spontaneous pneumothorax, air enters the pleural space without antecedent trauma.

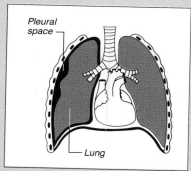

Tension pneumothorax
This type of pneumothorax occurs when a tear in the pleura permits air to leak into the pleural space but not to escape, leading to complete collapse of the lung and forcing the mediastinum to shift away from the affected side.

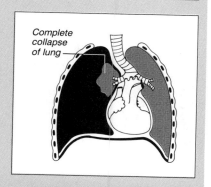

FactFinder

Causes of pneumothorax

The conditions and procedures listed below may trigger pressure changes that cause open, closed, or tension pneumothorax.

Open pneumothorax
• Penetrating chest injury, such as a gunshot or knife wound
• Insertion of a central venous catheter
• Chest surgery
• Transbronchial biopsy
• Thoracentesis or closed pleural biopsy.

Closed pneumothorax
Closed pneumothorax may be spontaneous, iatrogenic, or traumatic.

Spontaneous
• Asthma
• Pneumonia
• Air leakage from ruptured, congenital blebs adjacent to the visceral pleural space
• Rupture of emphysematous bullae
• Tubercular or cancerous lesions that erode into the pleural space
• Interstitial lung disease, such as eosinophilic granuloma

Iatrogenic
• Rupture resulting from barotrauma caused by high intrathoracic pressures during mechanical ventilation

Traumatic
• Blunt chest trauma.

Tension pneumothorax
• Penetrating chest wound treated with an airtight dressing
• Lung or airway puncture by a fractured rib associated with positive-pressure ventilation or as seen with flail chest trauma
• Mechanical ventilation after chest injury that forces air into the pleural space through damaged areas
• Mechanical ventilation with high-level positive end-expiratory pressure that causes alveolar blebs to rupture
• Chest tube occlusion or malfunction.

---

rax that releases only a small amount of air into the pleural space may cause no signs and symptoms.

Diagnostic test results
• Chest X-rays reveal air in the pleural space and, possibly, a mediastinal shift, which confirms the diagnosis.
• Arterial blood gas (ABG) studies may show hypoxemia, possibly accompanied by hypercapnia and respiratory acidosis. Arterial oxygen saturation levels may fall initially but typically return to normal within 24 hours.

NURSING DIAGNOSIS

Common nursing diagnoses for a patient with pneumothorax include:
• Anxiety related to pain, dyspnea, and feelings of impending doom
• Altered cardiopulmonary tissue perfusion related to decreased venous return and increased extrathoracic pressure
• Impaired gas exchange related to hypoventilation
• Ineffective breathing pattern related to restriction of the chest wall
• Pain related to lung collapse.

PLANNING

Based on the nursing diagnosis *anxiety*, develop appropriate patient outcomes. For example, your patient will:
• describe characteristics of anxiety
• identify measures to reduce anxiety
• report a decrease in his level of anxiety
• demonstrate reduced physical signs of anxiety.

Based on the nursing diagnosis *altered cardiopulmonary tissue perfusion*, develop appropriate patient outcomes. For example, your patient will:
• maintain blood pressure adequate for perfusion of vital organs
• show signs of improved LOC
• remain awake and alert.

Based on the nursing diagnosis *impaired gas exchange*, develop appropriate patient outcomes. For example, your patient will:
• maintain partial pressure of arterial oxygen within established limits
• maintain partial pressure of arterial carbon dioxide within established limits.

Based on the nursing diagnosis *ineffective breathing pattern*, develop appropriate patient outcomes. For example, your patient will:
• maintain a respiratory rate at rest of 20 breaths/minute or less
• demonstrate full, bilaterally equal breath sounds
• exhibit symmetrical chest wall motion
• report that dyspnea is absent.

Based on the nursing diagnosis *pain*, develop appropriate patient outcomes. For example, your patient will:
• initiate measures to increase his comfort level
• report a decrease in the amount and frequency of medication needed to reduce pain
• express feeling comfortable when moving, coughing, and breathing.

IMPLEMENTATION

Treatment focuses on alleviating the patient's anxiety and discomfort and maintaining adequate respiration. (See *Medical care of the patient with pneumothorax,* page 182.)

Nursing interventions

• Listen to your patient's fears and concerns. Explain all treatments and procedures. Offer reassurance when needed.
• Remain with your patient during periods of extreme stress and anxiety. Help the patient identify measures that promote relaxation. Encourage the patient and family members to initiate relaxation measures. Include them in care-related decisions whenever possible.
• Keep the patient as comfortable as possible and administer analgesics as necessary. The patient with pneumothorax usually feels most comfortable sitting upright. If your patient shows signs of hypoxemia, administer oxygen by face mask or nasal cannula.
• Watch for evidence of complications, including pallor, gasping respirations, and sudden chest pain. Carefully monitor vital signs at least every hour for indications of shock, increasing respiratory distress, or mediastinal shift. Listen for breath sounds over both lungs. Monitor ABG levels.
• Monitor the patient's LOC and mentation at least every 4 hours and more often if the patient's condition is unstable. Document his baseline LOC fully and precisely to ensure accurate reassessment.
• Watch for signs of tension pneumothorax, especially if the patient has not had chest tubes inserted. These signs include falling blood pressure and rising pulse and respiratory rates, which could be fatal without prompt treatment.

Medical care of the patient with pneumothorax

Treatment of spontaneous pneumothorax is conservative under these conditions:
• There are no signs of increased pleural pressure (indicating tension pneumothorax).
• Lung collapse is less than 30%.
• Dyspnea and other indications of physiologic compromise are absent. Conservative treatment consists of bed rest, oxygen administration, and careful monitoring of blood pressure and pulse and respiratory rates.

Reexpanding the lung
If more than 30% of the lung collapses, treatment seeks to reexpand the lung through placement of a thoracostomy tube in the second or third intercostal space in the midclavicular line. The thoracostomy tube connects to an under-water seal with low-pressure suction in a closed drainage system. Depending on the degree of severity, pneumothorax may require immediate removal of the air by needle aspiration (as an emergency procedure) before the chest tube is inserted.

Preventing recurrence
Recurring spontaneous pneumothorax requires thoracotomy and pleurectomy. These procedures prevent recurrence by causing the lung to adhere to the parietal pleura.

Other measures
Traumatic and tension pneumothorax require chest tube drainage; traumatic pneumothorax may also require surgical repair. Analgesics may be prescribed.

Chest tube insertion
• To facilitate chest tube insertion, place your patient in high Fowler's, semi-Fowler's, or the supine position, or have him lie on his unaffected side with his arms overhead. During chest tube insertion, ask him to control the urge to cough and gasp. However, once the chest tube is placed, encourage him to cough and breathe deeply at least once an hour to facilitate lung expansion.
• Change the dressings around the chest tube insertion site at least every 24 hours. Keep the insertion site clean, and watch for signs of infection. Be careful not to reposition or dislodge the tube.

Timesaving tip: Have a sterile petroleum gauze dressing on hand at the bedside. If the tube dislodges, immediately place the petroleum gauze dressing over the opening to prevent rapid lung collapse; however, use extreme caution. If the lung has a hole or tear (evidenced by bubbling in the water-seal chamber), tension pneumothorax may be created by a tight dressing placement.
• Watch for bubbling, a sign of continuing air leakage. This indicates the lung defect's failure to heal, which may necessitate surgery. Also, watch for increasing subcutaneous emphysema by palpating around the neck or at the tube's insertion site for crackling beneath the skin. For the patient receiving mechanical ventilation, watch for difficulty in breathing in time with the ventilator. Also watch for pressure changes on the ventilator gauges.

Discharge TimeSaver

Ensuring continued care for the patient with pneumothorax

Review the following teaching topics, referrals, and follow-up appointments to ensure that your patient is adequately prepared for discharge.

Teaching topics
Make sure that the following topics have been covered and that your patient's learning has been evaluated:
☐ explanation of pneumothorax, including its relationship to the underlying disorder
☐ need for deep breathing
☐ potential for recurrent symptoms
☐ need for immediate medical intervention should pneumothorax recur
☐ activity guidelines.

Referrals
Make sure that the patient has been provided with necessary referrals to:
☐ social services
☐ home health care agency.

Follow-up appointments
Make sure that the necessary follow-up appointments have been scheduled and that the patient has been notified:
☐ doctor or clinic
☐ diagnostic tests for reevaluation.

Thoracotomy

Monitor vital signs frequently after thoracotomy. Also, for the first 24 hours, assess respiratory status by checking breath sounds hourly. Every hour for the first 4 hours (and then per hospital protocol), observe the chest tube site for leakage and note the amount and color of drainage. Every 4 hours, monitor appropriate fluid levels in the water-seal and suction chambers on the closed drainage system; refill as needed. Ambulate the patient, as prescribed (usually on the first postoperative day), to promote deep inspiration and lung expansion.

Patient teaching

• Explain what pneumothorax is, what causes it, and all diagnostic tests and procedures. If your patient is having surgery or chest tubes inserted, explain why. Reassure him that the chest tubes will make him more comfortable.
• Encourage your patient to perform deep-breathing exercises every hour when awake.

• Discuss the potential for recurrent spontaneous pneumothorax and review its signs and symptoms. Emphasize the need for immediate medical intervention if these signs and symptoms occur. Also inform your patient to avoid activities that may result in pneumothorax due to extreme alterations in atmospheric pressure, such as traveling to very high altitudes (for example, in an airplane) and deep-water scuba diving. (See *Ensuring continued care for the patient with pneumothorax.*)

EVALUATION

When evaluating the patient's response to nursing care, gather reassessment data and compare this information with the patient outcomes specified in your plan of care.

Teaching and counseling

Begin by determining the effectiveness of your teaching. Consider the following questions:

• Does the patient understand the disorder, its possible complications, and its treatment?
• Does he know the signs and symptoms to report to the doctor?
• Can he identify activities that may result in pneumothorax and does he understand the need to avoid them?

Physical condition
Consider the following questions:
• Has the patient achieved a respiratory rate, an LOC, and ABG levels within established limits?
• Does he exhibit symmetrical chest wall motion?
• Does he demonstrate full, bilaterally equal breaths sounds?
• Does the patient report that dyspnea is absent?
• Does he express comfort with breathing, coughing, and moving?

Hemothorax

Hemothorax occurs when blood enters the pleural cavity from damaged intercostal, pleural, or mediastinal vessels (or occasionally from the lung's parenchymal vessels). Depending on the amount of blood and the underlying cause of bleeding, hemothorax can cause varying degrees of lung collapse.

Causes
Hemothorax usually results from either blunt or penetrating chest trauma. In fact, about 25% of patients with blunt or penetrating chest trauma experience hemothorax. Less often, hemothorax occurs as a consequence of thoracic surgery, pulmonary infarction, neoplasm, dissecting thoracic aneurysm, anticoagulant therapy, pneumonia, or pulmonary tuberculosis.

Complications of hemothorax may include mediastinal shift, ventilatory compromise, lung collapse and, without successful intervention, cardiopulmonary arrest.

During your assessment, obtain information about recent trauma, the underlying cause of hemothorax. Also assess for accompanying pneumothorax.

Health history
The patient may report chest pain and sudden difficulty breathing. Breathing difficulty may range from mild to severe, depending on the amount of blood in the pleural cavity.

Physical examination
Inspection typically discloses a patient with tachypnea, dusky skin color, diaphoresis, and hemoptysis (bloody, frothy sputum). If hemothorax progresses to respiratory failure, you may observe restlessness, anxiety, cyanosis, and stupor. The affected side of the chest may expand and stiffen; the unaffected side will rise and fall with the patient's gasping respirations.

Percussion may disclose dullness over the affected side of the chest; auscultation may detect decreased or absent breath sounds over the affected side. Depending on the volume of blood lost in hemothorax, the patient may develop tachycardia and hypotension.

Timesaving tip: Perform auscultation before palpation and percussion if your patient is experiencing respiratory distress.

Diagnostic test results
• Thoracentesis, performed for diagnosis and therapy, may yield blood or serosanguineous fluid. Fluid specimens may be sent to the laboratory for analysis.
• Chest X-rays may detect intrapleural fluid (as little as 200 to 300 ml) and mediastinal shift.

- Arterial blood gas (ABG) analysis may provide evidence of respiratory failure.
- Hemoglobin levels may be decreased, indicating blood loss.

NURSING DIAGNOSIS

Common nursing diagnoses for a patient with hemothorax include:
- Anxiety related to situational crisis and difficulty breathing
- Impaired gas exchange related to hypoventilation
- Ineffective breathing pattern related to restriction of chest wall
- Pain related to lung collapse and penetrating wounds
- High risk for infection related to traumatic chest wound
- High risk for fluid volume deficit related to injured pulmonary vessel.

PLANNING

Based on the nursing diagnosis *anxiety,* develop appropriate patient outcomes. For example, your patient will:
- identify the causes of his anxiety
- identify and use measures that are effective in reducing anxiety
- report experiencing less anxiety
- demonstrate fewer physical signs of anxiety
- report experiencing an increase in the ease of breathing.

Based on the nursing diagnosis *impaired gas exchange,* develop appropriate patient outcomes. For example, your patient will:
- maintain partial pressure of arterial oxygen (PaO_2) within established limits
- maintain partial pressure of arterial carbon dioxide ($PaCO_2$) within established limits.

Based on the nursing diagnosis *ineffective breathing pattern,* develop appropriate patient outcomes. For example, your patient will:

- maintain a respiratory rate at rest of 20 breaths/minute or less
- demonstrate full, bilaterally equal breath sounds during auscultation
- exhibit symmetrical chest wall motion
- report an absence of dyspnea.

Based on the nursing diagnosis *pain,* develop appropriate patient outcomes. For example, your patient will:
- describe characteristics of pain
- report a decrease in the amount and frequency of medication necessary to reduce pain
- report feeling comfortable when moving, coughing, and breathing.

Based on the nursing diagnosis *high risk for infection,* develop appropriate patient outcomes. For example, your patient will:
- maintain temperature within established range
- maintain white blood cell (WBC) count within established range
- remain free of pathogens, as evidenced by pleural fluid cultures
- maintain a clean chest wound with normal skin color and an absence of drainage.

Based on the nursing diagnosis *high risk for fluid volume deficit,* develop appropriate patient outcomes. For example, your patient will:
- exhibit normal skin turgor and mucous membranes
- maintain blood pressure, pulse rate, urine specific gravity, hemoglobin and hematocrit levels, and blood urea nitrogen (BUN) levels within established parameters
- maintain urine output greater than or equal to 30 ml/hour or 0.5 ml/kg/hour
- maintain or return to baseline level of consciousness (LOC)
- maintain cumulative intake and output within established limits.

Treatments

Medical care of the patient with hemothorax

In hemothorax, treatment aims to stabilize the patient's condition, stop the bleeding, evacuate blood from the pleural cavity, and reexpand the affected lung.

Mild hemothorax

Mild hemothorax usually clears in 10 to 14 days, requiring only observation for further bleeding.

Severe hemothorax

For severe hemothorax, treatment includes thoracentesis to remove blood and other fluids from the pleural cavity and then insertion of a chest tube into the sixth intercostal space in the posterior axillary line. The large diameter of a typical chest tube helps to prevent clot formation. Suction may also be used.

Other treatment measures

If the chest tube doesn't improve the patient's condition, the surgeon may need to perform a thoracotomy to evacuate blood and clots and to control bleeding.

Additional treatment measures for hemothorax include:
• autotransfusion, if the patient's blood loss approaches or exceeds 1,000 ml
• oxygen therapy
• I.V. therapy to restore fluid volume
• administration of analgesics.

IMPLEMENTATION

Treatment measures for the patient with hemothorax include monitoring vital signs, draining blood from the pleural cavity, replacing fluids, and helping the patient cope with the effects of trauma. (See *Medical care of the patient with hemothorax*.)

Nursing interventions

• Quickly check the patient's airway, breathing, and circulation; then inspect the wound site for bleeding.

Timesaving tip: Establish one or two I.V. sites using a large-bore catheter for rapid fluid or blood administration if needed.

• Administer I.V. fluids and blood transfusions, as ordered. If your patient has a massive hemothorax, prepare him for autotransfusion. (See *Using autotransfusion for chest wounds*.)

• Prepare your patient for a chest X-ray. Also obtain ABG values and hemoglobin and hematocrit levels to evaluate baseline gas exchange status and to help estimate blood loss.

• As ordered, give oxygen by face mask or nasal cannula.

• Use a central venous pressure line to monitor fluid replacement. A pulmonary artery line may be needed to assist with monitoring patient response to fluid replacement in elderly patients and in those with a history of cardiac problems. Also check skin turgor, mucous membranes, BUN, hemoglobin and hematocrit levels, urine specific gravity, and vital signs to monitor fluid volume status.

• Monitor the patient's urine output either every hour, every 2 hours, or every 4 hours, depending on the patient's hemodynamic status.

• Monitor vital signs diligently. Watch for increasing pulse and respiratory rates and falling blood pressure, which may indicate shock or massive bleeding. If danger signs are present, be ready to prepare your patient for surgery.

• Monitor ABG levels and breath sounds often. Be prepared to assist with endotracheal intubation if mechanical ventilation becomes necessary. Mechanical ventilation will be necessary if respiratory failure occurs.

• Watch for complications signaled by pallor and gasping respirations.

Using autotransfusion for chest wounds

Used most often in patients with chest wounds accompanied by hemothorax, an autotransfusion device aseptically collects and filters a patient's own blood, which can then be reinfused.

Autotransfusion eliminates the patient's risk for transfusion reaction or blood-borne disease, such as cytomegalovirus, hepatitis, and human immunodeficiency virus. It's contraindicated in patients with sepsis or cancer or if the collected blood becomes contaminated.

How autotransfusion works

A large-bore chest tube connected to a closed drainage system is used to collect the patient's blood from a wound or chest cavity. This blood passes through a filter, which catches most potential thrombi, including clumps of fibrin and damaged red blood cells (RBCs). The filtered blood passes into a collection device. The blood may be reinfused immediately. Or it may be processed in a commercial cell washer that reduces anticoagulated whole blood to washed RBCs for later infusion.

Assisting with autotransfusion

• Set up the blood collection system as you would any closed chest drainage system. Attach the collection device according to the manufacturer's instructions.
• If ordered, inject an anticoagulant, such as heparin or acid citrate dextrose (ACD) solution, into the self-sealing port on the connector of the patient's drainage tubing.
• During reinfusion, monitor the patient for complications, such as blood clotting, hemolysis, coagulopathies, thrombocytopenia, particulate and air emboli, sepsis, and citrate toxicity (from the ACD solution).

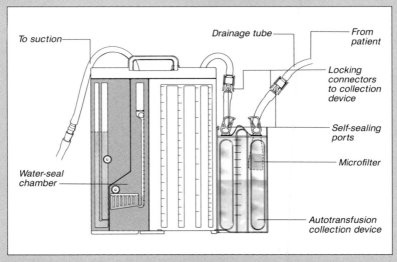

To suction

Drainage tube

From patient

Locking connectors to collection device

Self-sealing ports

Microfilter

Water-seal chamber

Autotransfusion collection device

• Administer antibiotics, as ordered, to decrease the potential for infection after penetrating chest trauma.

• Give pain medication, as prescribed, and record its effectiveness.

• Carefully observe the asymptomatic patient with a small hemothorax and prepare him for serial chest X-rays, as ordered. Monitor for signs of complications, and administer oxygen, as ordered. Anticipate the resolution of a small hemothorax within 14 days.

• If the patient is conscious, listen to his fears and concerns and offer reassurance. Remain with the patient during periods of stress and anxiety. Encourage him to identify actions that promote comfort and relaxation. Perform care measures to help the patient relax, and encourage the patient and family members to initiate relaxation measures as well.

• Encourage the patient and family members to participate in care-related decisions whenever possible.

• Note signs of improvement. These include reexpansion of the damaged lung on chest X-ray (with no recurrence of hemothorax on follow-up X-rays), decreased dyspnea and respiratory rate, full and equal breath sounds, symmetrical chest expansion, and stable vital signs.

Chest tube insertion

• Assist with chest tube insertion; for a smaller hemothorax, thoracentesis may be sufficient.

• Observe chest tube drainage carefully. Record the volume, color, and character of drainage at least hourly for 4 hours or until drainage is less than 100 ml/hour. Then document the finding either every 4 or 8 hours. Immediately report a chest tube that's warm and full of blood or a rapidly rising bloody fluid level in the drainage collection chamber. The patient may need emergency surgery.

• Follow your hospital's policy for milking the chest tube. If you can see bloody drainage or clots, milking may be permitted to keep the tube patent.

Timesaving tip: Keep petroleum gauze at the bedside in case the chest tube dislodges. If it does, place the gauze securely over the chest tube site, taking care not to cover the wound so tightly that tension pneumothorax results.

• Don't clamp the chest tube; this may create tension pneumothorax.

• Change the chest tube dressing as necessary using aseptic technique and according to hospital policy. Watch for signs of infection at the insertion site. Also assess any traumatic wound area for signs of infection. Monitor the patient's temperature, WBC count, and cultures for indications of infection.

• Avoid all tubing kinks because they act like clamps on the tube and may cause tension pneumothorax. Tape all chest tube connections, and tape the tube securely to your patient's chest.

Patient teaching

• Explain hemothorax to the patient and family members. Encourage them to ask questions, and answer all questions as honestly as you can.

• Teach the patient and family members about treatment for the disorder. Explain the rationale for chest tube therapy and hemodynamic lines. Teach the patient about mechanical ventilation, if necessary.

• Encourage your patient to perform deep-breathing exercises every hour when awake to promote adequate gas exchange.

• Instruct your patient not to cough during thoracentesis.

• If appropriate, provide preoperative and postoperative teaching. Discuss the need for early ambulation after surgery. (See *Ensuring continued care for the patient with hemothorax.*)

Discharge TimeSaver

Ensuring continued care for the patient with hemothorax

Review the following teaching topics, referrals, and follow-up appointments to ensure that your patient is adequately prepared for discharge.

Teaching topics
Make sure that the following topics have been covered and that your patient's learning has been evaluated:
□ explanation of hemothorax
□ need for deep-breathing exercises
□ need for ongoing antibiotic therapy
□ activity guidelines.

Referrals
Make sure that the patient has been provided with necessary referrals to:
□ social services
□ home health care agency.

Follow-up appointments
Make sure that the necessary follow-up appointments have been scheduled and that the patient has been notified:
□ doctor or clinic
□ diagnostic tests for reevaluation.

EVALUATION

When evaluating the patient's response to nursing care, gather reassessment data and compare this information with the patient outcomes specified in your plan of care.

Teaching and counseling
Begin by determining the effectiveness of your teaching. Consider the following questions:
• Does the patient express understanding of hemothorax, including its cause and potential complications?
• Does he understand the rationale for chest tube therapy and hemodynamic lines?
• Is he willing to perform deep breathing exercises?
• Can he successfully cope with anxiety caused by hemothorax? Has he identified the source of his anxiety?
• Can he identify and use effective measures to reduce anxiety?
• Does he express less anxiety?
• Does he exhibit fewer signs of anxiety?

• Do the patient and family members participate in care related decisions?

Physical condition
Next, evaluate the patient's physical condition, including an assessment of his pain. Consider the following questions:
• Are the his PaO_2 and $PaCO_2$ within established limits?
• Has he achieved a respiratory rate of 20 breaths/minute or less?
• Does he demonstrate full, bilaterally equal breath sounds?
• Does he exhibit symmetrical chest wall motion?
• Does he report that dyspnea is absent?
• Is he free of infection?
• Are his temperature and WBC count within appropriate ranges?
• Does analysis of his pleural fluid indicate an absence of pathogens?
• Does he maintain a chest wound with normal skin color and an absence of drainage?
• Does he exhibit normal skin turgor and mucous membranes?

• Are his blood pressure, pulse rate, urine specific gravity, hemoglobin and hematocrit levels, and BUN levels within established limits?

• Is his urine output greater than or equal to 30 ml/hour or 0.5 ml/kg/hour?

• Does he maintain or return to baseline LOC after treatment for hemothorax?

• Does he maintain cumulative intake and output within established limits?

Pain assessment
Consider the following questions:

• How does the patient describe his pain?

• After treatment, does he report a significant reduction in the amount and frequency of medication needed to reduce pain?

• Does he report feeling comfortable when moving?

• Is he able to cough and breathe without discomfort?

Caring for patients with pulmonary vascular disorders

Pulmonary embolism

An obstruction of the pulmonary arterial bed, a pulmonary embolism occurs when a mass — usually a migrating thrombus — lodges in a branch of the pulmonary artery. This obstruction causes a ventilation-perfusion mismatch, resulting in hypoxemia.

In roughly 10% of patients, the embolus causes pulmonary infarction. The risk of infarction is greatest for patients with chronic cardiac or pulmonary disease. Massive embolism (more than 50% obstruction of the pulmonary arterial circulation) and infarction can be rapidly fatal. (See *Key points about pulmonary embolism.*)

Causes

Pulmonary embolism most commonly results from migration of a thrombus originating in a deep vein in the legs. (*See How an embolus develops,* page 194.) Recent surgery (especially of the legs, pelvis, abdomen, or thorax) increases susceptibility. Prolonged bed rest may cause venous stasis, which heightens the risk of embolism.

Other less common causes of emboli include bone, air, fat, amniotic fluid, tumor cells, or a foreign object such as a needle, a catheter part, or talc (from drugs intended for oral administration that are injected I.V.).

ASSESSMENT

Your patient's signs and symptoms may be subtle or dramatic, depending on the extent of pulmonary involvement and the presence of hemodynamic complications.

Health history

Patients with pulmonary embolism often report sudden chest pain and dyspnea with no apparent cause. Further assessment may reveal that the chest pain is pleuritic (a sharp pain that worsens when the patient inhales).

Find out if the patient has a history of predisposing conditions, such as venous thrombosis, recent surgery (especially orthopedic surgery), cancer, a prolonged period of bed rest, or the use of oral contraceptives. (See *Risk factors for pulmonary embolism,* page 195.)

Physical examination

If you suspect pulmonary embolism, perform an abbreviated examination—a quick check of vital signs and auscultation of the patient's chest. This will often suffice to provide baseline values. Report your findings immediately to the doctor to allow for prompt treatment. Mortality from pulmonary embolism is highest during the first 2 hours. (See *Clinical findings in pulmonary embolism,* page 196.)

Inspection may reveal tachypnea, signs of anxiety, and a productive cough, possibly producing blood-tinged sputum. Chest splinting and massive hemoptysis may be evident but are less common. If the embolus is large, you may note cyanosis and syncope. If the patient has right ventricular failure, you may note distended neck veins. The patient may exhibit mental status changes, such as restlessness, irritability, and confusion.

Auscultating the chest may reveal wheezing and a transient pleural friction rub and crackles at the embolus site. You may also hear an S_3 and S_4 gallop and increased intensity of the pulmonic component of S_2.

Timesaving tip: Pulmonary embolism can cause heart failure. If you notice hypotension, distended neck veins, and heart sounds characteristic of heart failure, stop your assessment and immediately notify the doctor.

As you assess the patient's vital signs, you may note a slight fever, tachycardia, and tachypnea. You may use pulse oximetry to assess arterial oxygen saturation (SaO_2). SaO_2 may be normal or decreased, depending on whether the patient has underlying lung disease and on the size of the pulmonary embolism. Be alert for signs of circulatory collapse (for example, a weak, rapid pulse accompanied by hypotension and possibly restlessness, a change in level of consciousness [LOC], and cool, moist skin).

Diagnostic test results

The following tests may confirm a diagnosis of pulmonary embolism and reveal the extent of damage:
• Lung perfusion scan (lung scintiscan) may reveal the embolus.
• Ventilation scan (often performed at the same time as the lung perfusion scan) confirms the diagnosis.
• Pulmonary angiography, the most definitive test for pulmonary embolism, may indicate a defect in pulmonary vessel filling or flow. Either result indicates a pulmonary embolism. However, because of the test's risks, it's used only if the diagnosis can't be confirmed by other tests and if anticoagulants are contraindicated.
• Electrocardiography (ECG) distinguishes pulmonary embolism from myocardial infarction. If the patient has an extensive obstruction of the pulmonary vessels, ECG shows right axis deviation; right bundle-branch block; tall, peaked P waves; depressed ST segments; T-wave inversions (signaling right ventricular strain); and supraventricular tachyarrhythmias.
• Chest X-ray may be used to rule out other pulmonary diseases; however, this test is inconclusive during the first 1 to 2 hours after embolism occurs. Chest X-ray may also reveal areas of atelectasis, an elevated diaphragm, pleural effusion, and a prominent pulmonary artery. Occasionally, it shows

FactFinder

Key points about pulmonary embolism

• *Incidence:* Pulmonary embolism strikes more than 500,000 adults each year in North America. About 10% of cases are fatal.
• *Prognosis:* Mortality after the initial thromboembolism varies, according to the severity of the event and the patient's cardiopulmonary status. Patients who survive the initial event but fail to receive treatment risk potentially fatal recurrences.
• *Primary diagnostic methods:* Lung perfusion scan, ventilation scan
• *Treatment:* Oxygen, anticoagulants
• *Leading complication:* Pulmonary infarction
• *Other complications:* Atelectasis, pulmonary abscess, adult respiratory distress syndrome, hypotension, arrhythmias, heart failure, hepatic congestion, shock, ischemia of major organs, cardiac arrest (in massive pulmonary embolism)

the wedge-shaped infiltrate characteristic of pulmonary infarction.
• Arterial blood gas (ABG) analysis may reveal reduced partial pressure of oxygen in arterial blood (PaO_2), indicating hypoxemia. Partial pressure of carbon dioxide in arterial blood ($PaCO_2$) may also be reduced. Initially, results will indicate respiratory alkalosis; as damage progresses, results will indicate metabolic acidosis.
• Magnetic resonance imaging, although not a common procedure, may be performed to identify an embolus or changes in blood flow that indicate the presence of an embolus.

How an embolus develops

Typically, an embolus begins as a thrombus (blood clot) in a blood vessel. It may dissolve on its own, but trauma, abrupt muscle action, or changes in intravascular pressure may dislodge it from the vessel wall or break off one or more pieces.

The dislodged thrombus or fragment is carried by the blood to the heart's right side and enters the lung through the pulmonary artery. The mass — now called an embolus — may dissolve, continue to break apart, or grow. If it dissolves or becomes fragmented, phagocytes will digest the remains. If, however, the embolus enlarges, it may grow large enough to obstruct most or all of the pulmonary vasculature and cause death.

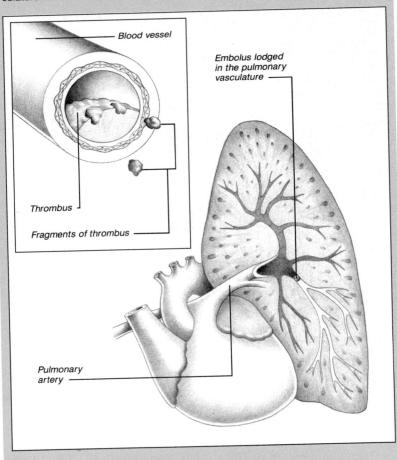

Blood vessel

Embolus lodged in the pulmonary vasculature

Thrombus

Fragments of thrombus

Pulmonary artery

NURSING DIAGNOSIS

Common nursing diagnoses for a patient with pulmonary embolism include:

• Impaired gas exchange related to ventilation-perfusion mismatch due to pulmonary embolism
• Decreased cardiac output related to right ventricular failure
• Pain related to the disorder
• Anxiety related to symptoms of acute respiratory distress and fear of death
• Knowledge deficit related to treatment and preventive measures.

PLANNING

Focus your nursing care on minimizing the effects of impaired gas exchange, relieving the patient's pain and anxiety, and teaching him and his family about pulmonary embolism.

Based on the nursing diagnosis *impaired gas exchange,* develop appropriate patient outcomes. For example, the patient will:
• maintain PaO_2 within an acceptable range
• maintain $PaCO_2$ at 35 to 45 mm Hg (or at acceptable baseline values)
• demonstrate clear breath sounds
• exhibit baseline LOC
• fail to develop cyanosis, cough, or hemoptysis
• report that dyspnea is absent.

Based on the nursing diagnosis *decreased cardiac output,* develop appropriate patient outcomes. For example, the patient will:
• maintain an acceptable pulse rate and rhythm
• maintain systolic blood pressure above 90 mm Hg
• maintain normal (or baseline) central venous pressure (CVP)
• not exhibit jugular vein distention
• maintain urine output of 30 ml/hour or more.

FactFinder

Risk factors for pulmonary embolism

During your assessment, confer with the patient, his family, or members of the health care team to determine if the patient's health history includes any of the following conditions, treatments, or other factors that increase his risk for pulmonary embolism.

Conditions
• Chronic lung disease
• Cardiovascular disease
• Infection
• Diabetes mellitus
• Thromboembolism
• Thrombophlebitis
• Vascular insufficiency
• Sickle cell disease
• Autoimmune hemolytic anemia
• Polycythemia
• Osteomyelitis
• Long-bone fracture
• Pelvic fractures or injuries
• Cancer
• Obesity
• Advanced age
• Burns
• Recent pregnancy

Treatments
• Recent surgery (especially if it involved the legs, pelvis, abdomen, or thorax)
• Prolonged bed rest or immobilization
• Orthopedic casts
• I.V. drug therapy

Other factors
• Manipulation or disconnection of central lines
• I.V. drug abuse
• Use of high-estrogen oral contraceptives

Assessment TimeSaver
Clinical findings in pulmonary embolism

Signs and symptoms of pulmonary embolism vary greatly, depending on the size and location of emboli, the degree of hemodynamic compromise, and the presence of perfusion deficit. In relatively minor cases, the patient will be asymptomatic. At worst, if the embolus lodges in the bifurcation of the main pulmonary artery, the patient may die as quickly as a victim of massive coronary artery occlusion.

Most common symptoms
- Pleuritic chest pain (in total occlusion of the pulmonary artery, chest pain may be accompanied by cyanosis and rapidly changing vital signs)
- Sudden dyspnea
- Cough with blood-tinged sputum
- Anxiety
- Tachypnea
- Tachycardia
- Restlessness
- Diaphoresis

Acute symptoms
- Crackles
- Low-grade fever
- Wheezes
- Pleural friction rub
- Dull percussion sounds
- Weak rapid pulse, hypotension (secondary to circulatory collapse)
- Transient unconsciousness, coma, or seizures (secondary to cerebral ischemia)
- Hemiplegia and other focal neurologic deficits (especially in elderly patients)

Based on the nursing diagnosis *pain,* develop appropriate patient outcomes. For example, the patient will:
- identify characteristics of his pain, including location and intensity, and factors that aggravate and alleviate the pain
- report that he no longer experiences pain or that his pain has diminished
- exhibit pain relief, as evidenced by an absence of muscular tension, grimacing, diaphoresis, or splinting.

Based on the nursing diagnosis *anxiety,* develop appropriate patient outcomes. For example, the patient will:
- perform relaxation techniques
- use support systems to assist with coping
- exhibit fewer physical symptoms of anxiety
- state that he feels less anxious.

Based on the nursing diagnosis *knowledge deficit,* develop appropriate patient outcomes. For example, the patient will:
- state the risk factors for pulmonary embolism
- express an understanding of anticoagulant therapy and its purpose, including dosage, route, adverse effects, precautions, and the importance of follow-up appointments
- identify measures to help prevent recurrence of pulmonary emboli
- state the warning signs that must be immediately reported to the doctor.

IMPLEMENTATION

Treatment for pulmonary embolism seeks to maintain cardiovascular and pulmonary function until the obstruction resolves and to prevent recurrence. (See *Medical care of the patient with pulmonary embolism.*)

Timesaving tip: When assessment reveals evidence of hypoxemia, your immediate priorities are to provide (or continue) oxygen therapy, maintain cardiac output, and relieve pain. These measures also help reduce anxiety and associated stress.

Treatments

Medical care of the patient with pulmonary embolism

Because most pulmonary emboli resolve in 10 to 14 days, treatment focuses on maintaining adequate cardiovascular and pulmonary function until the obstruction resolves and on preventing any recurrence. Appropriate treatments include:

• oxygen therapy to reverse ventilation-perfusion mismatch and relieve hypoxemia

• narcotic analgesics to alleviate apprehension and pain

• vasopressors to treat hypotension caused by an embolus

• anticoagulant therapy using heparin. If the embolus results from a dislodged thrombus, anticoagulants may inhibit the formation of new thrombi. Daily coagulation studies of partial thromboplastin time are necessary during treatment with heparin.

• ongoing anticoagulant therapy using warfarin. Therapy usually lasts 3 to 6 months, unless contraindicated by the presence of risk factors. Prothrombin time is monitored daily at first, then biweekly.

• thrombolytic therapy using urokinase, streptokinase, or alteplase. These thrombolytic agents can dissolve clots within 2 hours. They are pre-scribed for patients with massive pulmonary embolism and shock.

• antibiotic therapy. For patients with a septic embolus, antibiotics may be used instead of anticoagulants. Treatment requires concurrent evaluation of the source of infection, which is usually endocarditis.

• surgery. If the use of anticoagulants is contraindicated or the patient develops recurrent emboli during anticoagulant therapy, surgery may be necessary. Before surgery, angiography is used to locate the embolism and thereby confirm the diagnosis. During surgery, a device (such as an umbrella filter) is inserted into the vena cava to filter blood as it returns to the heart and lungs.

• antiembolism stockings. Used with or without sequential compression stockings, antiembolism stockings help to prevent venous thromboembolism following surgery.

• mechanical ventilation and corticosteroids. These interventions may be necessary for a patient with a fat embolus, if oxygen therapy alone is insufficient. A diuretic may be prescribed if pulmonary edema occurs.

Nursing interventions

Patients experiencing pulmonary embolism require immediate care to stabilize their condition, followed by measures to achieve relief of symptoms.

Initial care

• Administer prescribed oxygen by nasal cannula or face mask. If the patient has worsening dyspnea, check his ABG levels. If his breathing is severely compromised, anticipate providing en-dotracheal intubation with assisted mechanical ventilation.

• Monitor the patient's pulmonary and hemodynamic status closely throughout therapy.

• During the acute period, maintain bed rest and elevate the head of the bed to promote chest excursion. Help the patient perform activities to lessen dyspnea.

• If the patient has pleuritic chest pain, administer the prescribed analgesic and monitor his response.

• Anticipate anticoagulant therapy. Be prepared to start a peripheral I.V. with an appropriate gauge needle.

Ongoing care
• When the patient's condition permits, perform a more extensive assessment. Be sure to investigate risk factors.
• Explain all procedures to the patient and his family, and provide emotional support.
• Help the patient identify and practice effective coping techniques, such as relaxation.
• Administer prescribed heparin by I.V. push or by continuous drip. Monitor coagulation studies daily. (Effective therapy raises partial thromboplastin time to 2 to 2½ times normal.)
• During heparin therapy, don't give I.M. injections. Monitor the patient closely for signs of abnormal bleeding, such as epistaxis, petechiae, and hematuria. Check the patient's stools for occult blood.
• If thrombolytic drugs are prescribed (for example, if the patient's respiratory status is severely compromised, or he's hemodynamically unstable), administer them according to the established protocol. Remember that bleeding is a common adverse effect. If it occurs, notify the doctor and discontinue therapy.
• If needed, provide incentive spirometry to help the patient breathe deeply. Provide him with tissues and tape a disposal bag to the side rail of the bed.
• When the patient's condition is stable, encourage him to move about and help him perform isometric and range-of-motion exercises.
• If surgery is scheduled, help the patient prepare physically and emotionally. Augment the doctor's explanations by discussing the procedure with the patient and answering his questions. After surgery, monitor the patient carefully for complications. Implement measures to prevent venous stasis.

Patient teaching
• Explain how and where emboli form and how they obstruct the pulmonary circulation. Point out their risks.
• Describe all ordered diagnostic tests.
• Explain that coughing and deep breathing exercises help prevent atelectasis.
• If prescribed, explain anticoagulant therapy, including dosage and possible adverse effects and preventive measures. Make sure that the patient understands to take his medications exactly as prescribed. Tell him to talk with his doctor before taking any other medications — especially aspirin.
• Teach the patient the signs of bleeding (such as bloody stools, hematuria, bleeding gums, or unusually large bruises). Describe precautions to help prevent bleeding — for example, shaving with an electric razor rather than a blade, using a soft toothbrush, and being particularly careful to prevent bumps, scrapes, or falls.
• Stress that follow-up testing (such as the prothrombin test if the patient is taking an anticoagulant) is an essential part of monitoring response to therapy.
• Tell the patient to inform all of his health care providers (including his dentist) that he's receiving anticoagulants.
• If your patient is female and uses oral contraceptives, advise her to ask her gynecologist about alternative birth control measures.
• If your patient has a particularly high risk of emboli recurrence, teach him ways to prevent them — for example, by taking frequent walks and performing leg exercises. Explain that wearing support hose or antiembolism stockings will also help. Caution him against sitting with crossed legs or massaging his legs.
• Tell the patient to immediately report any calf pain or swelling. He should also report any signs or symptoms of recurrent pulmonary embolism, in-

Ensuring continued care for the patient with pulmonary embolism

Review the following teaching topics, referrals, and follow-up appointments to make sure that your patient is adequately prepared for discharge.

Teaching topics
Make sure that the following topics have been covered and that your patient's learning has been evaluated:
☐ causes, signs and symptoms, and associated risk factors
☐ guidelines for exercise and positioning
☐ anticoagulant therapy, including any adverse effects, and the need for careful monitoring
☐ need for and application of anti-embolism stockings
☐ signs and symptoms of recurring pulmonary embolism.

Referrals
Make sure that the patient has been provided with necessary referrals to:
☐ social services
☐ home health care agency.

Follow-up appointments
Make sure that the necessary follow-up appointments have been scheduled and that the patient has been notified:
☐ doctor
☐ diagnostic tests for reevaluation
☐ surgeon, if appropriate.

cluding dyspnea, tachypnea, chest pain (especially during deep breathing), apprehension, and a persistent nonproductive cough. (See *Ensuring continued care for the patient with pulmonary embolism*.)

EVALUATION

When evaluating the patient's response to your nursing care, gather reassessment data and compare this information with the patient outcomes specified in your plan of care.

Teaching and counseling
Begin by determining the effectiveness of your teaching and counseling. Consider the following questions:
• Does the patient understand the causes of pulmonary embolism and methods of preventing recurrent emboli?
• Does he understand all aspects of anticoagulant therapy, including its purpose, proper dosage, possible adverse effects and related precautions, and the importance of follow-up appointments?
• Is he using relaxation techniques to reduce his anxiety?
• Does he have a support system to help him cope?
• Can the patient describe the warning signs and symptoms that should be reported immediately to the doctor?
• Does he understand the dangers of bleeding and what precautions he can take to limit bleeding episodes?

Physical condition
Physical assessment and diagnostic tests will also help you evaluate the effectiveness of your care. If the patient complies with treatment, your ongoing assessment should indicate:
• ABG values within an acceptable range
• clear breath sounds
• comfortable breathing

- baseline LOC
- no evidence of cyanosis, cough, dyspnea, or hemoptysis
- baseline pulse rate and rhythm
- systolic pressure above 90 mm Hg (or an acceptable baseline value)
- no evidence of jugular vein distention
- CVP within normal limits (or acceptable baseline values)
- urine output of 30 ml/hour or more
- reduced pain as evidenced by a lack of muscular tension, grimacing, diaphoresis, and splinting
- fewer signs of anxiety.

Pulmonary edema

An abnormal fluid accumulation in the extravascular spaces of the lungs, pulmonary edema may occur as a chronic condition or develop quickly and become fatal rapidly. Acute pulmonary edema may progress to respiratory and metabolic acidosis with subsequent cardiac or respiratory arrest.

Causes

Cardiogenic pulmonary edema results from increased pulmonary artery wedge pressure (PAWP) due to left ventricular failure. This condition is brought on by arteriosclerosis, cardiomyopathies, hypertension, valvular heart disease, or fluid overload.

Noncardiogenic pulmonary edema results from increased capillary membrane permeability, usually related to adult respiratory distress syndrome.

Timesaving tip: You can quickly distinguish between cardiogenic and noncardiogenic pulmonary edema by checking the patient's PAWP. In cardiogenic pulmonary edema, fluid accumulates in the interstitial and alveolar spaces because of increased microvascular hydrostatic pressure, and *PAWP is high.* In noncardiogenic pulmonary edema, fluid accumulates because of increased capillary membrane permeability, and *PAWP is normal or low.*

This section will focus on cardiogenic pulmonary edema. (See *Looking at cardiogenic pulmonary edema.*) For information on noncardiogenic pulmonary edema, see "Adult Respiratory Distress Syndrome" in Chapter 4.

ASSESSMENT

The patient's medical history may provide information about predisposing factors. For example, the patient may have a history of chronic heart failure or a long-standing cardiomyopathy with deteriorating left ventricular function.

Health history

The patient may report a persistent cough, dyspnea on exertion, and cold symptoms. The patient with acute pulmonary edema may report a sudden onset of dyspnea that becomes severe quickly.

Timesaving tip: Characteristics of the patient's dyspnea can provide a quick insight into the severity of his heart disease. Typically, dyspnea becomes more disabling as heart failure progresses. Over time, it takes progressively less exertion to bring on dyspnea until symptoms occur even while the patient rests. In addition, patients with severe heart disease may complain of paroxysmal nocturnal dyspnea and orthopnea.

Physical examination

Physical findings will depend on the severity of the patient's pulmonary edema. In chronic, mild pulmonary edema, signs may be obscure. The patient may have difficulty breathing and exhibit some peripheral edema.

In acute pulmonary edema, signs and symptoms are unmistakable. The patient's breathing is visibly labored

Looking at cardiogenic pulmonary edema

In this type of pulmonary edema, the left ventricle's diminished function causes blood to pool in the left ventricle and atrium, eventually backing up into the pulmonary veins and capillaries. Rising capillary hydrostatic pressure pushes fluid into the interstitial spaces and alveoli.

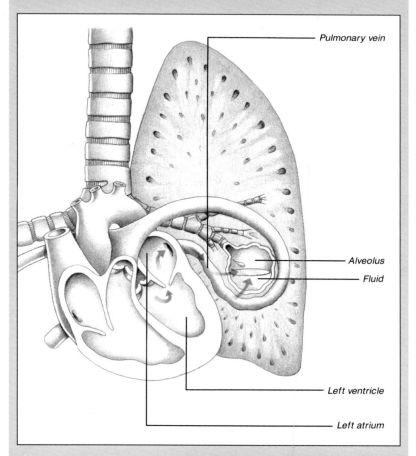

- Pulmonary vein
- Alveolus
- Fluid
- Left ventricle
- Left atrium

Assessment TimeSaver
Clinical findings in pulmonary edema

A quick review of signs and symptoms of the initial, advanced, and acute stages of cardiogenic pulmonary edema is presented below.

Initial stage
The initial stage results in pulmonary vascular congestion with the following signs and symptoms:
• anxiety
• restlessness
• tachypnea
• dyspnea
• orthopnea
• paroxysmal nocturnal dyspnea
• insomnia.

Advanced stage
The advanced stage results in interstitial pulmonary edema with the following signs and symptoms:
• tachycardia
• palpitations
• hypotension
• diaphoresis
• reduced lung compliance
• cough with frothy, often blood-tinged sputum
• pallor or cyanosis
• cool, mottled skin
• basilar crackles
• bronchial wheezing
• increased jugular vein distention
• diastolic gallop
• hypoxemia.

Acute stage
The acute stage results in alveolar pulmonary edema with the following signs and symptoms:
• decreased level of consciousness secondary to compromised cerebral perfusion
• pulmonary artery wedge pressure increased to 25 to 28 mm Hg
• tissue hypoxia with shock
• ventricular arrhythmias.

and rapid. He is quite apprehensive, restless, and unable to lie down. His cough may sound intense and produce frothy, bloody sputum. In advanced stages, the patient's level of consciousness (LOC) decreases and cyanosis is evident.

Palpation may reveal neck vein distention. In acute pulmonary edema, the patient's skin feels cool and moist or sweaty.

In chronic, mild pulmonary edema, auscultation of breath sounds may reveal a few crackles in the lung bases. In severe pulmonary edema, auscultation of breath sounds reveals crepitant crackles and wheezing throughout the lung fields.

Auscultation of heart sounds typically reveals an S_3 (diastolic gallop); however, this sound may be difficult to hear because of noisy respirations.

Signs of deterioration in the patient's condition include worsening tachycardia, reduced blood pressure, a thready pulse and, in advanced stages, diminished breath sounds. (See *Clinical findings in pulmonary edema.*)

Diagnostic test results
• Arterial blood gas (ABG) analysis usually shows decreased partial pressure of oxygen in arterial blood (PaO_2), indicating hypoxia. Partial pressure of carbon dioxide in arterial blood ($PaCO_2$) is variable. Results may also identify metabolic acidosis.
• Chest X-rays show diffuse haziness of the lung fields and may show cardiomegaly and pleural effusion.
• Pulse oximetry may reveal decreasing arterial oxygen saturation (SaO_2) levels.
• Pulmonary artery catheterization identifies left ventricular failure (indicated by an elevated PAWP).

NURSING DIAGNOSIS

Common nursing diagnoses for a patient with pulmonary edema include:
• Decreased cardiac output related to reduced stroke volume due to a mechanical, structural, or electrophysiologic cardiac disorder
• Impaired gas exchange related to ventilation-perfusion mismatch from pulmonary congestion
• Fluid volume excess related to pooling of blood in the pulmonary circulation and, possibly, the vena cava and systemic circulation
• Activity intolerance related to impaired gas exchange and associated reduced cardiac output
• Knowledge deficit related to the disorder and its treatment
• Anxiety related to pulmonary edema, respiratory distress, and fear of death.

PLANNING

Based on the nursing diagnosis *decreased cardiac output,* develop appropriate patient outcomes. For example, your patient will:
• achieve a systolic blood pressure of 90 mm Hg or higher
• achieve a heart rate of 60 to 100 beats/minute
• achieve acceptable (or maintain baseline) values for PAWP and central venous pressure (CVP)
• maintain baseline LOC
• experience no dizziness, syncope, arrhythmias, or chest pain
• exhibit warm, dry skin.

Based on the nursing diagnosis *impaired gas exchange,* develop appropriate patient outcomes. For example, your patient will:
• achieve PaO_2 within an acceptable range
• achieve a $PaCO_2$ between 35 and 45 mm Hg (or an acceptable baseline value)

• demonstrate clear breath sounds (or acceptable baseline sounds).

Based on the nursing diagnosis *fluid volume excess,* develop appropriate patient outcomes. For example, your patient will:
• maintain a daily output that exceeds intake until heart failure is resolved
• maintain a urine output of more than 30 ml/hour
• achieve and maintain baseline (or desired) weight
• exhibit acceptable, stable CVP and PAWP (if warranted) values (or acceptable baseline values)
• demonstrate clear breath sounds (or acceptable baseline sounds)
• maintain a respiratory rate of 12 to 20 breaths/minute.

Based on the nursing diagnosis *activity intolerance,* develop appropriate patient outcomes. For example, your patient will:
• identify activity limitations
• perform regular physical activity within his ability
• state that his tolerance for activity is at or approaching baseline
• plan rest periods each day
• demonstrate techniques for conserving energy while performing activities of daily living
• seek assistance with activities that produce fatigue.

Based on the nursing diagnosis *knowledge deficit,* develop appropriate patient outcomes. For example, your patient will:
• acknowledge all dietary restrictions such as sodium and fluid restrictions
• describe the prescribed medication regimen, including any adverse effects and preventive measures
• identify necessary lifestyle modifications and constructive coping mechanisms
• describe the signs and symptoms that require immediate intervention
• acknowledge the importance of attending all follow-up appointments.

Treatments

Medical care of the patient with pulmonary edema

Treatment for pulmonary edema focuses on reducing extravascular fluid, improving gas exchange and myocardial function and, when possible, correcting the underlying disorder. Treatment includes:

• oxygen therapy consisting of high concentrations of oxygen titrated to the patient's need. (Typically, the patient with pulmonary edema cannot tolerate a face mask.)

• a bronchodilator, such as aminophylline, to decrease bronchospasm and enhance myocardial contractility

• diuretics, such as furosemide, ethacrynic acid, or bumetanide, to increase urine output, thereby reducing circulatory blood volume and helping mobilize extravascular fluid

• mechanical ventilation, if the patient's arterial oxygen levels remain too low despite other therapeutic interventions. Mechanical ventilation can enhance arterial oxygenation and ventilation, improving the patient's acid-base balance. Mechanical ventilation with positive end-expiratory pressure is used to increase the functional residual capacity to improve oxygenation.

Treating myocardial dysfunction
Drugs used to address myocardial dysfunction include:

• positive inotropic agents, such as digitalis glycosides, dopamine, dobutamine, or amrinone, to enhance contractility

• antiarrhythmics, such as lidocaine, quinidine, procainamide, or calcium channel blockers, to address arrhythmias that may interfere with maintaining adequate cardiac output

• an arterial vasodilator, such as nitroprusside, to reduce peripheral vascular resistance, preload, and afterload

• morphine to dilate the systemic venous bed, thus promoting blood flow from the pulmonary circulation to the periphery. Morphine may also help reduce the patient's anxiety and dyspnea.

Treating acute pulmonary edema
Interventions used as emergency measures in cases of acute pulmonary edema include:

• oxygen therapy with mechanical ventilation, if necessary, to keep the partial pressure of oxygen in arterial blood above 60 mm Hg

• administration of diuretics and inotropics, as prescribed.

Based on the nursing diagnosis *anxiety*, develop appropriate patient outcomes. For example, your patient will:
• state that he feels less anxious about his illness
• exhibit fewer symptoms of anxiety or none at all.

IMPLEMENTATION

Treatment for pulmonary embolism includes drug therapy during the acute phase and then bed rest and activity restrictions. (See *Medical care of the patient with pulmonary edema.*)

Nursing interventions
Focus your nursing care on helping improve the patient's activity tolerance,

reducing his anxiety, and teaching him about his illness and the methods of treatment.

Acute care

• Assess the patient's airway, breathing, and circulation, and secure the airway.

• Administer supplemental oxygen to help the patient breathe more easily.

• Place the patient in high Fowler's position. In severe cases (and whenever possible), the patient should be sitting upright with his legs dangling freely.

• Establish an I.V. line for administration of prescribed medication. A central line may be warranted for monitoring and for administering medications.

• Insert an indwelling urinary catheter.

• Obtain vital signs and reassess them frequently.

Timesaving tip: Whenever possible, use an automatic cuff to monitor the patient's blood pressure.

• Anticipate assisting the doctor with insertion of an arterial line to monitor blood pressure and obtain blood samples.

• Draw blood for ABG analysis.

• Attach a pulse oximeter.

• Start continuous cardiac monitoring.

• Obtain a 12-lead electrocardiogram and a portable chest X-ray.

• Administer prescribed medications and note the patient's response. For example, about 20 minutes after giving a bolus injection of furosemide, tachypnea should decrease, and PaO_2 and urine output should increase. (Keep in mind, however, that these changes may take longer than 20 minutes to observe because the patient's left ventricle pumps ineffectively.)

• If morphine is administered, assess the patient carefully for hypoventilation. (Morphine may be reserved for use with intubated patients.)

• Anticipate giving vasodilators, such as I.V. nitroglycerin, if the patient responds poorly to oxygen and the first dose of a diuretic.

• Continue to monitor the patient's respiratory rate, pulse, and blood pressure, especially when changing the rate of drug administration.

• If the patient's systolic pressure falls below 90 mm Hg, administer inotropic drugs. Expect to administer dobutamine and dopamine in emergencies. *Monitor the patient carefully because both drugs can cause arrhythmias.*

Timesaving tip: Because dobutamine and dopamine are compatible, use a piggyback system to give them simultaneously through the same I.V. site.

• Carefully monitor arterial blood pressure and other hemodynamic indices, especially when amrinone, a powerful inotropic agent, is administered (usually short-term). Watch for adverse GI effects.

• If a digitalis glycoside is administered, monitor serum levels and observe the patient for signs of toxicity. Monitor serum potassium levels because hypokalemic patients are more likely to develop digitalis toxicity. Anticipate that this drug will be used for long-term therapy in chronic heart failure.

• Obtain a baseline weight.

• Help the patient relax to promote oxygenation, control bronchospasm, and enhance myocardial contractility.

• Stay with the patient and provide the calmest possible setting. Give him brief, clear explanations of the activities around him. Help him identify ways to cope with his anxiety. Provide emotional support to his family as well.

• Expect to initiate hemodynamic monitoring if the patient develops cardiogenic shock, responds poorly to treatment, or hasn't had the cause of his pulmonary edema identified. If the doctor inserts a pulmonary artery (PA) catheter, monitor PAWP, pulmonary artery diastolic pressure (PADP), and cardiac output. The goal is to maintain PAWP at 20 mm Hg or lower.

Timesaving tip: To avoid losing time when treating a patient with multiple I.V. and pressure-monitoring lines, color-code each line. For example, use a piece of red tape to label arterial lines, green tape to label PA catheter lines, yellow tape to label central venous catheter lines, and different colors for each medication line. On these tapes, note the medication being infused to help prevent drug incompatibility.

• Increasing acidosis, confusion, and a decreasing LOC are signs of advancing pulmonary edema. If these signs occur, be prepared to assist with intubation and mechanical ventilation. Positive end-expiratory pressure may be beneficial. If necessary, resuscitate the patient.

• Continue to assess the patient's condition frequently and document his response to treatment. Monitor ABG levels and pulse oximetry values, oral and I.V. fluid intake, and urine output. If the patient has a PA catheter, monitor PADP and PAWP as well. Check the cardiac monitor often. Report changes immediately.

• Monitor the patient for electrolyte depletion and complications of oxygen therapy (such as oxygen toxicity) and mechanical ventilation (such as pneumothorax or decreased cardiac output).

• If the patient can't clear his airway, provide suctioning to prevent further hypoxia.

Ongoing care
• Monitor ABG levels to maintain PaO_2 at 80 mm Hg or above and $PaCO_2$ at 35 to 45 mm Hg with a normal pH. Also, monitor SaO_2 to maintain a value above 95%.

• When the patient's condition stabilizes, monitor cardiopulmonary status every 2 to 4 hours or more frequently.

Assess blood pressure, apical and radial pulse rates and rhythms, respiratory rate, heart and breath sounds, and skin color.

• Monitor intake and output. Obtain daily weights. For consistency, weigh the patient at the same time each day on the same scale; he should also wear the same amount of clothing.

• Administer prescribed medications.

• Organize the patient's activities to maximize rest periods.

• If prescribed, help the patient adjust to fluid restrictions and explain their importance.

• Apply antiembolism stockings if prescribed.

• Report changes in the patient's condition immediately.

• Strictly enforce bed rest.

• Help the patient gradually increase his level of activity as his condition warrants.

Patient teaching
• Urge the patient to comply with the prescribed medication regimen to avoid recurrence of pulmonary edema.

• Explain all procedures to the patient and his family.

• Describe the early signs of fluid overload and emphasize the need to report them.

• Explain the reasons for sodium restrictions, and give the patient a list of high-sodium foods and drugs.

• Teach the patient about all prescribed medications and their possible adverse effects. Stress the importance of taking medications exactly as prescribed. Help simplify the drug regimen by suggesting that the patient write a schedule for medications. Recommend that he use a pillbox, which may allow him to organize up to one week's medications at a time. Suggest using an alarm clock to help take medications on time.

• If digitalis glycosides are prescribed, teach him how to monitor his pulse

Discharge TimeSaver

Ensuring continued care for the patient with pulmonary edema

Review the following teaching topics, referrals, and follow-up appointments to make sure that your patient is adequately prepared for discharge.

Teaching topics
Make sure that the following topics have been covered and that your patient's learning has been evaluated:
□ explanation of pulmonary edema, including its causes, symptoms, and complications
□ guidelines for rest and activity
□ medications, including dosage and possible adverse effects and preventive measures
□ sodium and fluid restrictions, as warranted
□ warning signs and symptoms that must be reported immediately, such as weight gain
□ importance of measuring weight daily (at the same time, on the same scale, and in similar clothing) and recording the results
□ prevention and detection of respiratory infection
□ sources of information and support.

Referrals
Make sure that the patient has been provided with necessary referrals to:
□ home health care agency
□ dietitian as needed.

Follow-up appointments
Make sure that the necessary follow-up appointments have been scheduled and that the patient has been notified:
□ doctor
□ diagnostic tests for reevaluation.

rate and warn him to report signs of toxicity. Encourage him to eat potassium-rich foods to reduce his risk of toxicity and cardiac arrhythmias.
• If a vasodilator is prescribed, explain the signs of hypotension and emphasize the need to refrain from drinking alcohol.
• Stress the need for regular checkups.
• Provide activity guidelines that coincide with the patient's cardiopulmonary status. Advise him to stay active but to avoid exhaustion.
• Encourage physical activity, such as walking, but suggest that he begin gradually. Consider his interests and current limitations when suggesting activities.
• Explain that he should plan most activities for the morning and include frequent rest periods throughout the day.
• Teach the patient techniques for simplifying work and conserving energy.

Help the patient delegate tasks that are too taxing to family and friends.
• Teach the patient relaxation techniques to help reduce anxiety.
• Suggest that he talk with his doctor about pneumonia and influenza vaccinations.
• Discuss sources of information and support. If appropriate, refer the patient to the local chapter of the American Heart Association or American Lung Association. (See *Ensuring continued care for the patient with pulmonary edema*.)

EVALUATION

When evaluating the patient's response to your nursing care, gather reassessment data and compare this information with the patient outcomes specified in your plan of care.

Teaching and counseling

Begin by evaluating the effectiveness of your teaching. Consider the following questions:

• Does the patient understand his disorder and its underlying causes?
• Does he understand sodium and fluid restrictions? Does he appear willing to comply with them?
• Can he describe the regimen of prescribed medications, including measures to avoid possible adverse effects?
• Does he appear willing to adhere to all prescribed treatments and lifestyle modifications?
• Can he state the signs and symptoms that require immediate intervention?
• Does he practice energy conservation techniques and plan daily rest periods?
• Does he identify activity limitations?
• Is he willing to seek assistance with tasks too taxing for his cardiopulmonary status?
• Does he appear less anxious?
• Has he stated his intention to attend all follow-up appointments?

Physical condition

Physical assessment and diagnostic tests will also help you evaluate the effectiveness of your care. If the patient complies with treatment, your ongoing assessment should indicate:

• CVP and PAWP (if warranted) values within acceptable limits (or at baseline) and stable
• heart rate of 60 to 100 beats/minute
• systolic pressure above 90 mm Hg
• freedom from dizziness, arrhythmias, chest pain, and cough
• warm, dry skin
• clear breath sounds (or acceptable baseline sounds)
• ABG levels within acceptable limits
• weight that is stable and has returned to baseline (or the target weight)
• unlabored respirations of 12 to 20 breaths/minute

• increased tolerance for physical activity.

Cor pulmonale

Cor pulmonale occurs in the final stages of chronic disorders that affect lung function or structure. In this disorder, pulmonary hypertension causes right ventricular hypertrophy and dilation and, occasionally, right ventricular failure. Because cor pulmonale accompanies late-stage irreversible pulmonary disease, the prognosis is poor. In addition to failure of both ventricles, other possible complications include hepatomegaly, edema, ascites, and pleural effusion. When polycythemia is present, cor pulmonale also increases a patient's risk of thromboembolism. (See *Understanding cor pulmonale.*)

Causes

The most common cause of cor pulmonale is chronic obstructive pulmonary disease (COPD). Other possible causes include:

• pulmonary diseases affecting airways, such as bronchial asthma
• disorders affecting the pulmonary parenchyma, such as pulmonary fibrosis, pneumoconiosis, cystic fibrosis, periarteritis nodosa, and tuberculosis
• vascular diseases, such as vasculitis, pulmonary embolism, or external vascular obstruction by a tumor or aneurysm
• chest wall abnormalities, including thoracic deformities
• conditions associated with obesity or living at high altitudes
• neuromuscular disorders, such as muscular dystrophy and poliomyelitis.

ASSESSMENT

Your assessment of a patient with cor pulmonale should include a thorough

Understanding cor pulmonale

In cor pulmonale, the heart labors under an increased workload caused by pulmonary hypertension. Normally, because of the low resistance in pulmonary blood vessels, the pulmonary vascular circuit is a low-pressure system. Pulmonary hypertension occurs when resting systolic pulmonary artery pressure (PAP) rises above 30 mm Hg and mean PAP rises above 18 mm Hg.

In an attempt to compensate, the right ventricle must exert more pressure to force blood through the pulmonary arteries. The additional workload leads to right ventricular hypertrophy. Eventually the compensatory mechanism begins to fail and an increasing amount of blood remains in the right ventricle at the end of diastole, causing right ventricular dilation. In chronic disease, right ventricular dilation may lead to right ventricular failure.

Signs and symptoms develop as right ventricular pressure increases, causing a rise in right atrial pressure and systemic venous congestion.

In response to hypoxemia already present with chronic obstructive pulmonary disease, the bone marrow produces more red blood cells, resulting in polycythemia. Increased blood viscosity may increase the workload of both ventricles, contributing further to heart failure.

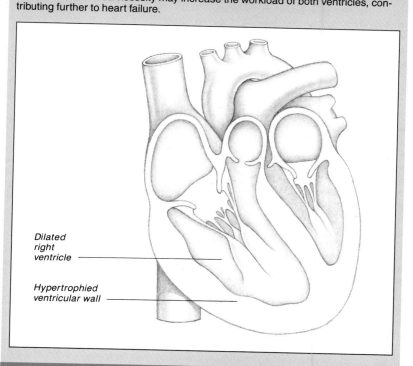

Dilated right ventricle

Hypertrophied ventricular wall

health history and physical examination, supported by a review of diagnostic test results.

Health history
As long as his heart is able to compensate for pulmonary hypertension, the patient with cor pulmonale may only report symptoms of the underlying disorder. Early complaints may include a chronic productive cough, dyspnea on exertion, wheezing, fatigue, and weakness. As cor pulmonale progresses, the patient may also report dyspnea at rest, tachypnea, orthopnea, dependent edema, weakness, and discomfort in the right upper quadrant of the chest.

Physical examination
Inspection may reveal dependent edema, distended neck veins, drowsiness, or changes in the patient's level of consciousness (LOC). Palpation may reveal tachycardia, a weak pulse, an enlarged and tender liver, hepatojugular reflux, and a prominent left parasternal lift. (See *Assessing for hepatojugular reflux.*)

Auscultation of the patient's breath sounds may provide information on the underlying pulmonary disorder. For example, if he has COPD, you may detect crackles, rhonchi, and diminished breath sounds.

When auscultating heart sounds, you may hear an S_3 (ventricular gallop) and a loud pulmonic component of S_2, signifying right ventricular failure.

Timesaving tip: To quickly check for an S_3, place the patient in the supine position and listen at the left sternal border of the fourth or fifth intercostal space.

If the patient has tricuspid insufficiency, you'll hear a pansystolic murmur at the lower left sternal border. The murmur's intensity increases when the patient inhales (distinguishing it from a murmur caused by mitral valve disease). At the left sternal border or over the epigastrium, you may hear an early right ventricular murmur that intensifies on inspiration. You may also hear a systolic pulmonary ejection sound. The presence of right ventricular murmur and systolic pulmonary ejection sound may indicate right ventricular failure.

Diagnostic test results
• Pulmonary artery catheterization reveals increased right ventricular pressure and increased pulmonary artery pressure (PAP) due to increased pulmonary vascular resistance. Both systolic pressures will be greater than 30 mm Hg. Pulmonary artery diastolic pressure will be above 15 mm Hg.
• Echocardiography or angiography shows enlargement of the right ventricle.
• Chest X-rays reveal enlargement of the main pulmonary artery and right ventricle.
• Arterial blood gas (ABG) analysis detects a decreased partial pressure of oxygen in arterial blood (PaO_2). PaO_2 is usually below 70 mm Hg and never above 90 mm Hg. Partial pressure of carbon dioxide in arterial blood ($PaCO_2$) may be variable.
• Electrocardiography (ECG) may indicate arrhythmias, such as premature atrial and ventricular contractions and atrial fibrillation during severe hypoxia. The patient's ECG may also show right bundle-branch block, right axis deviation, right ventricular hypertrophy, and prominent P waves and an inverted T wave in right precordial leads.
• Pulmonary function tests reflect the underlying pulmonary disease.
• Hematocrit is typically greater than 50%.
• Serum hepatic enzyme results show elevated levels of aspartate aminotransferase (formerly SGOT) with hepatic congestion and decreased liver function.

• Serum bilirubin level may be elevated if liver dysfunction and hepatomegaly are present.

NURSING DIAGNOSIS

Common nursing diagnoses for a patient with cor pulmonale include:
• Decreased cardiac output related to increased pulmonary vascular resistance
• Impaired gas exchange related to the underlying disorder
• Activity intolerance related to decreased cardiac output due to hypoxemic pulmonary disease
• Fluid volume excess related to right ventricular failure
• Knowledge deficit related to treatment of cor pulmonale and necessary lifestyle changes.

PLANNING

Focus your plan of care on reducing the patient's hypoxemia, increasing his exercise tolerance and, when possible, correcting the underlying condition.

Based on the nursing diagnosis *decreased cardiac output,* develop appropriate patient outcomes. For example, your patient will:
• maintain vital signs within specified limits
• exhibit baseline or reduced arrhythmias while at rest or during increased physical activity
• perform activities to tolerance levels
• maintain central venous pressure (CVP), pulmonary artery wedge pressure (PAWP), and PAP within specified limits.

Based on the nursing diagnosis *impaired gas exchange,* develop appropriate patient outcomes. For example, your patient will:
• maintain PaO_2 and $PaCO_2$ within specified limits
• maintain baseline LOC.

Assessment TimeSaver

Assessing for hepatojugular reflux

With the patient seated at a 30- to 45-degree angle, compress the abdomen over the liver for approximately 30 seconds while observing for an increase in jugular vein distention.

Significance of findings
An increase in jugular vein distention indicates hepatojugular reflux, a possible sign of right ventricular failure.

Abdominal compression increases venous blood flow and raises venous pressure. In a patient with right ventricular failure, the heart cannot compensate for this change. Instead, the compression increases the forward flow of blood to the right atrium, elevating pressure in (and distending) the jugular veins.

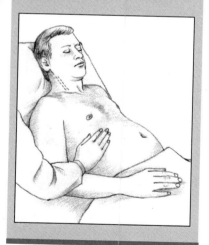

Based on the nursing diagnosis *activity intolerance,* develop appropriate patient outcomes. For example, your patient will:
• demonstrate a pulse rate during activity that's no more than 20 beats above baseline

• demonstrate a pulse rate that returns to baseline 5 minutes after activity

• demonstrate a respiratory rate that returns to baseline 5 to 10 minutes after activity

• demonstrate increased activity tolerance.

Based on the nursing diagnosis *fluid volume excess,* develop appropriate patient outcomes. For example, your patient will:

• maintain fluid intake and output within established limits

• maintain electrolyte levels within established limits

• maintain body weight within established limits

• maintain skin that is intact and free of infection.

Based on the nursing diagnosis *knowledge deficit,* develop appropriate patient outcomes. For example, your patient will:

• show understanding of a medication regimen, including possible adverse effects and precautions

• demonstrate how to use necessary equipment

• demonstrate how to perform recommended breathing exercises

• develop a plan for daily activities with rest periods

• express understanding of the need to modify diet and fluid intake

• express skill at identifying signs and symptoms of fluid and electrolyte imbalance and hypoxemia

• identify measures to prevent respiratory infection.

IMPLEMENTATION

Treatments seek to reduce hypoxemia, increase exercise tolerance and, when possible, correct the underlying condition. (See *Medical care of the patient with cor pulmonale.*)

Nursing interventions

Direct your nursing care toward providing respiratory support and helping the patient adjust to lifestyle changes and home care measures.

• Administer oxygen therapy, as directed.

• For patients with COPD, teach pursed-lip breathing exercises. Encourage the patient to rinse his mouth after receiving inhalation medications (to remove drug from the mouth).

• Watch for signs of respiratory failure (a change in pulse rate; deep, labored respirations; increased fatigue on exertion), and measure ABG levels if these signs occur.

• Provide bed rest during acute episodes.

• Plan care activities to avoid patient fatigue, and assist your patient with daily care needs.

• When the patient's condition permits, encourage activity to tolerance level. Identify and minimize factors that decrease the patient's activity tolerance.

• Listen to the patient's fears and concerns about his illness. Remain with him when he feels severe stress and anxiety. Encourage him to identify actions and care measures that promote comfort and relaxation. Include him in care-related decisions whenever possible.

• Plan a nutritious diet with the patient and a staff dietitian. Because the patient may tire easily, provide small, frequent feedings rather than three full meals. Avoid scheduling respiratory treatments immediately before or after meals.

• Assess the patient's fluid status by monitoring his intake and output, recording his daily body weight, and checking for evidence of dependent edema.

• If prescribed, limit the patient's fluid intake to 1,000 to 2,000 ml daily and provide a low-sodium diet. Explain the

Treatments

Medical care of the patient with cor pulmonale

Treatment for cor pulmonale includes drug therapy, oxygen therapy, and supportive measures.

Drug therapy
The following drugs may be prescribed for the patient with cor pulmonale:
• digitalis glycosides (digoxin) to increase cardiac output
• vasodilators, such as diazoxide, nitroprusside, or nitrates, and calcium channel blockers to reduce both pulmonary vasoconstriction and peripheral vascular resistance
• a diuretic such as furosemide to reduce edema
• antibiotics for an underlying respiratory tract infection. (Usually, sputum culture and sensitivity tests determine which antibiotic the patient receives.)

Oxygen therapy
The patient may need oxygen administered by mask or nasal cannula in concentrations ranging from 24% to 40%, depending on levels of partial pressure of oxygen in arterial blood. Relief of hypoxemia will decrease pulmonary

vascular resistance. In acute disease, therapy may also include mechanical ventilation.

Supportive measures
The patient may benefit from enforced bed rest, a low-sodium diet, and restricted fluid intake.

Additional measures
Occasionally, the patient with cor pulmonale may require a phlebotomy to decrease red blood cell mass. Small doses of an anticoagulant such as heparin can decrease the risk of thromboembolism.

Depending on the underlying cause, some treatment variations may be indicated. For example, the patient may need a tracheotomy if he has an upper airway obstruction. Or he may require corticosteroids if he has vasculitis or an autoimmune disorder.

need to restrict fluids, especially if the patient has underlying COPD. (Patients with COPD who don't have cor pulmonale are encouraged to drink up to 10 glasses of water daily.)
• Monitor serum potassium levels closely if the patient takes a diuretic. Low serum potassium levels can increase the risk of arrhythmias associated with digitalis therapy.
• Be alert for signs of digitalis toxicity, such as anorexia, nausea, vomiting, and seeing a yellow halo around an object.
• Monitor for cardiac arrhythmias.
• Watch for signs of thromboembolism.

• Reposition the bedridden patient often to prevent atelectasis.
• Consult with the social services department regarding home care services and oxygen equipment, if necessary.
• As needed, arrange for follow-up examinations.

Patient teaching
• Before discharge, make sure that the patient understands the need to maintain a low-sodium diet, weigh himself daily, and immediately report increased dependent edema. (See *Detecting peripheral edema*, page 214.)
• Instruct the patient to schedule frequent rest periods. Help the patient and

Teaching TimeSaver
Detecting peripheral edema

Teach the patient the following techniques for detecting peripheral edema:
• Tell him to press the skin over his shins with one finger, holding it for 1 to 2 seconds. Then check for a finger impression.
• Teach him to observe for puffiness in his hands, ankles, or feet or for marks from the elastic in socks or from rings on his fingers.
• Instruct him to weigh himself every day at about the same time, using the same scale and wearing the same amount of clothing. He should immediately report a weight gain of 2 to 3 lb (0.9 to 1.4 kg) over 1 to 2 days to his doctor.

his caregiver develop an activity schedule that enables the patient to function at maximum activity tolerance.
• Teach the patient and his family how to monitor pulse rate during activities, how to recognize the need for oxygen if prescribed, and how to use oxygen equipment properly.
• Because pulmonary infection usually exacerbates cor pulmonale (and COPD), advise the patient to watch for and immediately report early signs of infection, such as increased sputum production, a change in sputum color, increased coughing or wheezing, chest pain, fever, or tightness in the chest. Tell the patient to avoid crowds and people known to have infections, especially during influenza seasons.
• Urge the patient to discuss influenza and pneumonia immunizations with the doctor. Assist him to obtain the vaccinations, if appropriate.

• Warn the patient to avoid using non-prescription medications that cause drowsiness because they may depress respiratory drive.
• Teach him to check his radial pulse before taking digoxin or any other digitalis glycoside. Instruct him to notify the doctor if his pulse rate changes.
• Instruct the patient to add potassium-rich foods to his daily diet if he takes a potassium-wasting diuretic.
• If appropriate, discuss smoking cessation programs with the patient. Encourage him to quit smoking.
• Provide the patient and his family with additional sources of information and support, such as the local chapter of the American Lung Association. (See *Ensuring continued care for the patient with cor pulmonale.*)

EVALUATION

When evaluating the patient's response to your nursing care, gather reassessment data and compare this information with the patient outcomes specified in your plan of care. During your evaluation, remember that chronic cor pulmonale often signifies late-stage pulmonary disease and that the prognosis is often poor.

Teaching and counseling
Begin by determining the effectiveness of your teaching and counseling. Consider the following questions:
• Does the patient understand the importance of adopting a low-sodium diet?
• Is he willing to incorporate frequent rest periods into his daily schedule?
• Does he understand the need to report increased dependent edema?
• Does he plan to weigh himself daily?
• Can he demonstrate how to measure his pulse?
• Does he know the early signs of infection and the importance of reporting these signs immediately?

Ensuring continued care for the patient with cor pulmonale

Review the following teaching topics, referrals, and follow-up appointments to ensure that your patient is adequately prepared for discharge.

Teaching topics

Make sure that the following topics have been covered and that your patient's learning has been evaluated:
☐ explanation of cor pulmonale, including its causes, symptoms, and potential complications
☐ activity and rest guidelines
☐ medication therapy, including adverse effects and precautions
☐ dietary modifications and fluid restrictions
☐ self-assessment for excessive fluid retention
☐ warning signs and symptoms of deteriorating condition
☐ use of oxygen and suction equipment, if warranted
☐ breathing exercises
☐ smoking cessation
☐ prevention and detection of respiratory infection

☐ sources of information and support.

Referrals

Make sure that the patient has been provided with necessary referrals to:
☐ social services for consultation regarding equipment, medications, and home health care visits
☐ home health care agency
☐ medical equipment supplier for home oxygen
☐ occupational therapist for energy conservation techniques.

Follow-up appointments

Make sure that the necessary follow-up appointments have been scheduled and that the patient has been notified:
☐ doctor
☐ diagnostic tests for reevaluation.

• Does he understand his medication regimen, including possible adverse effects and precautions?

• Does he understand the importance of avoiding nonprescription drugs?

• Can he identify signs and symptoms of fluid and electrolyte imbalance and hypoxemia?

• Can he describe measures to prevent respiratory infection?

• Have the patient and his caregiver expressed plans to follow the prescribed treatment, to take measures to prevent complications, and to make necessary lifestyle changes?

• Have they successfully demonstrated how to manage respiratory equipment?

• Have they successfully demonstrated how to perform breathing exercises?

• Is the patient performing breathing exercises regularly?

• Is he planning to discuss obtaining appropriate immunizations and vaccinations with the doctor?

• If the patient was a smoker, has he quit or joined a smoking cessation program?

• Has he expressed fears and concerns about his illness?

Physical condition

A physical assessment and diagnostic tests will also help you evaluate the effectiveness of your care. Consider the following questions:

• Has the patient experienced an increase in arrhythmias during periods of rest or with increased activity?
• Is he able to perform activities to tolerance level?
• Does his pulse rate remain within 20 beats of baseline during activity? Does it return to baseline within 5 minutes after activity?
• Following activity, does his respiratory rate return to baseline within 5 to 10 minutes?
• Are his vital signs within specified limits?
• Is his LOC at baseline?
• Are CVP, PAWP, and PAP within specified limits?
• Are PaO_2 and $PaCO_2$ within specified limits?
• Is his fluid balance within an acceptable range? Are electrolyte levels within established limits?
• Is his skin intact and free of infection?
• Has he maintained body weight within established limits?

CHAPTER 8

Caring for patients with pulmonary infections

Pneumonia

Pneumonia is an acute infection of the lung parenchyma, typically accompanied by the accumulation of exudate in the bronchioles and alveoli. This disorder commonly results from a viral or bacterial infection or aspiration of a chemical irritant. Depending on the affected lung area, the infection is classified as bronchopneumonia (distal airways and alveoli), lobular pneumonia (part of a lobe), or lobar pneumonia (an entire lobe).

The prognosis is good for otherwise healthy individuals. However, infectious pneumonia most commonly occurs when one or more of the body's defense mechanisms is impaired. (See *Risk factors for pneumonia.*) Without proper treatment, pneumonia can lead to such life-threatening complications as septic shock, hypoxemia, and respiratory failure. The infection can spread within the patient's lungs or pleural space, causing a lung abscess or empyema. It may also spread to other parts of the body, causing bacteremia, endocarditis, pericarditis, or meningitis. Bacterial pneumonia is a leading cause of death in debilitated patients.

Causes

Pneumonia usually results from inhalation or aspiration of viruses, bacteria, *Mycoplasma,* fungi, or protozoa. It may also result from the hematogenous spread of bacteria within the body.

Pneumonia may occur secondary to initial lung damage, chest trauma, surgery, or specific systemic diseases. Pneumonia may also result from inhalation of foreign matter, such as vomitus or food particles, into the bronchi. This type of pneumonia is called aspiration pneumonia.

Prompt identification of the organism causing pneumonia helps to determine appropriate treatment, improves patient outcomes, and decreases the cost of treatment and length of stay in the hospital. The types of pneumonia that are most often acquired in the community include adenovirus, chicken pox, influenza, *Legionella,* measles, *Mycoplasma,* and *Streptococcus.* The types of pneumonia that are most often acquired in the hospital include *Klebsiella, Pseudomonas, Staphylococcus* and, in immunocompromised patients, *Legionella.* Patients with acquired immunodeficiency syndrome are at high risk for pneumonias — especially those caused by cytomegalovirus and *Pneumocystis carinii.* (See *Understanding types of pneumonias,* pages 220 to 224.)

ASSESSMENT

Focus your initial assessment on the major symptoms of pneumonia: chest pain, cough, sputum production, and chills. Then consider any associated complaints. Carefully review the patient's health history and physical examination findings. Include an assessment of risk factors for pneumonia. For a patient at risk for a hospital-acquired pneumonia, consider his environment to identify potential risk factors.

Health history

The patient may report pleuritic chest pain, cough, excessive sputum production, dyspnea, chills, fever, malaise, myalgia, and headache. If he has a viral infection, he may complain of GI problems, such as nausea or diarrhea.

Physical examination

During your inspection, the patient may be visibly shaking and appear flushed, dyspneic, anxious, and uncomfortable. If he is producing sputum, note its characteristics. Creamy yellow sputum suggests staphylococcal pneumonia; green sputum denotes pneumonia caused by a *Pseudomonas* organism; and sputum that looks like currant jelly indicates pneumonia caused by *Klebsiella*. If the sputum is clear, the patient doesn't have an infective process.

If hypoxemia is present, you may observe altered mentation (especially in elderly patients). The patient will exhibit cyanosis if hypoxemia is profound.

In advanced cases of pneumonia (all types), percussion of the affected area of the lung will reveal dullness. Auscultation may disclose crackles or rhonchi over the affected lung area. Commonly, bronchial breath sounds are present over areas of consolidation. Wheezing is uncommon. Both vocal and tactile fremitus is increased with lung consolidation. Measurement of vital signs typically reveals fever accompanied by tachycardia and tachypnea.

Diagnostic test results

The following tests may be used to confirm a diagnosis of pneumonia and identify its cause:

• Chest X-ray may reveal infiltrates.
• Gram stain and culture and sensitivity tests of sputum specimens may show acute inflammatory cells and may be used to help identify bacteria causing pneumonia.
• White blood cell (WBC) count may reveal leukocytosis in bacterial pneumonia; a normal or low WBC count may indicate viral or mycoplasmal pneumonia.
• Blood cultures may reveal bacteremia and thereby help determine the causative organism.
• Arterial blood gas (ABG) levels may vary, depending on the severity of the pneumonia and the underlying condition of the lung.
• Bronchoscopy, bronchoalveolar lavage, or transtracheal aspiration may be used to collect samples of respiratory secretions for culture or for the identification of causative factors.
• Samples of pleural fluid may be obtained for culture.
• Pulse oximetry may reveal a reduced arterial oxygen saturation (SaO_2) level.

Assessment TimeSaver

Risk factors for pneumonia

The following factors or conditions increase an individual's risk of developing pneumonia:
• elderly (over age 65)
• tracheostomy or nasogastric tube feedings
• chronic disease, such as cancer, chronic obstructive pulmonary disease, sickle cell disease, diabetes mellitus, heart disease, alcoholism, kidney disease, and liver disease
• immunosuppressive disorder or therapy
• upper abdominal or thoracic surgery
• impaired gag or swallowing reflex
• decreased level of consciousness
• exposure to noxious gases
• aspiration of substances
• atelectasis
• influenza
• prolonged bed rest
• smoking
• malnutrition
• poor oral hygiene.

NURSING DIAGNOSIS

Common nursing diagnoses for the patient with pneumonia include:
• Ineffective breathing pattern related to tachypnea, dyspnea, pleuritic pain, and hypoxemia
• Impaired gas exchange related to ventilation-perfusion mismatch secondary to increased pulmonary secretions and shunting

(Text continues on page 224.)

Understanding types of pneumonias

Cause	Signs and symptoms	Diagnostic test results	Treatment
Viral pneumonias			
Adenovirus Insidious onset; more often affecting young adults. Prognosis is good; usually clears with no residual effects; low mortality.	• Sore throat, fever, cough, chills, malaise, small amounts of mucoid sputum, retrosternal chest pain, anorexia, rhinitis, adenopathy, scattered crackles, rhonchi	• *Chest X-ray:* patchy distribution of pneumonia, more severe than indicated by physical examination • *White blood cell (WBC) count:* normal to slightly elevated	• Treat symptoms. • *Supportive:* rest, adequate hydration, nutrition
Chicken pox (varicella) Uncommon in children, but present in 30% of adults with varicella	• Characteristic rash, cough, dyspnea, cyanosis, tachypnea, pleuritic chest pain, hemoptysis and rhonchi 1 to 6 days after onset of rash	• *Chest X-ray:* shows more extensive pneumonia than indicated by physical examination, and bilateral, patchy, diffuse, nodular infiltrates • *Sputum analysis:* predominant mononuclear cells and characteristic intranuclear inclusion bodies	• *Supportive:* adequate hydration, oxygen therapy (for critically ill patients); acyclovir may be effective
Cytomegalovirus	• Difficult to distinguish from nonbacterial pneumonias • Fever, cough, shaking chills, dyspnea, cyanosis, weakness, diffuse crackles • In adults with healthy lung tissue, resembles mononucleosis and is generally benign; in neonates, occurs as devastating multisystemic infection; in immunocompromised patients, varies from clinically inapparent to fatal infection	• *Chest X-ray:* in early stages, variable patchy infiltrates; later, bilateral, nodular, and more predominant in lower lobes • Percutaneous aspiration of lung tissue, transbronchial biopsy, or open lung biopsy: typical intranuclear and cytoplasmic inclusions on microscopic examination; virus can be cultured from lung tissue	• *Supportive:* adequate hydration and nutrition, oxygen therapy, bed rest

Understanding types of pneumonias *(continued)*

Cause	Signs and symptoms	Diagnostic test results	Treatment
Viral pneumonias *(continued)*			
Influenza More common in elderly or debilitated patients. Prognosis is poor even with treatment; 50% mortality from cardiopulmonary collapse.	• Cough (initially nonproductive; later, purulent sputum), marked cyanosis, dyspnea, high fever, chills, substernal pain and discomfort, moist crackles, frontal headache, myalgia	• *Chest X-ray:* diffuse bilateral bronchopneumonia radiating from hilus • *WBC count:* normal to slightly elevated • *Sputum smear:* no specific organisms	• *Supportive:* for respiratory failure, endotracheal intubation and ventilator assistance; for fever, hypothermia blanket or antipyretics; for influenza A, amantadine
Measles (rubeola)	• Fever, dyspnea, cough, small amounts of sputum, coryza, rash, cervical adenopathy	• *Chest X-ray:* reticular infiltrates, sometimes with hilar lymph node enlargement • *Lung tissue specimen:* characteristic giant cells	• *Supportive:* bed rest, adequate hydration, antimicrobials; if necessary, assisted ventilation
Respiratory syncytial virus Most prevalent in infants and children; complete recovery in 1 to 3 weeks	• Listlessness, irritability, tachypnea with retraction of intercostal muscles, slight sputum production, fine moist crackles, fever, severe malaise and, possibly, cough or croup	• *Chest X-ray:* patchy bilateral consolidation • *WBC count:* normal to slightly elevated	• *Supportive:* humidified air, oxygen; antimicrobials commonly given until viral cause is confirmed; ribavirin by aerosol
Bacterial pneumonias			
Klebsiella	• Fever and recurrent chills; cough producing rusty, bloody, viscous sputum (currant jelly); cyanosis of lips and nail beds from hypoxemia; shallow, grunting respirations • More common among patients with chronic alcoholism, pulmonary disease, or diabetes; often acquired while in the hospital, but may be seen in the community	• *Chest X-ray:* typically (but not always) consolidation in the upper lobe that causes bulging of fissures • *WBC count:* elevated • *Sputum culture and Gram stain:* may show gram-negative cocci, *Klebsiella*	• *Antimicrobial therapy:* third-generation cephalosporin, such as cefotaxime, or an aminoglycoside (alternative)

(continued)

Understanding types of pneumonias *(continued)*

Cause	Signs and symptoms	Diagnostic test results	Treatment
Bacterial pneumonias *(continued)*			
Legionella pneumophila (Legionnaires' disease) Associated with contaminated water distribution systems	• Malaise, anorexia, headache, diarrhea, myalgia, followed by cough, dyspnea, chest pain, bradycardia, chills, fever higher than 102° F, (38.9° C), altered level of consciousness (LOC)	• *Chest X-ray:* reveals multilobar consolidation • *Direct immunofluorescent antibody staining* of sputum, bronchial washings or brushings, or pleural fluid may provide rapid diagnosis • *DNA probe:* newly available, fast, accurate • *Sputum culture:* identifies organism but takes much longer	• *Antimicrobial therapy:* erythromycin, rifampin
Pseudomonas aeruginosa Prognosis is poor; high mortality	• Productive cough with green, foul-smelling sputum; bradycardia; cyanosis; altered LOC • More common among hospitalized patients, especially those who are immunocompromised, are using respiratory equipment, or have tracheostomies	• *Chest X-ray:* reveals multiple infiltrates	• *Antimicrobial therapy:* may include penicillins (carbenicillin, ticarcillin) or aminoglycosides (gentamicin, tobramycin)
Staphylococcus	• Temperature of 102° to 104° F (40° C), recurrent shaking chills, bloody sputum, dyspnea, tachypnea, hypoxemia • Most often acquired during hospitalization • Should be suspected if the patient has cystic fibrosis or a viral illness, such as influenza or measles; is undergoing dialysis or surgery; or has a history of drug abuse	• *Chest X-ray:* multiple abscesses and infiltrates; frequently empyema • *WBC count:* elevated • *Sputum culture and Gram stain:* may show gram-positive staphylococci	• *Antimicrobial therapy:* nafcillin or oxacillin for 14 days if organism is penicillinase-producing • Vancomycin if organism is methicillin resistant • Chest tube drainage of empyema, if necessary

Understanding types of pneumonias *(continued)*

Cause	Signs and symptoms	Diagnostic test results	Treatment
Bacterial pneumonias *(continued)*			
Streptococcus (pneumococcal pneumonia) Most common of all pneumonias that are acquired outside the hospital	• Sudden onset of a shaking chill and sustained temperature of 102° to 104° F; tachypnea; shortness of breath; chest pain; often preceded by upper respiratory tract infection	• *Chest X-ray:* areas of consolidation, often lobar • *WBC count:* elevated • *Sputum culture:* may show gram-positive *Streptococcus pneumoniae*	• *Antimicrobial therapy:* penicillin G (erythromycin, if the patient is allergic to penicillin) for 7 to 10 days; therapy begins after taking culture specimens but before results are obtained.
Mycoplasmal pneumonia			
Mycoplasma pneumoniae Most common form of pneumonia acquired outside the hospital by young adults; also associated with mild respiratory infection in children	• Hacking cough (often unproductive), fever below 102° F, sore throat, headache, malaise	• *Chest X-ray:* reveals peripheral infiltrates • *Erythrocyte sedimentation rate:* elevated • *WBC count:* elevated • *Cold agglutinins:* may be positive, but test is not specific for this disease • *Complement fixation and culture of sputum:* confirm the diagnosis, but results are usually not available until after patient has recovered	• *Antimicrobial therapy:* erythromycin (recommended); doxycycline (alternative)
Protozoan pneumonia			
Pneumocystis carinii The incidence of *Pneumocystis carinii* pneumonia (PCP), an opportunistic infection, has increased significantly since the 1980s. Immunocompromised patients have the highest risk. PCP is especially prevalent in patients infected with human immunodeficiency virus; up to 90% of these patients contract PCP during their lifetime.	• Abrupt onset of symptoms; low fever, shortness of breath, and nonproductive cough may be accompanied by anorexia, fatigue, and weight loss; may progress to respiratory failure	• *Histologic tests:* demonstration of organism by staining of cells obtained from bronchoalveolar lavage or occasionally induced sputum • *Chest X-ray:* may show slowly progressive fluffy infiltrates and occasional nodular lesions or a spontaneous pneumothorax	• *Antimicrobial therapy:* Pentamidine or co-trimoxazole and corticosteroids in patients with acquired immunodeficiency syndrome • Pentamidine I.V. in patients with reaction to co-trimoxazole • Prednisone is added if patient is acutely ill or hypoxemic

(continued)

Understanding types of pneumonias *(continued)*

Cause	Signs and symptoms	Diagnostic test results	Treatment
Fungal pneumonias			
Aspergillus fumigatus (aspergillosis) ***Candida albicans*** (candidiasis) ***Histoplasma capsulatum*** (histoplasmosis) Most common in immunocompromised patients	• Persistent fever, dyspnea, tachypnea, cough, pleuritic chest pain, pleural friction rub	• *Chest X-ray:* may reveal nodular cavity formation • *Sputum smear:* may reveal a fungal organism; however, presence doesn't confirm diagnosis • *Needle or open-lung biopsy:* biopsy of lung tissue may be necessary to confirm a diagnosis	• *Antimicrobial therapy:* amphotericin B
Aspiration pneumonia (noninfectious)			
Aspiration of gastric or oropharyngeal contents into trachea and lungs	• Crackles, dyspnea, cyanosis, hypotension, tachycardia • Noncardiogenic pulmonary edema is possible if respiratory epithelium is damaged by contact with gastric acid	• *Chest X-ray:* location of areas of infiltrates varies according to position of patient at time of aspiration; diagnosis depends on area affected	• *Antimicrobial therapy:* used when there is evidence of bacterial infection; otherwise, anaerobic coverage may be started initially • *Supportive therapy:* oxygen therapy, suctioning, coughing, deep breathing, adequate hydration; I.V. corticosteroids may be used if patient has airway inflammation (wheezing, rhonchi)

• Ineffective airway clearance related to the production of thick sputum and the inability to mobilize secretions
• Pain related to excessive coughing and pleural inflammation
• Anxiety related to dyspnea
• Hyperthermia related to infection
• High risk for fluid volume deficit related to elevated body temperature
• Activity intolerance related to fatigue and dyspnea.

PLANNING

When caring for a patient with pneumonia, your goals are to control the patient's symptoms, avoid complications, and teach the patient about the disorder and its treatment.

Based on the nursing diagnosis *ineffective breathing pattern,* develop appropriate patient outcomes. For example, your patient will:
• achieve a respiratory rate within 5 breaths of the baseline rate

• demonstrate symmetrical chest expansion

• exhibit clear and bilaterally equal breath sounds (or a return to acceptable baseline breath sounds)

• state that he can breathe comfortably.

Based on the nursing diagnosis *impaired gas exchange*, develop appropriate patient outcomes. For example, your patient will:

• achieve a partial pressure of arterial oxygen of 80 to 100 mm Hg

• achieve a partial pressure of arterial carbon dioxide ($PaCO_2$) of 35 to 45 mm Hg (or return to an acceptable baseline value)

• achieve an SaO_2 of 93% to 97% (or return to an acceptable baseline value above 88%) and a pH of 7.35 to 7.45.

Based on the nursing diagnosis *ineffective airway clearance*, develop appropriate patient outcomes. For example, your patient will:

• produce a cough with thin, colorless mucus

• produce breath sounds that are clear during auscultation (or return to acceptable baseline breath sounds)

• achieve acceptable baseline ABG values.

Based on the nursing diagnosis *pain*, develop appropriate patient outcomes. For example, your patient will:

• report that his pain has subsided or stopped

• demonstrate increased comfort by no longer grimacing, holding his sides, or exhibiting muscular rigidity.

Based on the nursing diagnosis *anxiety*, develop appropriate patient outcomes. For example, your patient will:

• identify and use available support systems

• state that he feels less anxious

• exhibit a reduction in anxiety as evidenced by an improved ability to concentrate, a reduction in muscular tension, and normal autonomic activity.

Based on the nursing diagnosis *hyperthermia*, develop appropriate patient outcomes. For example, your patient will:

• maintain a body temperature within the normal range

• show no evidence of complications of hyperthermia

• state his willingness to take prescribed medications to eradicate the infection.

Based on the nursing diagnosis *high risk for fluid volume deficit*, develop appropriate patient outcomes. For example, your patient will:

• achieve fluid intake of 3,000 ml/day (if appropriate)

• maintain urine output of at least 30 ml/hour.

Based on the nursing diagnosis *activity intolerance*, develop appropriate patient outcomes. For example, your patient will:

• perform activities of daily living (ADLs) independently

• resume physical exercise gradually

• no longer experience undue fatigue or dyspnea after exertion

• demonstrate stable vital signs after exertion.

IMPLEMENTATION

Treatment for pneumonia focuses on minimizing the patient's discomfort and eradicating the infection. Typically, treatment involves medical interventions, such as drug therapy, and changes in lifestyle, such as bed rest, an increase in fluid intake, and dietary modifications. (See *Medical care of the patient with pneumonia*, page 226.)

Nursing interventions

• Obtain sputum specimens. Teach the patient how to produce a good sputum specimen. (See *Producing sputum specimens*, page 227.) Collect each specimen in a sterile container and deliver it

Treatments

Medical care of the patient with pneumonia

Medical care of the patient with pneumonia includes drug therapy and additional supportive measures.

Drug therapy

The most important initial intervention is to obtain a good quality sputum specimen. Specific drug therapy is chosen based on the organism that is identified. Initially, a broad-spectrum antibiotic is used to cover many potential organisms until a specific cause is identified. Although viral pneumonias are not affected by antibiotics, most patients are initially treated with antibiotics until the diagnosis is certain and it's clear that there is no complicating bacterial infection.

Antibiotic sensitivity studies are also obtained from the sputum culture to determine which antibiotic will be most effective for a specific organism. Organisms that are resistant to the usual antibiotic regimens are an increasing problem, particularly in immunocompromised patients who experience frequent infections and are given multiple courses of antibiotics. Because of a variety of possible causative organisms, therapy should be reevaluated early in the course of treatment — especially when treating immunocompromised patients, who have a high risk of serious infection.

Types of pneumonia and their common pharmacologic interventions include:

• streptococcal pneumonia: penicillin G (or erythromycin if the patient is allergic to penicillin)
• *Klebsiella pneumoniae* pneumonia: third-generation cephalosporin (treatment of choice); aminoglycoside (alternative)
• staphylococcal pneumonia: prompt treatment with nafcillin or oxacillin, vancomycin if organism is methicillin resistant

• *Legionella pneumophila* pneumonia: prompt treatment with erythromycin (rifampin may be given in conjunction with the erythromycin)
• *Mycoplasma pneumoniae* pneumonia: erythromycin or doxycycline (alternative)
• *Pneumocystis carinii* pneumonia: co-trimoxazole (treatment of choice); pentamidine (alternative); corticosteroids in patients with acquired immunodeficiency syndrome (may be added to treatment if the patient is acutely ill or hypoxemic)
• viral pneumonia: if influenza A virus is the cause, amantadine may be used; antivirals, such as acyclovir, may prove effective for some patients; otherwise, treatment focuses on symptoms, with antipyretics used for fever and analgesics for headache.

Supportive care

Treatment of all types of pneumonia also involves supportive care. Common interventions include:
• bed rest
• a high-calorie diet with foods that are easy to chew and swallow
• adequate fluid intake
• humidified oxygen therapy for hypoxemia
• bronchodilator therapy
• postural drainage and percussion to help mobilize secretions if patient has profuse secretions
• antitussives for cough
• analgesics to relieve pleuritic chest pain.

If the patient has severe pneumonia with respiratory failure, mechanical ventilation and, possibly, positive end-expiratory pressure are used to maintain adequate oxygenation.

promptly to the microbiology laboratory.

• Administer antibiotics parenterally, as prescribed, during the initial acute period. Afterward, administer oral antibiotics. Monitor the patient for any adverse reactions.

• Administer supplemental oxygen by Venturi mask or nasal cannula, as ordered, according to ABG levels. If the patient has an underlying chronic lung disease, carefully monitor his ABG levels and SaO_2. Watch for a rising $PaCO_2$ and decreasing Ph — signs of impending respiratory failure. If respiratory failure occurs, anticipate endotracheal intubation and mechanical ventilation.

• Maintain a patent airway. Encourage the patient to practice effective coughing and deep-breathing exercises at least every 2 hours. If necessary, use an incentive spirometer to promote effective breathing.

• If chest pain inhibits coughing, administer the ordered analgesic and teach the patient how to splint the painful area while coughing. Assess the patient's response to pain medication.

• Administer fluids. Unless contraindicated, administer oral fluids, parenteral fluids, or both, totaling 3,000 ml/day to prevent dehydration caused by fever and infection and to help liquefy secretions. Monitor the patient's intake and output.

• If auscultation reveals excessive secretions that are not being mobilized by coughing, perform postural drainage and percussion.

• If the patient has excessive secretions but is unable to cough effectively because of a weak cough or weak respiratory muscles, perform nasotracheal suctioning, as ordered. Before performing the procedure, always check the most current ABG results. If the patient is hypoxemic, be sure to hyperoxygenate before, during, and after suctioning. After coughing or suctioning, auscultate the patient's

Teaching TimeSaver
Producing sputum specimens

To teach a patient with suspected pulmonary infection how to produce a good sputum specimen, instruct him as follows:
• Explain that he needs to bring the sputum up from his lungs.
• Instruct him to inhale and exhale deeply three times, and then inhale quickly, cough forcefully, and expectorate into the sputum container.
• Make sure that he covers his nose and mouth with tissues when he coughs to avoid spraying organisms into the air.
• Allow him about 15 minutes to produce a specimen.
   If your patient can't expectorate sputum, a hypertonic saline aerosol mist may help him produce a good specimen. Instruct him to take several normal breaths of the mist, and then inhale deeply, cough, and expectorate. Remember, nasopharyngeal secretions and saliva aren't acceptable specimens.

breath sounds and note whether there is any improvement.

Timesaving tip: To dispose of a used suction catheter easily, quickly, and aseptically, wrap the catheter around your gloved hand, disconnect the catheter from the connecting tube, and then pull the glove off over the catheter. The catheter will be safely contained inside the disposable glove.

• Place the patient in semi-Fowler's position to make breathing easier. Help with hygienic needs during acute periods.

• If the patient can perform ADLs, encourage him to work slowly, rest often, and use supplemental oxygen if necessary for controlling hypoxemia during periods of physical exertion.

• After physical exertion, assess the patient's respiratory and pulse rates, respiratory effort, and use of accessory muscles. Note any evidence of cyanosis. Increase the patient's activity level gradually, based on your findings.

• Assess the patient's temperature at least every 4 hours. Administer antipyretics, as ordered. If the fever is excessive, assess the patient's level of consciousness and, if necessary, provide a hypothermia blanket.

• Provide a diet of soft foods that are high in calories and protein (to replenish calories and essential amino acids used to fight infection). If necessary, supplement oral feedings with nasogastric (NG) tube feedings or parenteral nutrition.

• Prevent aspiration during NG tube feedings by elevating the patient's head, checking the tube position for gastric retention, and administering the feeding slowly. Giving large volumes may cause vomiting.

• Control the spread of infection by disposing of secretions properly. Provide the patient with disposable tissues and explain the importance of using them to cover his nose and mouth when he sneezes or coughs. Tape a lined bag to the side of the bed for used tissues.

• Provide the patient with a quiet, calm environment and encourage frequent rest periods. Make sure that he has access to appropriate diversional activities.

• Listen to the patient's fears and concerns. Remain with him during periods of severe stress and anxiety. Explain all procedures thoroughly and calmly. If necessary, repeat instructions.

• Include the patient in decisions about his care. Encourage him to identify specific actions and care measures that make him feel comfortable and relaxed. Offer frequent reassurance; for example, point out signs of progress whenever possible.

• Include family members in all phases of the patient's care. Encourage visitation, but explain the patient's need for rest.

Patient teaching

• Teach the patient about pneumonia and its risk factors.

• Describe all diagnostic studies. Explain the reason for each study and how it will be conducted.

• Emphasize that getting adequate rest is crucial for full recovery and the prevention of relapse. Explain that the doctor will let him know when he can resume normal activities and return to work. Explain that he will have to resume activities gradually. Teach the patient techniques for conserving energy.

• Describe all prescribed medications. Stress the need to take the entire course of medication — even if he feels better. Explain that the patient is susceptible to recurrent respiratory infection. Describe possible adverse effects of the medications and ways to prevent them. Tell the patient what actions to take if he experiences an adverse reaction.

• Teach the patient diaphragmatic breathing exercises, techniques for coughing effectively, and proper use of the incentive spirometer. Encourage him to practice breathing exercises and effective coughing four times a day (or more often) for approximately 8 weeks.

• If warranted, teach the patient and his family about postural drainage, percussion, and vibration. Explain that these techniques help mobilize mucus in the lungs so it can be removed.

• If the patient will receive oxygen therapy at home, teach him how to use the equipment safely and effectively.

• Encourage the patient to drink 2 to 3 qt (2 to 3 liters) of fluid each day (unless contraindicated) to maintain adequate hydration and to keep mucus se-

Discharge TimeSaver

Ensuring continued care for the patient with pneumonia

Review the following teaching topics, referrals, and follow-up appointments to make sure that your patient is adequately prepared for discharge.

Teaching topics
Make sure that the following topics have been covered and that your patient's learning has been evaluated:
☐ the nature of pneumonia, including risk factors and complications
☐ diagnostic studies
☐ energy conservation techniques
☐ fluid intake
☐ medications, including their purpose, dosage, adverse effects, and the importance of completing the course of therapy
☐ procedure for coughing effectively
☐ warning signs and symptoms of a worsening condition
☐ sources of additional information and support.

Referrals
Make sure that the patient has been provided with necessary referrals to:
☐ social services
☐ home health care agency
☐ medical equipment supplier (oxygen equipment)
☐ smoking cessation program (if appropriate).

Follow-up appointments
Make sure that the necessary follow-up appointments have been scheduled and that the patient has been notified:
☐ doctor
☐ laboratory for further diagnostic tests.

cretions thin, thus making them easier to remove.
• Tell the patient to notify the doctor if he experiences chest pain, fever, chills, shortness of breath, hemoptysis, or increased fatigue.
• Advise the patient against the indiscriminate use of antibiotics for minor infections. This practice can result in colonization of the upper airways by bacteria that are resistant to antibiotics. Should pneumonia recur, the causative organisms may require treatment with a more toxic antibiotic.
• If the patient is at high risk for influenza or pneumococcal infection, encourage him to talk with his doctor about available vaccinations.
• Urge the patient to avoid irritants that stimulate secretions, such as cigarette smoke, dust, and significant environmental pollution. If appropriate, refer the patient to a local smoking ces-

sation program or to a branch of the American Lung Association or the American Cancer Society for further information and support.
• Discuss ways to avoid spreading the infection to others. Remind the patient to use a tissue when sneezing or coughing and to dispose of the tissues in a plastic (or lined) bag. Tell him to wash his hands thoroughly after handling contaminated tissues. (See *Ensuring continued care for the patient with pneumonia*.)

EVALUATION

When evaluating the patient's response to your nursing care, gather reassessment data and compare this information to the patient outcomes specified in your plan of care.

Teaching and counseling

Begin by determining the effectiveness of your teaching and counseling. During the course of evaluation, observe the patient's actions. Consider the following questions:

• Does the patient express an understanding of the nature of pneumonia?
• Is he prepared to follow the medical treatment plan and to practice energy-conserving techniques to prevent a relapse?
• Is he complying with the medication regimen? Does he express an understanding of the importance of taking the entire course of medication, even after he feels better?
• Is he using the incentive spirometer properly? Is he performing diaphragmatic breathing exercises and coughing effectively? Is he using postural drainage, percussion, and vibration to help mobilize and remove mucus from the lungs?
• Has he learned how to use oxygen equipment safely and effectively at home?
• Does he know the signs and symptoms that require prompt medical attention?
• Can he identify irritants in his environment that stimulate secretions?
• Can he describe ways to avoid spreading the infection?

Physical condition

A physical examination and diagnostic testing will also help you evaluate the effectiveness of your care. Look for indications that the patient's breathing has returned to normal by reassessing breath sounds and gas exchange. Auscultation should reveal clear lung sounds and ABG levels should be normal (or indicate a return to acceptable baseline values). The patient should no longer experience pain or anxiety. His temperature should be normal, and activity should not result in undue fatigue or dyspnea.

Lung abscess

A lung abscess is a pus-filled cavity in the lung formed by tissue necrosis. The affected area is often well defined, and the pus may be putrid or nonputrid. An abscess begins when bacteria localize in the lungs, causing necrosis and destruction of lung tissue. Hematogenous bacterial spread can result in multiple abscesses. (See *Looking at lung abscess.*)

Lung abscess may lead to complications such as localized bronchiectasis, empyema, or massive pulmonary hemorrhage (rare). However, antibiotic therapy has been effective in greatly reducing the incidence of lung abscess and related complications. With proper treatment, the prognosis is good.

Causes

Primary lung abscesses are most commonly caused by aspiration of anaerobic bacteria from the mouth. Factors that predispose a person to aspirate are alcoholism, anesthesia, seizures, neurologic disorders, esophageal disease, and drug overdose. Poor oral hygiene also may increase the likelihood of primary lung abscess.

Lung abscesses may also occur secondary to any bacterial pneumonia, especially those caused by *Staphylococcus* or gram-negative organisms. A fungus such as *Aspergillus* may cause a generalized infection leading to abscess formation. More commonly, fungi infect cavities that are already present in the lungs because of a disorder such as tuberculosis or pulmonary infarction. Malignant tumors may obstruct bronchial tubes and cause abscess formation distal to the obstruction.

Looking at lung abscess

A lung abscess is a suppurative inflammation of lung tissue with a well-defined border. This illustration shows the destruction of lung tissue caused by the abscess. As the abscess continues to develop, pressure increases and the infected tissue may rupture into the bronchus. This leads to drainage of pus, creating foul-smelling or bloody sputum.

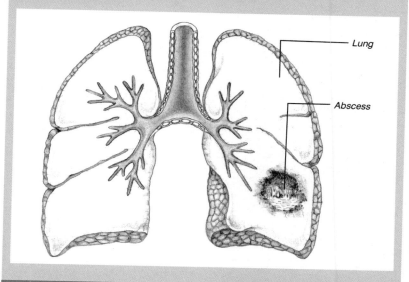

Lung

Abscess

During your assessment, look for the major signs of lung abscess: bloody, purulent, or foul-smelling sputum; sporadic fever; and dyspnea. Then consider associated complaints, such as pleuritic chest pain. The patient may appear chronically ill and malnourished and may have poor oral and dental hygiene. Carefully review the patient's health history, physical examination findings, and diagnostic test results.

Health history

The patient may report headaches, foul-tasting sputum, a generalized feeling of malaise, and anorexia with resulting weight loss. The health history may reveal a recent episode of pneumonia, influenza, or another associated disorder, such as a period of unconsciousness or other risk factor for aspiration.

Physical examination

During your inspection, you may note pallor, chills, malaise, and diaphoresis. Clubbing of the fingers may occasionally occur after 3 or 4 weeks. Percussion over areas of affected lung tissue may reveal dullness. On auscultation, you may hear inspiratory crackles and decreased breath sounds if the affected area is small or cavernous breath sounds if the abscess is large. A pleural friction rub may be present. Vital signs reveal tachycardia, tachypnea, and elevated temperature.

Diagnostic test results

The following tests are used to help confirm a diagnosis of lung abscess:
- Chest X-ray may reveal a localized infiltrate with one or more clear spaces that usually contain air and fluid. In the early stages of development, the abscess may appear as a solid mass until the liquefied material drains into a bronchus. Abscesses usually occur in the superior segments of lower lobes and the posterior segments of upper lobes. The right lung is affected more often than the left.
- Sputum culture produces normal aerobic flora if an anaerobic organism causes the abscess. *Staphylococcus* or gram-negative bacteria may be cultured if one of these is the causative organism.
- Sputum smear shows both aerobic and anaerobic organisms.
- White blood cell count may be elevated (above 10,000/mm^3).
- Computed tomography (CT) scanning may differentiate the type of lesion.

If an abscess fails to close within 4 to 6 weeks after appropriate treatment and the patient's condition permits, bronchoscopy may be used to provide a culture for identification of the causative organism and may indicate a drainage obstruction. (The use of bronchoscopy in the initial evaluation is controversial but may be indicated in patients who are not at risk for aspiration or who show evidence of an obstructive lesion on a CT scan.)

NURSING DIAGNOSIS

Common nursing diagnoses for the patient with lung abscess include:
- Altered nutrition: Less than body requirements, related to anorexia
- Activity intolerance related to dyspnea, excessive coughing, and fatigue
- Ineffective airway clearance related to excessive pulmonary secretions
- Pain related to abscess formation and excessive coughing.

PLANNING

Nursing care for the patient with a lung abscess focuses on controlling symptoms, preventing complications, and teaching the patient about the disorder and its treatment. Because of brief hospitalization and intensive home health care are common, optimal patient outcomes will probably be achieved at home rather than in the hospital.

Based on the nursing diagnosis *altered nutrition: less than body requirements,* develop appropriate patient outcomes. For example, your patient will:
- maintain his baseline weight or begin returning to an acceptable target weight
- maintain a high-calorie diet that is rich in protein and vitamin C.

Based on the nursing diagnosis *activity intolerance,* develop appropriate patient outcomes. For example, your patient will:
- demonstrate his ability to perform activities of daily living (ADLs)
- take frequent rest periods
- resume physical exercise gradually
- no longer exhibit undue fatigue or dyspnea after physical exertion
- exhibit normal vital signs after physical exertion.

Based on the nursing diagnosis *ineffective airway clearance,* develop appropriate patient outcomes. For example, your patient will:
- produce thin mucus with coughing

- exhibit clear breath sounds (or a return to acceptable baseline breath sounds) during auscultation
- achieve normal arterial blood gas (ABG) values (or acceptable baseline values)
- report decreased cough
- report that his dyspnea has diminished or disappeared.

Based on the nursing diagnosis *pain,* develop appropriate patient outcomes. For example, your patient will:
- report that his pain has diminished or stopped
- demonstrate increased comfort by no longer grimacing, holding his sides, or exhibiting muscle rigidity.

IMPLEMENTATION

Treatment for lung abscess focuses on minimizing the patient's discomfort and healing the abscess. (See *Medical care of the patient with lung abscess.*)

Nursing interventions
Your initial efforts should focus on stabilizing the patient's condition, helping him to breathe easier, and relieving his pain. Then turn your attention to providing both the patient teaching and ongoing care that are necessary to heal the abscess.

Initial care measures
- Administer antibiotics as prescribed and pain medication as needed. Show the patient how to reduce pain by splinting the painful area while coughing. Record the patient's response.
- Perform postural drainage and percussion. However, if the patient has a large abscess, be aware that postural drainage and percussion can mobilize purulent secretions in volumes too large for the patient to expectorate.

Timesaving tip: Before performing postural drainage and percussion, verify the exact location of the abscess by checking with the doc-

Treatments

Medical care of the patient with lung abscess

Treatment of lung abscess includes drug therapy, management of secretions, oxygen therapy and, in some cases, surgery.

Drug therapy
Drug therapy consists of prolonged antibiotic (penicillin G or clindamycin) therapy that continues until chest X-rays indicate that the abscess has healed or stabilized. Therapy typically continues for months, although signs and symptoms often disappear in a few weeks. Failure of an abscess to respond to antibiotic therapy suggests an underlying neoplasm or other obstruction.

Procedures
Other interventions include:
- postural drainage to help drain necrotic material into the larger airways, where the cough can remove it
- percussion to loosen secretions
- oxygen therapy to relieve hypoxemia.

Surgery
Although rare, surgery may be required in some instances. Surgery may involve:
- bronchoscopy to remove thick, tenacious sputum, if necessary
- resection of the lesion or lung (rare) if there is a poor therapeutic response or if the patient has massive hemoptysis, localized cancer, or bronchiectasis.

Rigorous follow-up, including serial chest X-rays, is necessary for the patient with lung abscess.

tor and referring to available X-rays. This information will help ensure proper positioning for effective postural drainage and ensure that percussion is performed over the affected area of the lung. Ineffective postural drainage and percussion is both uncomfortable for the patient and costly in terms of your time. Be sure to record the location of the abscess in your plan of care.

• Encourage the patient to perform deep-breathing and effective coughing exercises to loosen secretions. Encourage (or provide) frequent oral hygiene.

• Administer supplemental oxygen, according to ABG levels. Closely monitor ABG values and arterial oxygen saturation (SaO$_2$) throughout treatment.

Ongoing care

• Encourage frequent rest periods and provide a calm, quiet environment. Excessive coughing and repeated postural drainage and percussion can tire the patient.

• Encourage family visits, but emphasize the patient's need for rest.

• Encourage (or provide) frequent oral hygiene.

• During acute periods, help the patient with position changes and hygienic needs.

• If the patient can perform ADLs, encourage him to do so slowly and, if necessary, to use oxygen during physical exertion.

• After periods of physical exertion, assess the patient's respiratory and pulse rates, respiratory effort, and use of accessory muscles. Note any evidence of cyanosis. Gradually increase the patient's activity level, based on your findings.

• Continue to monitor vital signs, breath sounds, ABG values, and SaO$_2$.

• Make sure that the patient drinks enough fluids to help loosen secretions. Unless contraindicated, encourage him to drink 3,000 ml/day. Monitor his intake and output.

• Control the spread of infection by disposing of secretions properly. Provide the patient with tissues, and tape a lined bag to the side of the bed for used tissues.

• Provide a balanced diet that is high in calories and rich in protein and vitamin C. Small, frequent meals will help the patient conserve energy and prevent overexertion. If necessary, administer supplements and consult with the hospital dietitian. Weigh the patient at least once each week.

• Listen to the patient's fears and concerns. Remain with him during periods of extreme stress and anxiety.

• Encourage the patient to identify actions and personal care measures that make him feel more comfortable and relaxed. Then work with the patient to incorporate these measures into his daily routine.

• Provide strong emotional support to the patient, especially if there is a complicating underlying disease. Treatment may be lengthy, but if carefully followed, the patient can expect improvement.

• Whenever possible, include the patient in decisions about his care. Also, arrange to include family members in all phases of the patient's care.

• If surgery is required, provide preoperative and postoperative care.

Patient teaching

• Explain the nature of the disorder and, when appropriate, how it's associated to any underlying condition.

• Explain all medications to the patient and stress the need to take the entire course of medication, even if he feels better. Describe the possible adverse effects of antibiotics and discuss ways to prevent them. Explain what the patient should do if he experiences an adverse reaction.

• Explain each test and procedure.

Discharge TimeSaver

Ensuring continued care for the patient with lung abscess

Review the following teaching topics, referrals, and follow-up appointments to make sure that your patient is adequately prepared for discharge.

Teaching topics
Make sure that the following topics have been covered and that your patient's learning has been evaluated:
☐ nature of lung abscess
☐ medication therapy, including adverse effects, precautions, and the need to comply with the entire regimen
☐ diagnostic studies
☐ self-monitoring techniques
☐ guidelines for activity and rest
☐ deep-breathing and coughing exercises
☐ need for adequate hydration
☐ need for good oral hygiene
☐ importance of a high-calorie, high-protein, high-vitamin C diet
☐ warning signs and symptoms
☐ infection control measures
☐ postural drainage and percussion (if needed)
☐ pneumococcal and influenza vaccinations
☐ sources of information and support.

Referrals
Make sure that the patient has been provided with necessary referrals to:
☐ social services (financial assistance)
☐ home health care agency (especially if compliance with treatment regimen is questionable)
☐ medical equipment supplier (oxygen equipment)
☐ smoking cessation program.

Follow-up appointments
Make sure that the necessary follow-up appointments have been scheduled and that the patient has been notified:
☐ doctor
☐ laboratory for further diagnostic tests
☐ surgeon (if necessary).

• Teach the patient and family members how to perform postural drainage and percussion.
• Teach the patient productive coughing and deep-breathing techniques, and encourage him to practice them often. Tell him to cough secretions into tissues, deposit them in the bedside receptacle, and then wash his hands to prevent the spread of infection.
• Teach the patient and family members the safe and effective use of home oxygen equipment, if prescribed.
• Explain the importance of good oral hygiene.
• Discuss the importance of a nutritious diet that is high in calories and rich in protein and vitamin C. Consult with the hospital dietitian about dietary recommendations. Explain the benefits of eating smaller meals more often.
• Tell the patient to drink plenty of fluids to loosen secretions.
• Emphasize the importance of rest and teach the patient techniques for conserving energy. Provide activity guidelines in collaboration with the doctor.
• Tell the patient to notify the doctor if he experiences chest pain, fever, chills, shortness of breath, hemoptysis, or increased fatigue.
• Encourage the high-risk (immunocompromised) patient to ask his doctor about influenza and pneumococcal vaccinations.
• Urge the patient to avoid irritants that stimulate secretions, such as ciga-

rette smoke, dust, and significant environmental pollution. If necessary, refer him to a local smoking cessation program or a branch of the American Lung Association or the American Cancer Society for support and further information. (See *Ensuring continued care for the patient with lung abscess,* page 235.)

EVALUATION

When evaluating the patient's response to your nursing care, gather reassessment data and compare this information to the patient outcomes in your plan of care.

Teaching and counseling
Begin by determining the effectiveness of your patient teaching and counseling. Consider asking the following questions:
• Does the patient express an understanding of the nature of lung abscess?
• Is he willing to follow the medical treatment plan, get adequate rest, and take the entire course of medication?
• Does he understand the importance of good oral hygiene, deep-breathing techniques, and adequate fluid intake?
• Can he describe foods that are nutritious, high in calories, and rich in protein and vitamin C?
• Can the patient (or caregiver) demonstrate how to perform postural drainage and percussion?
• Does the patient know the signs and symptoms that require medical attention?
• Does he understand the importance of keeping follow-up appointments?

Physical condition
A physical examination and diagnostic testing will also provide data to help evaluate your patient's care. Look for the following:

• Weight should be stable or approaching the normal range (based on age and sex).
• Dyspnea and pain should be diminished.
• Activity tolerance should be improving and activities should no longer cause undue fatigue, dyspnea, or significant changes in vital signs.
• Auscultation should reveal clear breath sounds or a return to acceptable baseline breath sounds.
• Cough should produce thin mucus.
• ABG levels should be normal or return to acceptable baseline values.

Tuberculosis

Tuberculosis (TB) is an acute or a chronic infection characterized by pulmonary infiltrations, formation of granulomas (tubercles) with caseation, fibrosis, and calcification.

In advanced tuberculosis, necrosis and cavitation may be widespread. Although the primary focus of infection is the respiratory system (lungs), the bacteria responsible for tuberculosis may spread to other parts of the body. Possible sites of extrapulmonary tuberculosis include the pleura, meninges, joints, lymph nodes, peritoneum, genitourinary tract, and bowel. (See *Sites of tuberculosis.*)

Tuberculosis that affects the lungs (pulmonary tuberculosis) may cause massive damage to pulmonary tissue with inflammation and necrosis eventually leading to respiratory failure. Bronchopleural fistulas may develop and result in pneumothorax. Tuberculosis may also result in hemorrhage, pleural effusion, and pneumonia.

Causes
Tuberculosis is caused by *Mycobacterium tuberculosis*. Bacilli are transmitted from one host to another in droplet nu-

Sites of tuberculosis

Tuberculosis can have serious effects on many organs and body parts, which are shown in the illustration below.

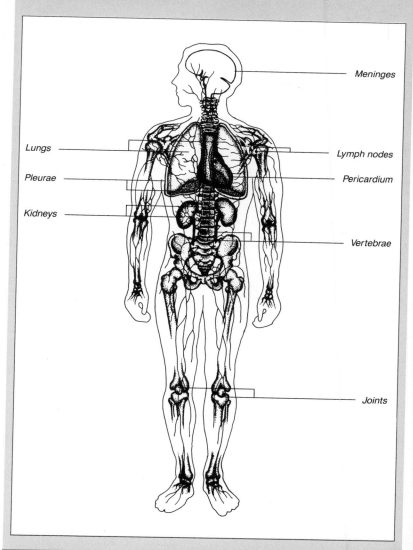

clei. When the host coughs, sneezes, or laughs, droplet nuclei are ejected. A new host may inhale the ejected bacilli, which become lodged in pulmonary alveoli. Cell-mediated immunity to the mycobacteria develops in 3 to 6 weeks and usually contains the infection, arresting the disease. In most instances, the host's immune system kills the bacilli or contains them in nodules called *tubercles.*

Tubercle formation is the hallmark of tuberculosis. Cytotoxic lymphocyte macrophages invade the area of infection and fuse to form giant cells that engulf the bacillus. This core is then covered by a layer of epithelioid cells, which is, in turn, covered by a layer of fibroblasts and lymphocytes.

The bacilli may lie dormant within the tubercle for years and then reactivate and spread, causing active infection. Conditions that increase a patient's risk of reactivation include gastrectomy, uncontrolled diabetes mellitus, Hodgkin's disease, leukemia, silicosis, and treatment with corticosteroids or other immunosuppressives. After reactivation, characteristic caseation of necrotic tissue results in debris that may spread throughout the lungs.

Rarely, infected individuals develop active disease within 1 year. Latent infection is more common. Patients who have tested positive for human immunodeficiency virus (HIV) are more likely than others to develop active disease immediately after infection with tuberculosis.

ASSESSMENT

Focus your assessment on the major symptoms of tuberculosis: progressive weakness and fatigue, anorexia, night sweats, and a cough. Then consider associated complaints. Carefully review the patient's health history, medication history, physical examination findings, and diagnostic test results.

Health history
Tuberculosis has an insidious onset. The patient with an active infection may complain of progressive weakness and fatigue, anorexia, weight loss, low-grade fever, and night sweats, occurring over a period ranging from weeks to months. The patient may also complain of a cough, possibly producing sputum streaked with blood. Pain or tightness in the chest may accompany the cough. A patient with laryngeal tuberculosis will report hoarseness.

During the health history, determine the patient's risk for tuberculosis and investigate possible exposure to tuberculosis (especially drug-resistant strains) and HIV. (See *Identifying high-risk patients.*)

Medication history
Ask the patient if he has ever received bacille Calmette-Guérin (BCG) vaccine. This vaccine, which contains attenuated tubercle bacilli, is intended to promote resistance to tuberculosis. (Although not routinely administered in North America, BCG is often prescribed in many countries.) After several years, those vaccinated with BCG will have a negative skin test or a diminished positive reaction. If your patient received the BCG vaccine, he should be screened for tuberculosis. If testing proves positive, a follow-up chest X-ray and evaluation for tuberculosis are appropriate.

Physical examination
During the initial physical examination, look for signs of active tuberculosis. Physical findings may vary greatly, depending on the severity of pulmonary involvement. Percussion may reveal dullness over the affected area of the lung, signifying consolidation or the presence of pleural fluid. Auscultation may reveal crepitant crackles, bronchial breath sounds, wheezes, and whispered pectoriloquy.

Assessment TimeSaver

Identifying high-risk patients

The incidence of tuberculosis in North America has increased dramatically since the mid-1980s and once again poses a significant health threat. A combination of social, cultural, and medical factors contributes to the spread of tuberculosis. These factors include the spread of acquired immunodeficiency syndrome, a growing homeless population, poverty, drug abuse, prison overcrowding, immigration from countries with high tuberculosis rates, cuts in public health funding, and increasingly drug-resistant strains of tuberculosis.

Epidemiology
The greatest incidence of tuberculosis occurs in the 25 to 44 age-group. This age group also has the highest incidence of human immunodeficiency virus (HIV) infection. However, the incidence is also higher in children under age 15 and in Black and Hispanic populations. Tuberculosis is twice as common in men as in women and four times more likely to affect nonwhites than whites.

High-risk groups
Arrange tuberculosis testing and place the patient on acid-fast bacilli isolation if your assessment leads you to suspect tuberculosis and your patient falls into one or more of the following high-risk groups:
• HIV-infected individuals (and those at risk for HIV infection)
• individuals who have had close contact with a person with active infectious tuberculosis
• individuals with conditions that increase the risk of active tuberculosis after infection, such as silicosis, diabetes mellitus, chronic renal failure, or cancer (especially Hodgkin's disease, leukemia, and lymphomas)
• individuals whose weight is 10% below ideal
• individuals receiving prolonged therapy with corticosteroids or other immunosuppressants

• individuals born in countries with a high prevalence of tuberculosis
• substance abusers, such as alcoholics, I.V. drug users, and cocaine or crack users
• residents of long-term care facilities, nursing homes, prisons, mental institutions, homeless shelters, or other congregate housing settings
• medically underserved, low-income populations, such as racial and ethnic minorities, homeless people, and migrant workers
• health care workers and others who provide services to any high-risk group.

High risk for drug-resistant tuberculosis
The following groups are at high risk for drug-resistant strains of tuberculosis:
• individuals who have a history of preventive treatment or treatment for active tuberculosis
• individuals born in countries in Africa, Asia, Central America, or South America (areas with a high incidence of tuberculosis)
• residents of areas in North America with high rates of drug-resistant tuberculosis (New York City and Florida, for example)
• patients with *Mycobacterium tuberculosis* in their sputum specimens after 3 months of drug therapy.

Interpretation

Interpreting results of the Mantoux test

When interpreting the results of the Mantoux test, consider the patient's risk for tuberculosis.

An induration of **5 mm or more** may be considered a positive test if the patient:

• has had recent, close contact with a person with active infectious tuberculosis.

• has a chest X-ray showing pulmonary fibrotic lesions that might be old, healed tuberculosis lesions.

• is infected with human immunodeficiency virus (HIV) or has a high risk of HIV infection.

An induration of **10 mm or more** may be considered a positive test if the patient has one or more of the following risk factors for tuberculosis:

• a medical condition that increases the risk of active disease once infection has occurred

• born in Asia, Africa, Central America, or South America

• Black, Native American, or Hispanic *and* a member of a low socioeconomic, medically underserved group

• I.V. drug user

• resident or staff member of a congregate living arrangement (for example, a long-term care facility, prison, or nursing home)

• health care worker exposed to tuberculosis

• very young or very old.

An induration of **15 mm or more** may be considered a positive test in all other patients with no risk factors.

Note: A positive skin test indicates that the patient has been infected with *Mycobacterium tuberculosis*. It does not necessarily indicate active disease.

Induration indicating absence of infection

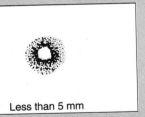

Less than 5 mm

Induration suggesting infection

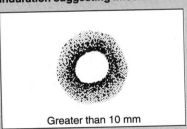

Greater than 10 mm

Diagnostic test results

• Tuberculin skin testing, the primary screening tool, may reveal that the patient has been infected with tuberculosis at some point; however, it doesn't indicate active disease.

Multipuncture, or tine, tests are usually used only when the probability of infection is low. Intradermal tuberculin skin testing using the Mantoux method (Aplisol, Tubersol) is preferred. This test involves an intradermal injection of 0.1 ml of intermediate-strength purified protein derivative (PPD) containing 5 tuberculin units into the forearm. Results are interpreted 48 to 72 hours later. (See *Interpreting results of the Mantoux test.*) Patients with immune system impairment may require

Interpretation

Distinguishing inactive tuberculosis from active pulmonary tuberculosis

	Inactive tuberculosis	Active pulmonary tuberculosis
Tuberculosis organisms present in the body	Yes	Yes
Infected with tuberculosis	Yes	Yes
Tuberculosis skin test positive	Yes	Yes
Chest X-ray	Usually normal	Usually abnormal
Sputum smears or cultures	Negative	Usually positive
Symptoms	None	Cough, fever, night sweats, weight loss
Infectious	No	Often, especially before treatment

anergy testing to verify results of the Mantoux test.

Companion skin tests (controls) are administered at least once, usually for candidiasis, mumps, or tetanus. Positive reactions to one or more of these tests indicate that the patient can mount a cell-mediated immune response, indicating that a negative reaction to PPD is probably accurate.

• Chest X-rays may show lesions that vary in size, shape, and density (with or without cavitation), anywhere in the lungs, especially in HIV-positive and other immunocompromised patients. They also may show upper lobe infiltrates. Scar tissue and calcium deposits may be evident in infected individuals without evidence of active disease.

Chest X-rays may be inconclusive in distinguishing between active and inactive tuberculosis, and they do not confirm the diagnosis. A negative chest X-ray will usually rule out pulmonary tuberculosis, but not active disease in other organs. (See *Distinguishing inactive tuberculosis from active pulmonary tuberculosis.*)

• Sputum smear for acid-fast bacilli (AFB), if positive, provides a presumptive diagnosis of tuberculosis. Sputum culture is used to confirm the diagnosis; however, results take 2 to 12 weeks. If you suspect tuberculosis, expect to obtain at least three sputum specimens, on consecutive days, for smear and culture.

Because of the increased incidence of drug-resistant strains of *M. tuberculosis,* drug-sensitivity testing on initial sputum specimens is essential. Other specimens may be cultured when nonpulmonary tuberculosis is suspected.

• Computed tomography or magnetic resonance imaging scans may be used to evaluate lung damage or confirm a difficult diagnosis.

• Bronchoscopy may be performed if the patient has trouble producing an adequate sputum specimen spontaneously or by induced sputum collection.

Several diagnostic tests may be necessary to distinguish tuberculosis from diseases that may mimic it, such as lung cancer, lung abscess, pneumoconiosis, and bronchiectasis.

NURSING DIAGNOSIS

Common nursing diagnoses for patients with tuberculosis include:
• Noncompliance related to failure to adhere to treatment regimen, resulting in the spread of disease
• Altered nutrition: Less than body requirements, related to anorexia, infection, or adverse effects of drug therapy
• Knowledge deficit related to the treatment and prevention of tuberculosis
• Fatigue related to infection and associated weight loss
• Impaired social interaction related to stigma associated with the diagnosis and isolation precautions
• Altered protection related to a decrease in ability to guard self from the disease (particularly common in immunocompromised patients).

PLANNING

Nursing care for the patient with tuberculosis focuses on controlling the patient's symptoms, controlling the infection, avoiding complications, and teaching the patient about the infection and the importance of strict compliance with the treatment regimen.

Based on the nursing diagnosis *noncompliance,* develop appropriate patient outcomes. For example, your patient will:
• complete an effective course of drug therapy
• attend scheduled follow-up appointments and obtain regularly ordered sputum specimens
• cover his mouth and nose when laughing, coughing, or sneezing
• express an understanding of the importance of refraining from drug or alcohol abuse.

Based on the nursing diagnosis *altered nutrition: less than body requirements,* develop appropriate patient outcomes. For example, your patient will:

• experience no further weight loss
• express an understanding of the importance of a nutritious diet that is rich in calories and protein.

Based on the nursing diagnosis *knowledge deficit,* develop appropriate patient outcomes. For example, your patient will:
• express a desire to learn about tuberculosis and its treatment
• seek and obtain accurate information about tuberculosis
• communicate an understanding of how tuberculosis is contracted and managed and how to prevent a recurrence
• communicate an understanding of the importance of completing treatment as prescribed, even after feeling better.

Based on the nursing diagnosis *fatigue,* develop appropriate patient outcomes. For example, your patient will:
• incorporate rest periods into his daily routine
• practice energy conservation techniques when performing activities of daily living (ADLs)
• report experiencing less fatigue as treatment progresses
• resume ADLs gradually
• return to his normal level of activity before treatment ends (within 6 months), except in very advanced disease.

Based on the nursing diagnosis *impaired social interaction,* develop appropriate patient outcomes. For example, your patient will:
• express feelings of anxiety, frustration, or sadness
• communicate with caregivers
• interact with family members and friends
• participate in at least one enjoyable activity each day
• state that he feels less isolated
• increase his level of social interaction after discharge.

Based on the nursing diagnosis *altered protection,* develop appropriate patient outcomes. For example, the patient will:

• express an understanding of his need for HIV risk assessment and counseling

• express an understanding of the importance of being tested for HIV (if indicated)

• acknowledge the importance of modifying his use of alcohol or drugs

• experience an absence of adverse reactions to prescribed therapy

• maintain adequate liver function as evidenced by test results within normal limits.

IMPLEMENTATION

Treatment for tuberculosis seeks to reduce the patient's discomfort, destroy the infectious organism as quickly as possible, and avoid promoting drug-resistant organisms. (See *Medical care of the patient with tuberculosis,* page 244.)

Nursing interventions
Patients with tuberculosis require immediate care to combat the disease and ongoing care to prevent the emergence of drug-resistant organisms.

Initial care
Your first priority will be to institute precautions to prevent the transmission of tuberculosis. Precautions will vary depending on the clinical setting. (See *Quick review of CDC recommendations for preventing transmission of tuberculosis,* page 245.)

• To protect yourself, other health care workers, and other patients, obtain sputum specimens in a small room or booth containing an exhaust fan, high-efficiency particulate air filters, or ultraviolet air disinfection (ideally, all three). If this is not possible, wear a particulate respirator and collect the specimen in a private room.

• Patients with suspected tuberculosis and suspicious signs and symptoms lasting 3 weeks or more should be placed on AFB isolation precautions — don't wait for confirmation of the diagnosis. AFB isolation precautions include the use of an isolation room with negative air pressure and exhaust ventilation to the outside. Upper room irradiation is preferred if other environmental controls are not available.

• Make sure that all visitors and hospital staff members wear a particulate respirator or a tightly fitting submicron filtering mask while in the patient's room. Standard masks are not effective because AFB particles can pass through the mask material. Unless the patient is unable or unwilling to cover his nose and mouth when he coughs or sneezes, he does not have to wear a mask in his room, but he should wear a mask if he is transported outside his room.

• Place a covered trash can near the patient's bed, or tape a lined bag to the bedside, for his used tissues.

• Keep all doors to the room closed while the patient is on AFB precautions.

• Implement universal precautions.

• Local health officials must be informed of suspected cases of tuberculosis by the appropriate person at your hospital, often the infection-control nurse or the patient's doctor. Make sure they are notified of initial reports of positive smears within 24 hours so they can begin the process of investigating the patient's close contacts. Keep the infection-control nurse informed of all developments, including the patient's degree of compliance with therapy.

Additional measures
After precautionary measures have been taken, you may continue with other interventions.

Medical care of the patient with tuberculosis

Antitubercular therapy may consist of daily oral doses of isoniazid, rifampin, pyrazinamide, or ethambutol for 6 to 9 months. In most cases, the patient is no longer infectious after 2 to 4 weeks of therapy and may resume normal activities while continuing to take medication until cured. However, a patient infected with the human immunodeficiency virus (HIV) or drug-resistant tuberculosis may require alternate treatment regimens.

Multiple-drug regimens
Multiple-drug regimens are designed to destroy the organism quickly while preventing the emergence of drug-resistant organisms.

Currently, a 6-month regimen is recommended for HIV-negative patients. It consists of daily doses of isoniazid, rifampin, and pyrazinamide for the first 2 months. Ethambutol or streptomycin may be prescribed if isoniazid resistance is suspected. For the next 4 months, the patient receives isoniazid and rifampin daily or twice a week.

An HIV-positive patient may undergo a 9-month regimen, which consists of daily doses of isoniazid, rifampin, and pyrazinamide for the first 2 months. Ethambutol or streptomycin may be used if tuberculosis has spread throughout the body or into the central nervous system or if drug-resistant tuberculosis is suspected. For the next 7 months, the patient receives isoniazid and rifampin daily or twice weekly.

If the patient's sputum cultures are negative, treatment continues for 3 months if the patient is HIV-negative and 6 months if the patient is HIV-positive.

If the patient is noncompliant, the regimen may be changed to administration of high doses twice a week under direct supervision of the health care team.

Treating drug-resistant strains
Patients with drug-resistant tuberculosis may require second-line drugs, such as cycloserine, ethionamide, or para-aminosalicylic acid (PAS). Other alternative drugs include kanamycin, amikacin, capreomycin, ciprofloxacin, ofloxacin, and clofazimine.

Surgical intervention
Surgery, although not common, may be performed to remove as much of the disease as possible. Surgery may be considered if the patient has localized disease and the infecting organism is resistant to several drugs. In most instances, surgery is combined with aggressive antibiotic therapy.

• Provide the patient with appropriate enjoyable diversions and activities. Check on him frequently and make sure that the call button is conveniently located.
• Listen to the patient's concerns and fears and provide emotional support. Encourage communication with friends and relatives, especially while AFB isolation precautions are in effect.

• Administer prescribed medications. Observe the patient for adverse reactions and take steps to prevent them. For example, isoniazid and ethambutol, which may cause nausea, could be given with food.

Ongoing care
• Make sure that the patient gets plenty of rest. Schedule alternating periods of

Quick review of CDC recommendations for preventing transmission of tuberculosis

The Centers for Disease Control and Prevention (CDC) has issued the following recommendations for preventing the transmission of tuberculosis. These guidelines are applicable to all health care settings.

• Identify persons who have tuberculosis and are at high risk for active tuberculosis early and initiate preventive treatment promptly.
• Identify persons with *active* tuberculosis early and treat them promptly.
• Develop and maintain appropriate ventilation, including enhanced ventilation in facilities serving populations with a high prevalence of tuberculosis.
• Use supplemental environmental approaches, such as high-efficiency filtration or germicidal ultraviolet irradiation.

• Sterilize critical items; clean semicritical items with high-level disinfectants (or sterilize) and noncritical items with low-level disinfectants.
• Maintain active surveillance for tuberculosis among both patients and hospital personnel.
• Perform periodic screening and testing for tuberculosis if exposure to an infectious tuberculosis patient has occurred.

rest and light activity to promote health, conserve energy, and reduce oxygen demand. Explain that fatigue will fade as treatment progresses.
• Provide the patient with a nutritious high-calorie diet. Encourage small, frequent meals to help the patient conserve energy. (Also, small, frequent meals may encourage the anorectic patient to eat more.) If the patient asks for supplements, consult with the dietitian.
• Provide supportive care and help the patient adjust to any lifestyle changes necessitated by his illness.
• Include the patient in decisions about his care. Encourage family members to participate in the patient's care whenever possible.
• Monitor the patient's respiratory status. Auscultate breath sounds frequently.
• Monitor the patient's weight at least once each week. Report any weight loss of 2 lb (0.9 kg) or more.
• Begin discharge planning early. Consult with the social services department about evaluating the patient's living conditions. Arrange for follow-up home health care visits, if appropriate.
• It's essential to monitor the patient's compliance with therapy after discharge. If noncompliance is a continuing problem, the patient may be required to take medication under the direct supervision of a health care professional.
• Refer the patient to sources of information and support in the community, for example, the American Lung Association or a local health department.
• If the patient is an alcoholic or drug addict, refer him for appropriate counseling and treatment and recommend that he attend a self-help group, such as Alcoholics Anonymous. Alcohol and drug abuse frequently hinder compliance with treatment and can lead to the recurrence and spread of tuberculosis.
• If the patient is at high risk for HIV infection, refer him to appropriate counseling and testing.

Patient teaching

Effective patient teaching is essential. If the patient complies with treatment, the prognosis is good. If not, there is a high risk that the infecting organism will become drug-resistant and that more pulmonary destruction will occur.

• Explain the nature of the disease, how it spreads, and how it's prevented.

• Teach the patient to cover his mouth and nose when laughing, coughing, and sneezing, even when alone in a room.

• Teach the patient how to obtain a good specimen. Explain that the sputum must come from his lungs. Tell him to inhale and exhale deeply three times; then inhale swiftly and cough forcefully; and, finally, expectorate into the sputum container. If these efforts fail, he may need the help of a hypertonic saline aerosol mist. Instruct him to take several normal breaths of the aerosol mist and then inhale deeply, cough, and expectorate into the sputum container.

• If ordered, explain the use of bronchoscopy to obtain bronchial washings, brushings, and biopsy specimens.

• Teach the patient the importance of strict compliance to the medication regimen for the entire prescribed period. Describe possible adverse effects. Tell the patient to report any adverse reactions immediately.

• Teach the patient and family members the signs and symptoms of recurring tuberculosis.

• Advise family members that anyone exposed to the patient should receive a tuberculin test and, if necessary, a chest X-ray and prophylactic drug therapy (typically, isoniazid for 6 months unless organism is isoniazid resistant or the patient is HIV-positive).

• If your patient is taking rifampin, explain that the drug will temporarily make bodily secretions appear orange. Reassure him that this is harmless. If your patient is female and taking oral contraceptives, warn her that rifampin may make the contraceptive less effective. If your patient is receiving methadone, the dose may need to be adjusted while he is taking rifampin.

• Explain the importance of rest and discuss energy conservation techniques. Advise a gradual return to normal activities as he starts to feel better.

• Discuss the signs and symptoms that require medical assessment, including increased bouts of coughing, hemoptysis, unexplained weight loss, fever, and night sweats.

• Stress the importance of adopting a balanced diet that is high in calories and protein.

• Explain respiratory and universal precautions. Tell him to take precautions against spreading the disease (such as covering his mouth when coughing) until the doctor tells him that he is no longer contagious (usually after negative results are found on three consecutive sputum smears.) Explain the need to notify health care providers, such as his dentist or eye doctor, of his condition so that they can institute infection-control precautions.

• Teach the patient precautionary measures that will help him avoid spreading the infection, such as coughing and sneezing into tissues and then disposing of the tissues properly. Stress the importance of the patient washing his hands thoroughly in hot, soapy water afterward.

• Emphasize the importance of scheduling and keeping follow-up appointments. Monthly (or more frequent) sputum testing is critical to monitor his response to therapy and determine the duration of therapy. If sputum tests continue to be positive after 3 months, suspect drug resistance or noncompliance with drug therapy.

• If your patient is a recent immigrant, provide the patient and his family members with information on the

Discharge TimeSaver

Ensuring continued care for the patient with tuberculosis

Review the following teaching topics, referrals, and follow-up appointments to make sure that your patient is adequately prepared for discharge.

Teaching topics
Make sure that the following topics have been covered and that your patient's learning has been evaluated:
□ nature of tuberculosis, including symptoms, complications, management, and prevention
□ guidelines for activity and rest
□ prescribed medications, including adverse effects, precautions, and the importance of compliance
□ importance of a high-calorie, balanced diet
□ warning signs and symptoms
□ infection-control measures
□ importance of follow-up care and testing
□ need for close contacts to be tested
□ sources of information and support.

Referrals
Make sure that the patient has been provided with necessary referrals to:
□ social services
□ public health nurse
□ dietitian
□ alcohol or drug treatment program (if indicated).

Follow-up appointments
Make sure that the necessary follow-up appointments have been scheduled and that the patient has been notified:
□ doctor
□ home health care agency
□ community outreach worker
□ laboratory for further diagnostic tests.

health care system in your country. (See *Ensuring continued care for the patient with tuberculosis.*)

EVALUATION

When evaluating the patient's response to your nursing care, gather reassessment data and compare this information to the patient outcomes in your plan of care.

Teaching and counseling
Begin by determining the effectiveness of your teaching and counseling. Consider asking the following questions:
• Does the patient understand the nature of tuberculosis and its treatment and prevention?

• Is he willing to follow the treatment plan, institute infection-control measures, and complete the medication regimen?
• Does the patient cover his mouth when laughing, coughing, and sneezing?
• Does he understand the possible adverse effects of the medications?
• Is he able to expectorate sputum?
• Does he know the signs and symptoms of recurring tuberculosis?
• Does he understand the importance of keeping follow-up appointments?
• Has he identified (names and addresses) individuals who may have been exposed to his illness?
• Do family members who may have been exposed to active infectious tuberculosis know what steps to take?

Physical condition

A physical examination and diagnostic testing will also help evaluate the effectiveness of your care. Look for the following signs:

• stable body weight (or approaching a desired target weight)
• clear breath sounds
• productive cough (thin mucus)
• less fatigue as treatment progresses
• a return to a normal level of activity
• decreased feelings of isolation
• normal ABG values for the patient's age
• negative results of sputum specimen tests within 3 months.

CHAPTER 9

Caring for patients with environmental disorders

Silicosis

A fibrotic lung disease, silicosis results from the inhalation of silica dust. Silica occurs naturally in the majority of the rocks that form the earth's surface. Depending on its severity, onset, and progression, silicosis is classified as acute, accelerated, or chronic. Chronic silicosis is further subdivided into simple and complicated forms. (See *Key points about silicosis.*)

Complications occur in about 20% of patients. In chronic complicated silicosis, massive pulmonary fibrosis may occur. (See *Looking at progressive massive fibrosis,* page 252.) Pulmonary fibrosis, in turn, may lead to cor pulmonale and ventricular or respiratory failure. Other complications of silicosis may include bronchiectasis, spontaneous pneumothorax, pulmonary hemorrhage, pulmonary hypertension, pleural adhesions, malnutrition, and increased susceptibility to tuberculosis and bronchopneumonia.

Some patients develop rheumatoid arthritis, systemic lupus erythematosus, or scleroderma, suggesting an autoimmune link to silicosis development.

Causes
Silicosis results from chronic inhalation of fine silica dust that collects in the lungs.

ASSESSMENT

The patient with silicosis is often asymptomatic. Learning about his occupation may provide you with the first clues to the disorder. Note if he has had long-term exposure to silica dust. (See *Identifying silicosis risk,* page 253.) Also inquire about his smoking history. Because smoking impairs mucociliary clearance, a smoker is more likely than a nonsmoker to suffer from a silica-induced disorder as well as from such co-existing conditions as chronic bronchitis and emphysema.

Health history
The patient may report dyspnea on exertion, which he may attribute to "being out of shape" or "slowing down with age." If the disease has progressed to chronic complicated silicosis, the patient may report having a dry or slightly productive cough, especially in the morning. Fever is rare. Other complaints may include fatigue, back and retrosternal pain, hemoptysis, cyanosis, and trouble eating, sleeping, or speaking.

Physical examination
A patient with chronic silicosis may show no signs on physical examination. A patient with advanced silicosis may show signs indistinguishable from nonspecific chronic obstructive pulmonary disease. During your initial observation, you may note hyperpnea with tachypnea, caused by lung restriction. Inspection may reveal decreased chest expansion.

Timesaving tip: If the patient exhibits lethargy or confusion, suspect advanced silicosis. To distinguish silicosis from advanced chronic bronchitis and pulmonary emphysema, look for evidence of reduced lung volume from fibrosis.

Percussion of the patient's chest may reveal areas of increased and decreased resonance over the lungs. Auscultation may reveal fine to medium crackles, diminished breath sounds, and an intensified ventricular gallop on inspiration — a hallmark of cor pulmonale.

Diagnostic test results
• A patient's history of industrial exposure to silica and a chest X-ray that shows changes suggestive of silicosis

FactFinder

Key points about silicosis

When caring for a patient with silicosis, be aware of the different types of silicosis, risk factors, treatments, and preventive measures.

Types of silicosis

• *Chronic silicosis* occurs after 20 to 40 years of exposure and may be described as either simple or complicated. In simple silicosis, small, rounded nodules are scattered throughout the upper lobes of the lungs. In complicated silicosis, nodules form conglomerate masses of fibrous tissue that obliterate normal lung tissue.

• *Accelerated silicosis* produces effects similar to those of complicated silicosis, but it progresses more rapidly with extensive lung involvement. It usually results from a shorter, more concentrated exposure to silica.

• *Acute silicosis* may develop after several months to several years of exposure to silica dust. In this form of the disorder, alveoli become filled with proteinaceous material. Acute silicosis is characterized by rapid deterioration.

Risk factors

• Silicosis results from prolonged exposure to high concentrations of airborne, respirable silica dust (particles less than 5 microns in diameter).

• An individual's susceptibility to silicosis depends on the dust concentration (typically in the workplace), the number of years of exposure, and the individual's response.

• The threshold limit value or "acceptable" level of silica dust in the workplace is 100 mg/m³, according to the Occupational Safety and Health Administration (OSHA).

• High-risk groups include workers who mine, process, or manufacture products containing silicates, such as ceramics, sandstone building materials, and cement.

• Also at risk are people who work with powdered silica (silica flour), which is used in making paints, porcelain, scouring soaps, and wood fillers and in mining gold, lead, zinc, and iron.

Treatment and preventive measures

• No cure exists for silicosis. Instead, therapy focuses on alleviating symptoms.

• Eliminating exposure is the only way to prevent the disease or, in patients with diagnosed silicosis, to prevent further damage. Eliminating exposure may prevent progressive massive fibrosis. Leaving a high-risk job, however, isn't an option for most people, especially since silicosis doesn't usually become manifest until 10 to 20 years after exposure.

• If the patient continues to work in a high-risk environment, he should use a particulate-filtering mask and work at a site with an advanced circulation system capable of filtering silica dust.

---

are the two most important diagnostic indicators.

• Chest X-ray in *simple silicosis* will reveal small, discrete, nodular lesions throughout both lungs, with concentrations in the upper zones. The hilar lung nodes may appear enlarged and show eggshell calcification. In *complicated*

silicosis, chest X-ray will show one or more conglomerate masses of dense tissue.

• Pulmonary function tests in complicated silicosis reveal reduced forced vital capacity (FVC). Forced expiratory volume in 1 second (FEV_1) declines, but the ratio of FEV_1 to FVC is normal

Looking at progressive massive fibrosis

In the advanced stages of silicosis, silicotic nodules coalesce to form regions of dense fibrosis leading to progressive massive fibrosis. Progressive massive fibrosis is most often found in the upper lobes of the lung.

Fibrotic regions erode and obliterate lung parenchyma, occasionally causing the upper lobes to contract. Pleural adhesions are common.

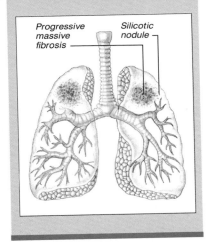

Progressive massive fibrosis

Silicotic nodule

or elevated. The diffusing capacity of the lung for carbon monoxide (DLCO) is decreased. If the patient has obstructive disease (emphysematous silicotic areas), FEV_1 will decline.

• The results of arterial blood gas (ABG) analysis in simple silicosis are essentially normal. In more advanced stages, the partial pressure of arterial oxygen (PaO_2) may be normal when the patient is at rest but declines when he exercises. The partial pressure of arterial carbon dioxide ($PaCO_2$) is normal during exercise; however, hyperventilation may cause it to drop below normal, even when the patient rests. In both chronic simple silicosis and chronic complicated silicosis, the PaO_2 level may be significantly below normal. If restrictive lung disease develops, the PaO_2 level may be elevated if the patient has severe alveolar ventilatory impairment.

• High-resolution computed tomography scan and electron spin resonance spectroscopy may reveal changes in the lung parenchyma during early stages.

NURSING DIAGNOSIS

Common nursing diagnoses for patients with silicosis include:
• Impaired gas exchange related to ventilation-perfusion mismatch and decreased oxygen diffusing capacity
• Ineffective breathing pattern related to dyspnea and decreased vital capacity
• Altered nutrition: Less than body requirements, related to diminished food intake and increased metabolic demands
• Anxiety related to possible occupational change, physical deterioration, or death
• Activity intolerance related to dyspnea and reduced oxygen supply
• High risk for infection related to altered alveolocapillary membranes and cell-mediated immunity and to malnutrition.

PLANNING

Based on the nursing diagnosis *impaired gas exchange,* develop appropriate patient outcomes. For example, your patient will:
• maintain adequate ventilation as indicated by $PaCO_2$ level
• maintain adequate PaO_2 level
• maintain clear breath sounds
• maintain optimal mental status.

Based on the nursing diagnosis *ineffective breathing pattern*, develop appropriate patient outcomes. For example, your patient will:
• maintain respiratory rate within 5 breaths of baseline
• maintain adequate ABG levels
• achieve optimal lung expansion with adequate ventilation.

Based on the nursing diagnosis *altered nutrition: less than body requirements*, develop appropriate patient outcomes. For example, your patient will:
• maintain his weight or return to his target weight
• receive specified caloric intake daily
• not experience adverse reactions to enteral or parenteral nutrition.

Based on the nursing diagnosis *anxiety*, develop appropriate patient outcomes. For example, your patient will:
• use support systems to improve his ability to cope
• demonstrate fewer signs of anxiety
• if currently employed in a high-risk industry, state a plan of action to modify contact with the hazardous environment.

Based on the nursing diagnosis *activity intolerance*, develop appropriate patient outcomes. For example, your patient will:
• express an understanding of the relationship between silicosis and activity intolerance
• identify an appropriate plan for increasing his level of activity
• demonstrate an ability to use energy-conserving techniques while performing activities of daily living
• maintain blood pressure and pulse and respiratory rates within specified limits when active.

Based on the nursing diagnosis *high risk for infection*, develop appropriate patient outcomes. For example, your patient will:
• maintain baseline temperature and heart rate

Assessment TimeSaver

Identifying silicosis risk

To determine if your patient is at risk for silicosis, find out if he has ever worked in any of the following occupations:
• mining, processing, and handling diatomite (a light, friable siliceous material formed from algae remains and used in the manufacture of filters)
• manufacturing filters for inorganic and organic liquids
• manufacturing bricks and cement used for heat and sound insulation
• mining gold, tin, copper, platinum, or mica
• quarrying granite, slate, or pumice
• tunneling for sewers and roads; excavating sandstone
• stonecutting and polishing; cleaning and carving of masonry
• manufacturing abrasives using crushed sand, sandstone, or quartzite; abrasive blasting
• manufacturing glass and enameling
• processing products that use quartz
• working in iron and steel foundries
• manufacturing china, porcelain, stoneware, and earthenware
• building and dismantling kilns, steel furnaces, ovens in gas-making plants, and boiler houses
• cleaning and scaling boiler flues and fireboxes.

• remain free of infection as evidenced by a lack of pathogen growth in cultures
• maintain clear, odorless respiratory secretions and a productive (though not incapacitating) cough.

IMPLEMENTATION

Treatment focuses on relieving the patient's symptoms, managing hypoxe-

Treatments

Medical care of the patient with silicosis

Treatment may include measures to relieve respiratory symptoms, maintain oxygenation, and eliminate respiratory tract infection.

Relieving respiratory symptoms
• Daily bronchodilating aerosols
• Increased fluid intake to at least 3 qt (3 liters) daily

Maintaining oxygenation
• Oxygen administration by cannula or mask
• Mechanical ventilation

Eliminating respiratory infection
• Antibiotic administration
• Physical activity as tolerated
• Detecting and treating tuberculosis infections

mia and cor pulmonale, preventing respiratory tract irritation and infection, and monitoring for signs of tuberculosis. (See *Medical care of the patient with silicosis*.)

Nursing interventions
• Assess for changes in baseline respiratory function, changes in sputum quality and quantity, restlessness, increasing tachypnea, and changes in breath sounds. Report significant findings to the doctor.
• Monitor oxygenation with pulse oximetry and ABG analysis.
• Administer oxygen by cannula or mask as prescribed. In severe cases, anticipate mechanical ventilation if the patient's respiratory rate increases to more than 30 breaths/minute, his PaO_2 level falls below 55 mm Hg despite oxygen therapy, or his $PaCO_2$ increases.

• Provide inhaled bronchodilators as prescribed.
• Provide steam inhalation therapy as needed.
• Perform postural drainage, chest percussion, and vibration of the involved lobes several times a day to help clear secretions.
• Schedule respiratory therapy at least 1 hour before or after meals. Provide oral care after bronchodilator therapy and periodically thereafter if supplemental oxygen is administered.
• Make sure the patient drinks at least 3 qt (3 liters) each day to loosen secretions. Maintain accurate intake and output records.
• Encourage the patient to participate in appropriate daily activities. Plan alternating periods of rest and activity to help him conserve energy.
• Administer prescribed medications. Monitor the patient for possible adverse reactions.
• Provide a high-calorie, high-protein diet and encourage him to eat small, frequent meals that include soft foods.
• Monitor for complications, such as tuberculosis infection, bacterial infection, and cor pulmonale.
• Administer prescribed antibiotics if the patient develops a respiratory tract infection.
• Help him adjust to the lifestyle changes associated with chronic illness.
• Answer all questions and encourage the patient to express his concerns about the illness.
• Provide support during periods of extreme stress and anxiety.
• Include the patient and his family in decisions about care whenever possible.

Patient teaching
• Advise the patient to avoid crowds and people with known infections. Suggest that he discuss influenza and

pneumococcus immunizations with his doctor.

• Warn the patient of the risk of tuberculosis and explain skin testing. Also, teach him to recognize the signs of tuberculosis infection: cough, fever, hemoptysis, malaise, night sweats, and weight loss.

• If the patient will receive oxygen at home, discuss the reasons for treatment and the proper use of the equipment. If a transtracheal catheter is to be used, demonstrate how to care for the equipment.

• Teach the patient controlled coughing and deep-breathing techniques. Whenever possible, avoid using codeine mixtures, which suppress the cough reflex.

• Teach the patient and members of his family how to perform postural drainage and chest percussion. Explain that he should remain in each position for 10 minutes and then receive percussion. Afterward, the patient should use productive coughing techniques to remove secretions.

• Thoroughly explain all medications. Describe proper administration and possible adverse effects.

• Encourage the patient to follow a high-calorie, high-protein diet and to drink plenty of fluids to prevent dehydration and help loosen secretions.

• If the patient smokes, encourage him to quit. Refer him to a local smoking cessation program.

• Provide the patient and members of his family with appropriate referrals to support services. (See *Ensuring continued care for the silicosis patient.*)

EVALUATION

When evaluating the patient's response to your care, gather reassessment data and compare this information to the patient outcomes specified in your plan of care.

Discharge TimeSaver

Ensuring continued care for the silicosis patient

Review the following teaching topics, referrals, and follow-up appointments to make sure that your patient is adequately prepared for discharge.

Teaching topics
Make sure that the following topics have been covered and that the patient's learning has been evaluated:
☐ nature of silicosis, including its process, risk factors, and complications
☐ signs and symptoms that should be reported to the doctor immediately, including shortness of breath, cough, fever, sputum production, and hemoptysis
☐ activity guidelines
☐ nutrition and hydration guidelines
☐ prescribed medications and possible adverse effects
☐ proper use of supplemental oxygen and safety measures
☐ sources of support and information.

Referrals
Make sure that the patient has been provided with necessary referrals to:
☐ social services
☐ home health care agency
☐ medical equipment supplier
☐ smoking cessation program (if applicable).

Follow-up appointments
Make sure that the necessary follow-up appointments have been scheduled and that the patient has been notified:
☐ doctor
☐ diagnostic tests for reevaluation, including chest X-ray, pulmonary function tests, arterial blood gas analysis, or co-oximetry.

Teaching and counseling

Begin by evaluating the effectiveness of your teaching and counseling. Note statements by the patient indicating his understanding of the condition, including its progression and possible complications. Listen for indications that he intends to make necessary changes in his lifestyle. Consider the following questions:
• Has the patient made appropriate plans to increase his level of activity?
• Is he able to identify causes of fatigue and willing to employ energy-conserving methods?
• Is he willing to use support systems to help with coping?
• Does he report feeling less anxious?

Physical condition

Physical examination and diagnostic test results will also help to evaluate the effectiveness of care. If treatment has been effective, you should note the following:
• ABG levels within acceptable limits
• pulse, blood pressure, and respiratory rate, depth, and pattern within established limits
• clear breath sounds
• clear mentation
• adequate nutritional status, as evidenced by weight within established limits
• absence of signs and symptoms of tuberculosis or other infection.

Asbestosis

In this disorder, pulmonary fibrosis and pleural fibrosis result from long-term inhalation of asbestos fibers. Asbestosis may progress to such complications as pleural effusion, pulmonary hypertension, or cor pulmonale. Impaired oxygenation may lead to respiratory failure. In addition, exposure to asbestos has been linked to GI, bronchial,

and lung cancers. (See *Key points about asbestosis.*)

Causes

Asbestosis results from the embedding of inhaled asbestos fibers in lung tissue and visceral pleura. In most patients, the disorder appears after 15 to 20 years of regular exposure to asbestos.

ASSESSMENT

During your assessment, investigate the patient's work history to uncover possible sources of asbestos exposure.

Health history

The patient with pleuropulmonary asbestosis is usually asymptomatic. When symptoms are present, the patient may complain of dyspnea on exertion. If extensive interstitial and pleural fibrosis is present, he may complain of dyspnea at rest and, if fibrosis is extensive, a dry cough. If he smokes cigarettes, the cough may be productive. Also, the patient may complain of pleuritic or retrosternal pain. The medical history may reveal recurrent respiratory tract infections.

Physical examination

Inspection may reveal tachypnea and finger clubbing. Auscultation may reveal characteristic dry crackles in the lung bases.

Diagnostic test results

The following tests help establish the diagnosis.
• Chest X-ray may show fine, irregular, linear, diffuse pulmonary infiltrates, or a rounded, regular nodular pattern. In extensive fibrosis, the lung may have a characteristic honeycombed or ground-glass appearance. Pleural thickening and calcification and bilateral obliteration of costophrenic angles may be evident. In advanced stages of the disease, X-ray may show

an enlarged heart with a classic "shaggy" border.

• Pulmonary function tests may identify decreased vital capacity, decreased forced vital capacity (FVC), decreased total lung capacity and, when fibrosis is advanced, reduced diffusing capacity of the lung for carbon monoxide (DLCO). Forced expiratory volume in 1 second (FEV$_1$) may be decreased or within the normal range. The ratio of FEV$_1$ to FVC remains at baseline. The progression of the disease can be estimated by determining the degree of reduction in vital capacity and DLCO.

• Arterial blood gas (ABG) analysis may reveal decreased partial pressure of arterial oxygen (PaO$_2$) and decreased partial pressure of arterial carbon dioxide (PaCO$_2$) due to hyperventilation.

• Bronchoalveolar lavage may reveal the presence of asbestos fibers. Macrophage and leukocyte cell counts of the lavage fluid may give evidence of the progression of the disease.

• High-resolution computed tomography scan and electron spin resonance spectroscopy may reveal evidence of changes in the lung parenchyma in early stages of the disease.

NURSING DIAGNOSIS

Common nursing diagnoses for the patient with asbestosis include:

• Impaired gas exchange related to ventilation-perfusion mismatch and decreased lung capacity

• Ineffective breathing pattern related to dyspnea and decreased vital capacity

• Altered nutrition: Less than body requirements, related to poor dietary habits and increased metabolic demands

• Anxiety related to the diagnosis and interruption in work, physical deterioration, and possible death

FactFinder

Key points about asbestosis

• *Causative agents.* Asbestos refers to a group of fibrous mineral silicates, especially magnesium and iron. Products that may contain asbestos include acoustic products, brake linings, clutch casings, cement, floor tiles, fire-fighting suits, fireproof paints, insulation, and roofing materials.

• *Populations at risk.* Employees or former employees of companies that mine asbestos minerals or manufacture, install, or remove products containing asbestos — for example, construction, demolition, insulation, pipe fitting, and ship fitting firms — are at risk for developing asbestosis. Family members of these workers are also at risk because they may inhale fibers shaken from work clothes. Other people may be exposed to dust from asbestos building materials in schools, factories, or other buildings.

• *Exposure and disease development.* The probability of developing asbestosis depends on the concentration of asbestos in dust, the duration of exposure, and the patient's response. Usually, it takes 15 to 20 years of occupational exposure to develop asbestosis. Given the large number of workers exposed to asbestos (27.5 million in the United States between 1940 and 1979), many more patients will develop asbestosis and related problems during the next decade.

• *Safety concerns.* Although an "acceptable" threshold limit value (TLV) has been defined for asbestos, the safe level of exposure isn't known. For example, a study of pipefitters found that many developed asbestosis after exposure to only one-fifth the TLV. Another study found that almost every member of a group of insulation workers developed asbestosis within 30 years of exposure.

• Activity intolerance related to disability and decreased oxygen supply
• High risk for infection related to interstitial and pulmonary tissue alterations, altered cell-mediated immunity, and malnutrition.

PLANNING

Based on the nursing diagnosis *impaired gas exchange,* develop appropriate patient outcomes. For example, your patient will:
• maintain adequate ventilation
• maintain PaO_2 and $PaCO_2$ levels within an acceptable range
• maintain optimal breath sounds.

Based on the nursing diagnosis *ineffective breathing pattern,* develop appropriate patient outcomes. For example, your patient will:
• maintain respiratory rate within 5 breaths of baseline
• attain adequate ABG levels
• report feeling comfortable when breathing
• achieve maximum lung expansion with adequate ventilation.

Based on the nursing diagnosis *altered nutrition: less than body requirements,* develop appropriate patient outcomes. For example, your patient will:
• maintain weight or achieve targeted weight
• maintain the specified daily caloric intake
• experience no adverse reactions to enteral or parenteral nutrition.

Based on the nursing diagnosis *anxiety,* develop appropriate patient outcomes. For example, your patient will:
• experience fewer physical symptoms of anxiety
• state his intention to adopt the specified changes in lifestyle
• express willingness to seek help from health professionals, counselors, or support groups in dealing with his worsening physical limitations and with anxiety or depression.

Based on the nursing diagnosis *activity intolerance,* develop appropriate patient outcomes. For example, your patient will:
• express an understanding of his condition, including its progression, treatment, and complications
• develop an appropriate plan to increase his level of activity
• demonstrate techniques for conserving energy while performing activities of daily living
• maintain blood pressure and pulse and respiratory rates within specified parameters.

Based on the nursing diagnosis *high risk for infection,* develop appropriate patient outcomes. For example, your patient will:
• maintain temperature and heart rate within acceptable limits
• remain free from infection (as evidenced by a lack of pathogen growth in cultures)
• exhibit clear and odorless respiratory secretions and a productive (though not incapacitating) cough.

IMPLEMENTATION

Treatment for asbestosis focuses on relieving signs and symptoms of respiratory distress and preventing infections and other complications. (See *Medical care of the patient with asbestosis.*)

Nursing interventions
• Assess for changes in respiratory function, including changes in sputum quality and quantity, restlessness, increased tachypnea, and changes in breath sounds. Report any changes to the doctor immediately.
• Monitor blood gas status, including pulse oximetry and ABG values.
• Administer oxygen by cannula or mask as prescribed. In severe cases, anticipate mechanical ventilation if the patient's respiratory rate increases to more than 30 breaths/minute, his PaO_2

level falls below 55 mm Hg with a fraction of inspired oxygen of 21%, and his PaCO₂ level increases.
- Perform postural drainage, chest percussion, and vibration of the involved lobes several times a day.
- Schedule respiratory therapy at least 1 hour before or after meals. Provide oral care after bronchodilator therapy and periodically thereafter if supplemental oxygen is administered.
- Provide the patient with a high-calorie, high-protein diet of soft foods. Encourage him to take small, frequent meals.
- Make sure the patient receives enough fluids to loosen secretions. Monitor and record intake and output.
- Encourage the patient to participate in appropriate daily activities. Advise him to conserve energy by alternating periods of rest and activity.
- Administer prescribed medications. Monitor the patient for possible adverse reactions.
- Watch for complications, such as pulmonary hypertension, infection, or cor pulmonale.
- Help the patient adjust to lifestyle changes necessitated by chronic illness. Answer all questions and encourage him to express his concerns. Stay with the patient during periods of extreme stress and anxiety.
- Include the patient and members of his family in decisions about care whenever possible.

Patient teaching
- Advise the patient to avoid crowds and people with known infections. Suggest that he discuss influenza and pneumococcus immunizations with his doctor.
- If the patient will receive home oxygen therapy, explain the reasons for treatment and demonstrate the proper use of equipment. If a transtracheal catheter is needed, teach proper catheter care and precautions.

Treatments

Medical care of the patient with asbestosis

Care includes both preventive measures for patients at risk for asbestosis and therapeutic measures for those who have already developed the disorder.

Preventive measures
People in occupations that expose them to asbestos should use all available precautions. Patients with a 10-year or longer history of exposure to asbestos should undergo annual diagnostic chest X-rays and pulmonary function studies of vital capacity. Smoking cessation helps prevent cancers associated with or exacerbated by asbestosis.

Therapeutic measures
- Bronchodilator therapy and inhaled mucolytics coupled with fluid intake of at least 3 qt (3 liters) each day may help relieve respiratory symptoms.
- Hypoxemia requires oxygen administration by cannula or mask. Mechanical ventilation may be used if the patient can't maintain a PaO₂ above 55 mm Hg with oxygen therapy or if his PaCO₂ is acutely elevated.
- If the patient has cor pulmonale, diuretic agents and digitalis glycoside preparations may be prescribed. He may also need to restrict his salt intake.
- Antibiotic therapy helps treat respiratory tract infections.

- Teach the patient techniques for effective coughing and deep breathing and explain that they will ease breathing and help remove secretions.
- Teach the patient and members of his family how to perform postural drainage and chest percussion. Explain

Discharge TimeSaver

Ensuring continued care for the patient with asbestosis

Review the following teaching topics, referrals, and follow-up appointments to make sure that your patient is adequately prepared for discharge.

Teaching topics
Make sure that the following topics have been covered and that your patient's learning has been evaluated:
☐ the nature of asbestosis, including its process, risk factors, and complications
☐ signs and symptoms to report to the doctor
☐ activity guidelines
☐ nutrition and hydration guidelines
☐ prescribed medications, including possible adverse effects
☐ proper use of supplemental oxygen at home, including safety measures
☐ sources of information and support.

Referrals
Make sure that the patient has been

provided with necessary referrals to:
☐ social services
☐ occupational retraining
☐ home health care agency
☐ medical equipment supplier
☐ smoking cessation program (if necessary).

Follow-up appointments
Make sure that the necessary follow-up appointments have been scheduled and that the patient has been notified:
☐ doctor
☐ diagnostic tests for reevaluation, including chest X-rays, computed tomography scan, pulmonary function test, arterial blood gas analysis, or co-oximetry.

---

that the patient should remain in each position for 10 minutes and then receive percussion. Afterward, the patient should use productive coughing techniques to remove secretions.
• Thoroughly explain all medications. Discuss proper administration and possible adverse effects.
• Encourage the patient to adhere to a high-calorie, high-protein diet and to drink plenty of fluids to prevent dehydration and help loosen secretions.
• Teach the patient to use pursed-lip breathing to alleviate shortness of breath due to small-airway obstruction.
• If the patient smokes, encourage him to stop. Refer him to a local smoking cessation program.
• Provide referrals to other appropriate support services.

• If the patient risks further exposure to asbestos, teach him the importance of wearing a mask and using other protective devices to reduce the risk. (See *Ensuring continued care for the patient with asbestosis.*)

EVALUATION

When evaluating the patient's response to your care, gather reassessment data and compare this information to the patient outcomes specified in your plan of care.

Teaching and counseling
Begin by evaluating the effectiveness of your teaching and counseling. Note statements by the patient indicating his understanding of the condition, its progression, and the possible complica-

tions. Consider the following questions:

• Is the patient willing to adopt necessary lifestyle changes?
• Has he developed a plan to increase his activity level?
• Does he use energy-conserving techniques during activities?
• Does the patient state that he feels less anxiety? Is he willing to use coping strategies and support systems, such as psychosocial counseling groups or work rehabilitation clinics, to reduce anxiety? Do his appearance and behavior suggest reduced anxiety?

Physical condition

Physical examination and diagnostic test results will also help to evaluate the effectiveness of care. Note whether the following criteria have been achieved:

• adequate ABG values
• optimal breath sounds
• respiratory rate, depth, and pattern within acceptable limits
• weight approaching targeted level
• an absence of signs or symptoms of infection.

Coal worker's pneumoconiosis

This progressive nodular pulmonary disease results from the inhalation of coal dust. *Simple* coal worker's pneumoconiosis is characterized by pinpoint black nodules (coal macules) and focal emphysema. It may evolve into *complicated* pneumoconiosis, or progressive massive fibrosis, which is characterized by the formation of fibrous tissue masses and pigmented nodules greater than 1 cm in diameter in one or both lungs.

Pulmonary tuberculosis often accompanies the disorder and may hasten its progress. Although exposure to coal dust alone may cause chronic

bronchitis and airway obstruction, smoking significantly increases the risk of complications, which include malnutrition, chronic bronchitis, bronchopneumonia, bronchiectasis, spontaneous pneumothorax, and emphysema. As the disease progresses, pulmonary hypertension and cor pulmonale may occur. Silicosis may also coexist with coal worker's pneumoconiosis because coal workers may need to cut through silica-containing rock.

Causes

Coal worker's pneumoconiosis results from accumulation of coal dust particles in the lung, overwhelming airway clearance mechanisms. The disease is triggered by an immune response.

ASSESSMENT

In both simple and complicated pneumoconiosis, assessment will reveal exposure to coal dust. Occupational exposure may have occurred during the mining or handling of lignite, anthracite, or bituminous coal; kaolin; mica; or silica. (See *Risk factors for coal worker's pneumoconiosis,* page 262.) Since most people with coal worker's pneumoconiosis are asymptomatic, diagnosis is based on a history of exposure to coal dust and on positive chest X-ray findings.

Health history

If the patient is a nonsmoker and has simple coal miner's pneumoconiosis, he will most likely be asymptomatic. If he has the complicated form of the disease, he may complain of dyspnea on exertion and a persistent cough. In some cases, the patient's cough produces inky-black sputum (melanoptysis) caused by avascular necrosis and cavitation. If concurrent bronchial and pulmonary infections are present, he may report sputum that is either coal-

Whether or not a mine worker exposed to coal dust will develop coal worker's pneumoconiosis depends upon several factors, described below:

• *Duration of exposure.* Development of the disorder usually requires 10 to 15 years of occupational exposure to coal dust.
• *Severity of exposure.* In the United States, federal regulations mandate that respirable dust levels in underground coal mines not exceed 2 mg/m³. Before enactment of these regulations in 1969, miners were commonly exposed to higher dust levels. Workers in the area where coal is cut, known as the coal face, were exposed to especially high concentrations of coal dust.
• *Size of coal particles.* Coal particles must be less than 5 microns wide to enter the lung.
• *Type of coal.* Risk is greatest for workers who mine older coal with a higher percentage of carbon. Anthracite mining in the eastern United States is associated with the highest incidence of coal worker's pneumoconiosis. Bituminous mining is considered less hazardous.

flecked, thick yellow or green, or milky or clear gray.

Physical examination

Inspection may reveal a barrel chest. Chest percussion may disclose hyperresonant lungs with areas of dullness. Auscultation may disclose diminished breath sounds, crackles, rhonchi, and wheezes.

Diagnostic test results

• In simple coal worker's pneumoconiosis, chest X-ray may show small opacities, possibly in all lung zones but more prominent in the upper lung zones. In complicated coal worker's pneumoconiosis, chest X-ray may reveal larger opacities, some with cavitation.
• In simple coal worker's pneumoconiosis, pulmonary function studies indicate normal vital capacity. The ratio of residual volume to total lung capacity is normal.

In the complicated form of the disease, studies indicate decreased vital capacity, decreased forced expiratory volume in 1 second, and increased residual volume. Also, diffusing capacity of the lung for carbon monoxide significantly declines, reflecting alveolar septal destruction and pulmonary capillary obliteration.
• Arterial blood gas (ABG) analysis reveals normal partial pressure of arterial oxygen (PaO_2) in simple coal worker's pneumoconiosis and a decreased PaO_2 in the complicated form of the disease. In the simple form, partial pressure of arterial carbon dioxide ($PaCO_2$) may decline if the patient is hyperventilating due to hypoxemia and may increase if the patient has impaired alveolar ventilation.

NURSING DIAGNOSIS

Common nursing diagnoses for the patient with complicated coal worker's pneumoconiosis include:
• Impaired gas exchange related to ventilation-perfusion mismatch and decreased oxygen diffusion capacity
• Ineffective breathing pattern related to dyspnea, airway obstruction, and loss of elastic recoil of the lung
• Activity intolerance related to dyspnea and decreased oxygen supply.

PLANNING

Based on the nursing diagnosis *impaired gas exchange,* develop appropriate patient outcomes. For example, your patient will:
• maintain adequate ventilation as evidenced by normal $PaCO_2$ and PaO_2 levels
• maintain optimal breath sounds.

   Based on the nursing diagnosis *ineffective breathing pattern,* develop appropriate patient outcomes. For example, your patient will:
• maintain a respiratory rate within 5 breaths of the baseline rate
• maintain adequate ABG levels
• achieve optimal lung expansion with adequate ventilation.

   Based on the nursing diagnosis *activity intolerance,* develop appropriate patient outcomes. For example, your patient will:
• express an understanding of the disorder and its relationship to activity intolerance
• develop an appropriate plan to increase his level of activity
• develop skill in conserving energy while performing activities
• maintain acceptable values for pulse rate, blood pressure, and respiratory rate during activities.

IMPLEMENTATION

Treatment of the patient with coal worker's pneumoconiosis focuses on relieving the patient's symptoms and teaching him about the disorder and care measures. (See *Medical care of the patient with coal worker's pneumoconiosis,* page 264.)
• Assess for changes in the patient's respiratory function. Document any changes in breath sounds, increasing tachypnea, or restlessness. Report significant changes immediately.

• Observe, document, and report changes in the quality or quantity of the patient's sputum.
• Monitor blood gas status, including pulse oximetry and ABG levels.
• Administer oxygen by cannula or mask as prescribed. Anticipate mechanical ventilation if the patient's respiratory rate exceeds 30 breaths/minute, his PaO_2 falls below 55 mm Hg with a fraction of inspired oxygen of 21%, and his $PaCO_2$ increases.
• Perform postural drainage, chest percussion, and vibration several times daily.
• If the patient requires incentive spirometry, encourage him to sit or assume semi-Fowler's position to promote optimal lung expansion.
• If the patient is receiving inhalation therapy, perform oral care after the treatments and periodically during the day.
• Watch for complications, such as respiratory infection, cor pulmonale, or tuberculosis.
• Administer prescribed medications and record the patient's response.
• Make sure the patient receives adequate hydration to loosen secretions. Maintain accurate intake and output records.
• Provide the patient with a high-calorie, high-protein diet of soft foods.
• Help the patient conserve energy and prevent fatigue by providing small, frequent meals and scheduling respiratory treatments at least 1 hour before or after meals.
• Encourage the patient to participate in appropriate daily activities. Plan alternating periods of rest and activity.
• Help the patient adjust to lifestyle changes necessitated by chronic illness.
• Encourage him to express his concerns. Include the patient and members of his family in decisions about care whenever possible.

Treatments

Medical care of the patient with coal worker's pneumoconiosis

Therapy for coal worker's pneumoconiosis emphasizes preventing exacerbation of the illness and alleviating its symptoms.

Preventive measures
• Eliminating the patient's exposure to coal dust
• Smoking cessation, if appropriate
• Immunization against pneumococcal infection and influenza

Therapeutic measures
• Bronchial hygiene, including systematic hydration, humidification of inspired air, postural drainage, and percussion
• Drug therapy to ease air exchange and promote breathing comfort. For example, theophylline, aminophylline, or oral or inhaled sympathomimetics (such as albuterol or metaproterenol) may be prescribed for acute episodes of reversible bronchospasm. If the patient shows evidence of persistent bronchospasm and airway inflammation, corticosteroids (such as oral prednisone or inhaled beclomethasone) may be used to suppress the inflammatory response in the airway.
• Antibiotic therapy to treat respiratory infections (including tuberculosis)
• Diuretic agents, digoxin, and sodium restrictions to treat cor pulmonale, if necessary
• Appropriate drug therapy, if tuberculosis is detected
• Incentive spirometry to improve alveolar ventilation
• Nocturnal or continuous oxygen therapy administered by cannula or mask to treat hypoxemia
• Mechanical ventilation for patients who develop respiratory failure

Patient teaching
• Advise the patient to avoid crowds and people with known infections.
• Suggest that he discuss influenza and pneumococcus immunizations with his doctor.
• Teach the patient how to use pursed-lip breathing to control shortness of breath.
• If home oxygen therapy is prescribed, explain its purpose and teach the patient how to use the equipment.
• Teach techniques for effective coughing and deep breathing to promote ventilation and remove secretions.
• Teach the patient and members of his family how to perform postural drainage and chest percussion. Explain that the patient should remain in each position for 10 minutes and then re-ceive percussion. Afterward, he should use productive coughing techniques to remove secretions.
• Demonstrate how to use an incentive spirometer and explain its purpose.
• Discuss the medication regimen. Describe dosages, possible adverse effects, and the purpose of each prescribed drug.
• Encourage the patient to adopt a high-calorie, high-protein diet. Emphasize that he should drink plenty of fluids to prevent dehydration and help loosen secretions.
• If the patient smokes, urge him to stop. Explain how smoking increases his risk of complications. If necessary, refer him to a local smoking cessation program.
• As appropriate, provide information about preventing coal worker's pneu-

Discharge TimeSaver

Ensuring continued care for the patient with coal worker's pneumoconiosis

Review the following teaching topics, referrals, and follow-up appointments to make sure that your patient is adequately prepared for discharge.

Teaching topics
Make sure that the following topics have been covered and your patient's learning has been evaluated:
☐ nature of coal worker's pneumoconiosis, including its risk factors and possible complications
☐ signs and symptoms that should immediately be reported to the doctor
☐ activity guidelines
☐ nutrition and hydration guidelines
☐ prescribed medications, including possible adverse effects
☐ proper, safe use of supplemental oxygen, if prescribed for home use
☐ sources of support and information.

Referrals
Make sure that the patient has been provided with necessary referrals to:
☐ social services
☐ occupational rehabilitation
☐ home health care agency
☐ medical equipment supplier
☐ smoking cessation program if applicable.

Follow-up appointments
Make sure that the necessary follow-up appointments have been scheduled and that the patient has been notified:
☐ doctor
☐ diagnostic tests for reevaluation, including chest X-ray, pulmonary function tests, arterial blood gas analysis, or co-oximetry.

---

moconiosis. If the patient must return to a hazardous work environment, emphasize the importance of wearing an effective respirator. (See *Ensuring continued care for the patient with coal worker's pneumoconiosis.*)

EVALUATION

When evaluating the patient's response to your care, gather reassessment data and compare this information to the patient outcomes specified in your plan of care.

Teaching and counseling
Begin by evaluating the effectiveness of your teaching and counseling. Note statements by the patient indicating his understanding of the condition, including its progression and possible com-

plications. Listen for indications that the patient intends to make necessary lifestyle changes. Consider the following questions:
• Does the patient understand home care measures and the medication regimen?
• Are the patient and family members aware of the patient's nutrition and hydration needs?
• Does the patient know how to avoid infections?
• Is he planning to obtain immunizations?
• Has he taken steps to increase his level of activity?
• Does he demonstrate skill at conserving energy during activities?

Physical condition

Physical examination and diagnostic tests will also provide information for evaluation. Note whether the following parameters have been attained:

• acceptable pulse and respiratory rates and blood pressure
• optimal breath sounds
• adequate oxygenation and ventilation, as evidenced by optimal ABG levels
• maximal lung expansion with comfortable breathing.

Smoke inhalation injury

A patient who inhales smoke or toxic fumes during a fire may experience thermal injuries, chemical injuries, or both. Early detection and aggressive treatment of smoke inhalation injuries are crucial to ensuring the survival of any patient exposed to a fire.

Thermal injuries result from inhaling steam or superheated air. Thermal injuries may cause burning or irritation in the upper respiratory tract and may lead to laryngeal edema and airway obstruction.

Chemical injuries result from inhaling noxious chemicals contained in smoke and gases (for example, smoke from a building fire or fumes from burning chemicals). They affect both the upper and lower respiratory tracts. (See *Toxic gases in house-fire smoke.*) Smoke inhalation injuries can also result from inhalation of particulates, such as ash or soot.

Carbon monoxide (CO) toxicity, which frequently accompanies smoke inhalation injury, poses special problems because it binds with hemoglobin in place of oxygen, thus preventing adequate transport of oxygen from the lungs to the rest of the body's tissues. It is commonly seen in patients who attempt suicide by inhaling automobile exhaust fumes as well as in burn victims. Anyone who inhales substantial levels of CO risks cardiopulmonary failure, central nervous system damage, and death. Older patients, children, and patients with preexisting anemia or cardiopulmonary disease are especially susceptible to the effects of CO toxicity.

Your assessment findings will vary, depending on the type of gas inhaled and the nature of the injury (cutaneous burns, upper airway burns or irritation, or lower airway involvement).

Physiologic changes that result from acute injury to the alveolocapillary membrane may be delayed for 1 or 2 days or even longer. Therefore, after taking a health history, performing a physical examination, and reviewing diagnostic test results, be sure to follow up on your findings.

Health history

You may learn the patient was injured in a fire in a building, automobile, or other enclosed space. If the patient is not conscious, consult witnesses to the fire, family members, or emergency personnel. Find out the duration of exposure, whether or not the patient received treatment at the site of the fire, and if he has any preexisting cardiopulmonary conditions. If possible, obtain descriptions of the environment and materials involved in the fire.

If the patient is conscious, he may complain of chest pain, respiratory distress, disorientation, dizziness, nausea, sleepiness, muscular twitching, or stiffness.

Physical examination

First look for evidence of cutaneous burns or soot, especially around the mouth and nose. The patient may exhibit a broad range of symptoms that

Toxic gases in house-fire smoke

Because house-fire smoke consists of potent mucosal irritants and bronchoconstrictors, inhalation may lead to direct airway and parenchymal lung injury. The following chart lists toxic gases that may be emitted during a housefire and their potential effects on the patient.

Gas	Sources	Effects
Carbon monoxide	• Organic matter	• Tissue hypoxia
Carbon dioxide	• Organic matter	• Narcosis
Nitrogen dioxide	• Wallpaper • Wood	• Bronchial irritation • Dizziness • Progressive hypoxemia • Pulmonary edema
Hydrogen chloride	• Plastics (polyvinylchloride)	• Severe mucosal irritation • Increased airway resistance • Restricted lung volume • Altered intracellular pH • Protein denaturation • Cell destruction • Increased capillary permeability
Hydrogen cyanide	• Wool, silk, nylon • Polyurethane	• Headache • Respiratory failure • Coma • Tissue hypoxia
Benzene	• Petroleum • Plastics	• Mucosal irritation • Coma
Aldehydes	• Wood • Cotton • Paper	• Severe mucosal damage • Upper airway irritation or obstruction • Pulmonary edema • Extensive lung damage
Ammonia	• Nylon	• Mucosal irritation • Altered intracellular pH • Protein denaturation • Cell destruction • Increased pulmonary capillary permeability
Chlorine	• Cleaning solutions (especially when mixed with ammonia, vinegar, or other acids) • Water-purification products	• Severe mucosal irritation • Increased pulmonary capillary permeability • Tissue hypoxia • Headache • Altered level of consciousness

FactFinder
Complications of smoke inhalation injury

Smoke inhalation injuries commonly cause tissue hypoxia, methemoglobinemia, hypoxemia, and metabolic acidosis (all of which may reflect carbon monoxide, chlorine, or cyanide toxicity). Pulmonary edema may develop up to 72 hours after injury (even if the patient is asymptomatic initially). It may be compounded by hypoproteinemia and by the action of vasoactive mediators released by injured tissues. Also, alveolar and interstitial edema may be aggravated by massive fluid resuscitation.

Other possible complications of smoke inhalation injury include:
• asthma and pneumonia
• cerebral edema
• cor pulmonale and myocardial ischemia
• bronchiolitis fibrosa obliterans
• chemical pneumonitis and surfactant damage
• interstitial fibrosis
• disseminated intravascular coagulation
• neuropsychiatric sequelae, such as parkinsonism, hearing and speech disturbances, or changes in personality
• microembolization
• shock, coma, and death.

vary in severity. Symptoms that indicate upper airway involvement are hoarseness, stridor, and painful swallowing. The patient should be watched carefully for evidence of airway obstruction due to sudden edema. Inspection of the throat and nose may reveal erythema, singed hairs, edema, and ulceration. Cough, cyanosis, tachypnea, and carbonaceous sputum are also signs that lung injury from smoke inhalation has occurred. However, it is

possible that the patient may be asymptomatic. (See *Complications of smoke inhalation injury*.)

Auscultation may disclose crackles and inspiratory or expiratory wheezing.

Carbon monoxide toxicity
Signs and symptoms of the inhalation of sublethal amounts of CO are primarily related to cerebral hypoxia and include headache, confusion, fatigue, dizziness, and visual disturbances that may progress to ataxia, hallucinations, combativeness, or coma.

Timesaving tip: CO inhalation causes flushing, which may mask pallor or cyanosis in a patient experiencing hypoxemia and tissue hypoxia. Physical examination is unreliable in detecting the severity of CO poisoning; therefore, if CO poisoning is suspected (as it should be whenever smoke inhalation is possible), promptly treat the patient with 100% oxygen.

Diagnostic test results
The following tests help establish the nature and extent of smoke inhalation injury. Because effects may be delayed in smoke inhalation injury, initial chest X-ray and arterial blood gas (ABG) analysis findings may be normal. Continued monitoring is essential.

• Serial chest X-rays may illustrate the progression of pulmonary damage. Initial results may be clear or reveal areas of hyperinflation. Bilateral pulmonary edema or diffuse patchy infiltrates may appear hours or days later. Complete whiteout may develop 4 to 7 days later, indicating adult respiratory distress syndrome (ARDS).

• Initial ABG levels may indicate slight respiratory alkalosis due to tachypnea. Twenty-four to 48 hours after the injury, findings may indicate hypoxemia, hypocapnia or hypercapnia, and a widened alveolar-arterial gradient. If ARDS develops, hypoxemia will be severe despite high levels of inspired oxygen.

ABG results and pulse oximetry may be misleading in CO poisoning. Most labs routinely calculate the arterial oxygen saturation (SaO_2) based upon the partial pressure of arterial oxygen (PaO_2), but in CO poisoning, the actual SaO_2 may be very low despite an adequate PaO_2 because of the high affinity of hemoglobins for CO over oxygen.

• Blood carboxyhemoglobin (COHb) measurements may be used to identify and monitor CO toxicity. (See *Understanding blood carboxyhemoglobin measurements,* page 270).

• Transnasal fiber-optic bronchoscopy or laryngoscopy may disclose the level of injury and provide visual evidence of edema, ulceration, inflammation, and necrosis. Mucosal changes distal to the larynx often correlate with respiratory difficulty.

• Radionuclide lung ventilation-perfusion scintiphotography may be used to diagnose smoke inhalation injury; however, the results may provide false-positives in patients with previous pulmonary disease. A radionuclide scan that shows a normal distribution with normal clearance of the radioactive tracer virtually excludes the diagnosis of smoke-induced distal airway damage.

• Pulmonary function studies may indicate decreased forced vital capacity and decreased forced expiratory volume in 1 second. Minute volumes are normal or decreased. The diffusing capacity of the lungs for CO may be normal. The inspiratory portion of the flow volume loop may indicate upper airway obstruction.

• Pulse oximetry measurements may be used to monitor SaO_2. The optimal range is 98% to 100%. Pulse oximetry readings are also misleading because the technology does not allow for the distinction between oxyhemoglobin and COHb. A co-oximeter can distinguish between hemoglobin saturated with oxygen and that which is saturated with CO. However, co-oximetry may not be readily available.

• Plasma lactic acid (lactate) concentration higher than 16 mg/dl in a patient who does not have severe burns indicates metabolic acidosis secondary to CO, chlorine gas, or cyanide toxicity, a common form of toxic injury resulting from the burning of synthetic products. CO and cyanide prevent cellular use of oxygen, causing severe oxygenation problems.

• Urine cyanide concentration identifies the severity of cyanide inhalation. A normal reading is 0.05 mcg/ml; a toxic level is 0.5 mcg/ml; and concentrations of 1 mcg/ml or greater are acutely toxic.

NURSING DIAGNOSIS

Common nursing diagnoses for the patient with smoke inhalation injury include:

• Impaired gas exchange related to airway obstruction, ventilation-perfusion mismatch, and injury to the gas-exchange surface

• Ineffective breathing pattern related to pain, excessive secretions, and anxiety

• Ineffective airway clearance related to upper airway edema, obstruction, or increased secretions

• High risk for infection related to impaired respiratory defense mechanisms.

PLANNING

Based on the nursing diagnosis *impaired gas exchange,* develop appropriate patient outcomes. For example, your patient will:

• maintain adequate ventilation as evidenced by normal partial pressure of arterial carbon dioxide ($PaCO_2$) levels

Interpretation

Understanding blood carboxyhemoglobin measurements

Blood carboxyhemoglobin measurements are used to determine the concentration of carbon monoxide (CO) in a patient's blood. Normal levels are below 5%. Higher levels may be associated with various signs and symptoms, as described below:

• 10% — hyperventilation (Note, however, that smokers and people who live in polluted cities may tolerate 10% carboxyhemoglobin levels.)
• 15% to 20% — headache and confusion
• 20% to 40% — fatigue, disorientation, dizziness, visual disturbances, chest pain or arrhythmias from myocardial ischemia
• 40% to 60% — ataxia, hallucinations, combativeness, and coma (secondary to cerebral hypoxia)
• 60% or greater — death.

Alternatively, the laboratory may report the patient's CO concentration in terms of partial pressure of carbon monoxide (PCO), measured in millimeters of mercury (mm Hg).

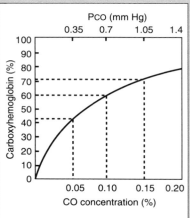

• achieve PaO_2 level within acceptable range (75 to 100 mm Hg)
• maintain clear breath sounds.

Based on the nursing diagnosis *ineffective breathing pattern,* develop appropriate patient outcomes. For example, your patient will:
• maintain respiratory rate within 5 breaths of baseline
• achieve maximum lung expansion with adequate ventilation.

Based on the nursing diagnosis *ineffective airway clearance,* develop appropriate patient outcomes. For example, your patient will:
• demonstrate ability to keep airway clear of excessive secretions
• maintain adequate airway free of pharyngeal and laryngeal edema

• maintain normal ventilation free of tracheobronchial obstruction.

Based on the nursing diagnosis *high risk for infection,* develop appropriate patient outcomes. For example, your patient will:
• maintain temperature and heart rate within acceptable limits
• remain free from infection (as evidenced by a lack of pathogen growth in cultures)
• exhibit clear and odorless respiratory secretions and a productive (though not incapacitating) cough.

IMPLEMENTATION

Treatment of smoke inhalation injury focuses on preventing complications and restoring the patient's respiratory function. Therapy typically includes providing adequate oxygenation and carefully monitoring the patient's respiratory status to prevent respiratory failure. (See *Medical care of the patient with smoke inhalation injuries,* pages 272 and 273 .)

Nursing interventions

• Carefully and periodically assess for signs of impending airway obstruction (stridor, anxiety, labored breathing). Maintain high-flow, humidified oxygen to the patient's airway.

• Assist with the initiation of hyperbaric oxygen therapy, if prescribed.

• At regular intervals, perform chest auscultation for stridor, crackles, rhonchi, and wheezing to monitor possible deterioration in respiratory status from airway obstruction, inability to clear secretions, bronchospasm, and pulmonary edema.

• Frequently assess your patient's level of consciousness to detect neuropsychiatric sequelae caused by the inhalation of CO or another noxious gas. Observe for signs of disorientation, parkinsonism, gait disturbances, hearing disturbances, speech disturbances, and personality changes (such as depression, moodiness, irritability, aggressiveness, and impulsiveness).

• Monitor vital signs frequently at first, then periodically, to assess core temperature fluctuations, arrhythmias, hypotension, or hypertension and to detect early indications of complications.

• Administer bronchodilators, corticosteroids, analgesics, and antibiotics as prescribed.

• Frequently turn and reposition your patient to facilitate pulmonary hygiene and skin and muscle care, especially when surface burns are present.

• Assist the patient to cough and clear secretions.

• Carefully titrate the patient's fluid resuscitation rate to correspond with his progress.

• Maintain adequate hydration, avoiding overhydration and underhydration. In inhalation injuries, hypovolemia may underperfuse the injured lung and increase the ventilation-perfusion mismatch. Overhydration increases the risk of pulmonary edema and pneumonia.

• If the patient's condition is critical, measure urine output hourly.

• Monitor results of laboratory tests to help guide oxygen therapy. Be especially alert for decreases in PaO_2, which may signal the onset of ARDS or infection.

• Obtain spirometry and flow volume measurements to detect changes in the airways.

• Assist your patient in the grieving process if family members, pets, or property were injured or lost.

Mechanical ventilation

• Monitor the patient's hemodynamic status.

• Monitor ABG levels. Your goal is to keep the fraction of inspired oxygen and positive end-expiratory pressure (PEEP) as low as possible while maintaining acceptable PaO_2, $PaCO_2$, and SaO_2 levels. A PaO_2 level falling below 70 mm Hg indicates hypoxemia. A $PaCO_2$ level falling below 35 mm Hg indicates hypocapnia. An increasing pH (above 7.45) and a decreasing $PaCO_2$ level (below 35 mm Hg) indicate respiratory alkalosis. Trends in results are more important than specific findings because the patient's airway may deteriorate or CO may fail to increase when exposure ends.

In CO inhalation injuries, PaO_2 and SaO_2 levels cannot be used as absolute guides to measuring oxygenation because CO interferes with hemoglobin's oxygen-carrying capacity.

• Make sure the endotracheal tube is adequately secured. Oral or nasal reintubation may be impossible because of edema.

Treatments

Medical care of the patient with smoke inhalation injuries

Treatment for smoke inhalation injury will depend on the severity of injury, materials present in the fire, and the presence or absence of carbon monoxide (CO) toxicity and other complications.

Treating moderate upper airway injury

Treatment may be initiated based on visual inspection of the patient's upper airway and on arterial blood gas measurements that indicate possible injury. Common measures include:
• maintaining a patent airway
• administering humidified oxygen, bronchodilators, and racemic epinephrine (if necessary)
• providing pulmonary toilet and chest physiotherapy
• continuing supplemental oxygen (usually at 100%) until carboxyhemoglobin (COHb) levels return to normal.

Treating severe injury

The patient may need to undergo the following interventions for severe cough, bronchoconstriction, or hypoxemia:
• immediate ventilatory support
• orotracheal or nasotracheal intubation, if the patient exhibits progressive respiratory distress and persistent hypoxemia (despite an adequate airway and oxygen therapy) or upper airway obstruction
• mechanical ventilation with positive end-expiratory pressure to provide adequate oxygenation and prevent extensive alveolar collapse

• endotracheal intubation and mechanical ventilation if fiber-optic bronchoscopy identifies erythema, edema, and ulceration at the vocal cord level in patients at risk for obstruction. (Endotracheal intubation is preferred over tracheostomy when the airway injury is not at the larynx level.)
• bronchodilators (theophylline, aminophylline) for bronchoconstriction. (Note that bronchodilators must be chosen carefully because burn victims often have a sinus tachycardia as a baseline cardiac rhythm and many bronchodilators cause tachycardia as an adverse effect.)

Treating CO toxicity

Patients with impaired consciousness are routinely treated for exposure to CO. Interventions include 100% oxygen or hyperbaric oxygen therapy, especially if COHb saturation levels exceed 50%. Whenever CO exposure is suspected, 100% oxygen should be routinely administered. Administering 100% oxygen reduces the half-life of COHb from 4 hours to about 50 minutes. A hyperbaric chamber further reduces the half-life to 22 minutes. Prompt hyperbaric chamber treatment may also decrease the incidence of late-occurring neuropsychiatric effects of CO poisoning. The doctor may also

• If the patient has facial and nasal burns, secure the knots of the endotracheal tube's strings to prevent pressure on the nasal septum. (Otherwise, cartilage loss and a severe cosmetic defect can result.)

• Use strict sterile technique when suctioning the endotracheal tube.
• Use a closed suctioning system for its aseptic quality, to maintain PEEP levels, and to prevent additional alveolar collapse.

prescribe methemoglobinemia antidotes, such as methylthionine blue or toluidine blue.

Additional interventions
• Cyanide antidotes, such as sodium thiosulfate or hydroxocobalamin, may be administered to counteract the effects of hydrogen cyanide poisoning. Other antidotes that may be prescribed, depending on the materials present in the fire, include organophosphate antidotes (such as atropine or oximes) and heavy metal chelators (such as dimercaptopropane sulfonate or dimercaptosuccinic acid).
• Antibiotics may be administered to treat infection. Cultures of sputum, urine, blood, and wounds are obtained prior to antibiotic therapy and at regular intervals during extended hospitalization.
• Corticosteroid therapy may be prescribed to counter the risk of delayed toxic pulmonary edema or to decrease cerebral edema or bronchospasms; however, its use is controversial.
• Repeated bronchoscopies and regional lavage with directed suctioning (in addition to frequent pulmonary toilet and suctioning) may be used to remove sloughed bronchial tissues.

• During suctioning, monitor the electrocardiogram and SaO_2 level to detect hypoxemia and bradycardia.

Patient teaching
• When appropriate, provide the patient with explanations about his condition and its causes. Many patients can't recall the inhalation incident, especially if a fire was involved.
• Teach your patient how to use a Yankhauer suction apparatus, if necessary. Burns and inhalation injuries to the face and oropharynx cause copious amounts of oral secretions. The ability to clear the airway may provide feelings of autonomy and help reduce anxiety.
• Teach the patient techniques for productive coughing and deep breathing and explain that they promote ventilation and remove secretions.
• Show the patient how to use an incentive spirometer properly and explain its purpose.
• Discuss the medication regimen with the patient and members of his family. Review dosages, possible adverse effects, and the purposes of prescribed drugs.
• Encourage the patient to follow a high-calorie, high-protein diet and to drink plenty of fluids to prevent dehydration and help loosen secretions.
• If the patient smokes, urge him to stop because it adds to the carbon dioxide in the lungs. Provide him with information and refer him for counseling.
• Teach patients and family members to recognize signs and symptoms of complications requiring immediate medical attention: airway obstruction (difficult or noisy breathing), neurologic complications (headaches, personality changes, loss of consciousness), worsening respiratory function (dyspnea, cough, infection, increase or change in sputum). (See *Ensuring continued care for the patient with smoke inhalation injuries,* page 274.)

EVALUATION

When evaluating the patient's response to your care, gather reassessment data and compare this information to the

Ensuring continued care for the patient with smoke inhalation injuries

Review the following teaching topics, referrals, and follow-up appointments to make sure that your patient is adequately prepared for discharge.

Teaching topics
Make sure that the following topics have been covered and that your patient's learning has been evaluated:
☐ the nature and process of the injury, including associated risk factors and possible complications
☐ specific therapies prescribed for burn injuries
☐ signs and symptoms that should be reported to the doctor
☐ activity guidelines
☐ nutrition and hydration guidelines
☐ information about prescribed medications, including possible adverse effects
☐ proper, safe use of supplemental oxygen, if prescribed for home use
☐ sources of support and information.

Referrals
Make sure that the patient has been provided with necessary referrals to:
☐ social services
☐ posttrauma support group or emergency shelter, as indicated
☐ home health care agency
☐ medical equipment supplier.

Follow-up appointments
Make sure that the necessary follow-up appointments have been scheduled and that the patient has been notified:
☐ doctor
☐ diagnostic tests for reevaluation, including chest X-rays and pulmonary function tests.

patient outcomes specified in your plan of care.

Teaching and counseling
Begin by evaluating the effectiveness of your teaching and counseling. Consider asking the following questions:
• Does the patient understand his condition and its possible complications?
• Is he implementing steps to maintain adequate ventilation, nutrition, and hydration?
• Do the patient and members of his family understand the medication regimen and other home care measures?

Physical condition
Physical examination and diagnostic tests will provide additional evaluation information. If treatment has been successful, you should note the following outcomes:

• blood pressure, pulse rate, and respiratory rate within specified limits
• breath sounds that have returned to normal
• optimal ABG levels
• maximal lung expansion and comfortable breathing
• normal body temperature.

CHAPTER 10

Caring for patients with cancer

Lung cancer

An uncontrolled growth of abnormal cells in the lung, this cancer usually originates on the wall or epithelium of the bronchial tree. That's why the disorder is often referred to as bronchogenic carcinoma.

Lung cancer represents the most common cause of cancer death for both men and women. Because symptoms rarely occur in the disease's early stages, the prognosis for most patients is poor. Roughly 85% of all patients succumb to the disease within 5 years of diagnosis.

Researchers believe that lung cancer develops slowly over 10 to 30 years after inhalation of a cancer-producing substance, or a carcinogen. This exposure may be one-time or prolonged. Lung cancer's first symptoms sometimes occur in a totally different part of the body, the result of metastasis. The most common sites of metastasis are the contralateral lung, liver, brain, cervical nodes, scalene nodes, skin, adrenal gland, kidneys, and bones.

Causes
Cigarette smoking ranks as the major cause of lung cancer, accounting for about 80% of tumors. Male smokers possess a 10 times greater risk of the disorder than male nonsmokers; female smokers, a 5 times greater risk than female nonsmokers. However, nonsmokers of both sexes can also be at risk because of inhalation of secondhand smoke. (See *Risk factors for lung cancer.*)

Classification
Many types of lung cancer exist. The four most common types are squamous cell (epidermoid) carcinoma, small-cell (oat cell) carcinoma, adenocarcinoma, and large-cell (anaplastic) carcinoma. (See *Major types of bronchogenic carcinomas,* pages 278 and 279.)

All types of lung cancer metastasize via the lymphatic system early in their course. However, complications resulting from lung cancer and the extent of metastasis will vary, depending on the cell type involved. (See *Complications of lung cancer,* page 280.)

Lung cancers may also be classified by the degree of malignancy of the cells. They're classified in levels I to IV, with level I the least malignant and least likely to spread and level IV the most malignant and having the least resemblance to normal tissue.

To guide therapy, doctors use a method of staging tumors called the TNM system (Tumor size, Nodal involvement, Metastatic progress). The TNM classification system provides an accurate tumor description that's adjustable as the cancer progresses. Staging allows reliable comparison of treatment and survival rates among large groups of patients. It also identifies nodal involvement and metastasis. (See *Staging lung cancer,* page 281.)

ASSESSMENT

Because symptoms rarely occur in early stages, lung cancer is often advanced at the time of diagnosis. When symptoms do appear, they vary considerably, according to the tumor's size, location, and cell type, and whether the patient has any underlying pulmonary disease. As a result, your assessment should include careful consideration of the patient's health history (including known risk factors), physical examination findings, and diagnostic test results.

Health history
The most common complaint is a persistent cough. The patient may also complain of hemoptysis, dyspnea, mild or severe chest pain, or hoarseness (due

to pressure from the tumor or tumor-bearing lymph nodes on the laryngeal nerve). If the cancer is advanced, the patient may report anorexia, weight loss, weakness, and fatigue.

Be sure to assess the patient for risk factors. If he smokes cigarettes, determine the extent of his use and how long he's been smoking. Long-time, heavy smokers possess the highest risk for lung cancer.

You can quantify a patient's smoking history by calculating his accumulated "pack years." To do so, multiply the number of packs he smokes daily by the number of years that he has smoked. For example, a patient who has smoked one pack of cigarettes daily for 40 years has accumulated 40 pack years. A patient who has smoked two packs a day for 20 years has accumulated the same number of pack years.

Physical examination

Observation may reveal dyspnea during mild exertion (when walking, for example), during heavy exertion, or even when resting.

Inspection may disclose alterations in the patient's breathing pattern. If the patient is experiencing pleuritic chest pain, his breathing may be rapid and shallow and he may use accessory muscles to minimize the pain.

Inspection may also reveal finger clubbing, edema (face, neck, and upper torso), dilated veins in the chest and abdomen (superior vena cava syndrome), weight loss and muscle wasting, and signs of anxiety.

Auscultation may disclose decreased or absent breath sounds, wheezing, and pleural friction rub (with pleural effusion). If metastasis has occurred, palpation may reveal enlarged lymph nodes and an enlarged liver. Percussion may reveal dullness over areas of tumor growth or pleural effusion.

FactFinder

Risk factors for lung cancer

Exposure to known carcinogens (cancer-producing substances) is the greatest risk factor for lung cancer.

Carcinogens
Carcinogens that are associated with lung cancer include:
• cigarette smoke (either direct inhalation or passive inhalation of smoke from someone else's cigarette)
• radon gas (occurs naturally in some regions and can leak from the ground and collect in buildings)
• asbestos
• arsenic
• chromium
• coal and petroleum by-products
• iron oxides
• nickel
• vinyl chloride.

Additional risk factors
Other factors that increase lung cancer risk include:
• family history of lung cancer (doubles an individual's risk)
• vitamin A deficiency
• living in an urban area (higher incidence).

Diagnostic test results

• Chest X-ray is the primary diagnostic tool in lung cancer. In most patients, it shows an advanced lesion and indicates tumor size and location. (It can, in fact, detect a lesion up to 2 years before symptoms appear.)
• Magnetic resonance imaging reveals tumors, including their size and location, and the invasion or compression of vascular structures by a tumor.
• Cytologic analysis of a sputum specimen is 75% reliable, helping to support a diagnosis of lung cancer. Sputum specimens must be obtained from

Major types of bronchogenic carcinomas

Four major types of bronchogenic carcinoma account for 95% of all primary lung cancers.

Adenocarcinoma
Characterized by enlarged cuboidal or columnar cells with prominent nuclei and excessive cytoplasm, this tumor usually develops in the peripheral submucosa and forms gland-like structures or sacs. This is the most common lung cancer in women. Distant metastasis is common.

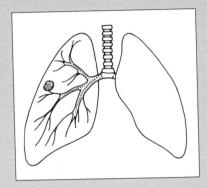

Squamous cell (epidermoid) carcinoma
This carcinoma is characterized by intracellular keratinization, intracellular bridges, and shrunken nuclei. Because this carcinoma usually is centrally located in the large bronchi, exfoliated tumor cells are often detected in bronchial secretions. Squamous cell carcinoma is the most common lung cancer in men. Metastasis is primarily local.

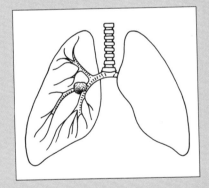

the tracheobronchial tree; they mustn't contain postnasal secretions or saliva.
• Bronchoscopy may be used to identify the tumor site. During this procedure, the doctor passes a fiberoptic instrument through the trachea into a bronchus. Bronchoscopic washings provide material for cytologic and histologic study. (See *Understanding bronchoscopy*, page 283.)

• Needle biopsy of the lungs uses biplanar fluoroscopy to locate peripheral tumors and then withdraw a tissue specimen for analysis. This procedure confirms the diagnosis in 80% of lung cancer patients.
• Tissue biopsy of metastatic sites (including supraclavicular and mediastinal nodes and pleura) helps assess the cancer's extent. The disease is staged based on these histologic findings.

Large-cell (anaplastic) carcinoma
Large-cell carcinoma is marked by cellular and nuclear enlargement with well-defined cytoplasmic boundaries. Multinucleated giant cells may be present. This carcinoma grows peripherally in any area of the lung. Early, extensive metastasis is common, resulting in a poor prognosis for most patients.

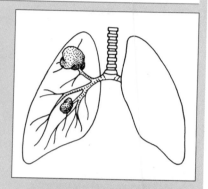

Small-cell carcinoma
Small-cell carcinomas (of which oat cell carcinoma is the most common) are composed of densely packed cells with prominent nuclei and very little cytoplasm. Typically, cells are arranged in clusters, nests, or ribbons. Small-cell carcinomas usually grow in central submucosa and involve the mediastinal nodes. These tumors are characterized by rapid growth and early, extensive metastasis; consequently, the prognosis is poor.

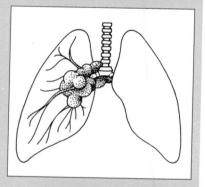

• Thoracentesis, the insertion of a needle through the chest wall and into the pleura to remove pleural fluid, allows chemical and cytologic detection of malignant cells.
• Chest tomography, bronchography, esophagography, and angiocardiography (contrast studies of the bronchial tree, esophagus, and cardiovascular tissues) may be used to characterize the disease or support a diagnosis.

• Bone scan may be used to confirm metastasis. If results are abnormal, bone marrow biopsy may be ordered (common for patients with small-cell carcinoma).
• Computed tomography scan of the brain, liver function studies, and gallium scans of the liver and spleen may be used to detect metastasis.

FactFinder
Complications of lung cancer

Complications may be associated with bronchial obstruction, local spread of the tumor, or distant metastasis.

Bronchial obstruction
Complications associated with bronchial obstruction due to tumor growth include:
• atelectasis
• pneumonia
• lung abscess.

Local spread of the tumor
Complications associated with local spread of the primary tumor to other intrathoracic structures include:
• tracheal obstruction
• esophageal compression with dysphagia
• phrenic nerve paralysis with hemidiaphragm elevation and dyspnea
• sympathetic nerve paralysis with Horner's syndrome
• compression of the eighth cervical and first thoracic nerves with ulnar and Pancoast's syndrome (shoulder pain radiating to the ulnar nerve pathways)
• lymphatic obstruction with pleural effusion
• hypoxemia.

Distant metastasis
Distant metastasis to the brain, bones, liver, and supraclavicular lymph nodes is common. Complications of distant metastasis include:
• anorexia and weight loss (sometimes leading to cachexia)
• clubbing of fingers
• hypertrophic osteoarthropathy
• ectopic hormone syndromes or hypercalcemia (both are medical emergencies).

• Mediastinoscopy allows for biopsy of lymph nodes behind the breastbone to search for cancer cells.
• Thoracoscopy may be used when fluid has collected between the lungs and the chest wall or examination of the fluid doesn't show cancer cells.

Common nursing diagnoses for a patient with lung cancer include:
• Pain related to pressure from the tumor, lung surgery, or metastatic disease
• Impaired gas exchange related to the destruction of lung tissue
• Ineffective airway clearance related to an obstructive tumor and ineffective cough
• Activity intolerance related to hypoxemia and malnutrition
• Anxiety related to dyspnea and fear of death
• Knowledge deficit related to the disease, treatments, and sources of support
• Altered nutrition: Less than body requirements, related to difficult or painful swallowing, surgery, or metastasis.

PLANNING

Focus your nursing care on controlling the patient's pain, reducing his anxiety, promoting rest, providing appropriate diversions, and teaching the patient and family members about lung cancer.

Based on the nursing diagnosis *pain,* develop appropriate patient outcomes. For example, your patient will:
• report that his pain has been relieved or adequately controlled
• demonstrate improved comfort, as evidenced by reduction in tachycardia, restlessness, facial grimacing, and muscular tension
• identify factors that influence his comfort.

Staging lung cancer

The following is the TNM (tumor, node, metastasis) system of staging lung cancer, developed by the American Joint Committee on Cancer.

T for primary tumor
T refers to the extent of the primary tumor, and depends on its size, depth of invasion, and surface spread.

TX — tumor can't be assessed; or sputum or bronchial washings contain malignant cells, but tumor is undetected by X-ray or bronchoscopy

T0 — no evidence of a primary tumor

Tis — carcinoma in situ

T1 — tumor 3 cm or less in diameter surrounded by normal lung or visceral pleura; no bronchoscopic evidence of cancer closer to center of body than lobar bronchus

T2 — tumor larger than 3 cm in diameter; or one that involves the main bronchus and is 2 cm or more from the carina; or one that invades the visceral pleura; or one that is accompanied by atelectasis or obstructive pneumonitis that extends to the hilar region but doesn't involve the entire lung

T3 — tumor of any size that extends into neighboring structures, such as the chest wall, diaphragm, or mediastinal pleura; or tumor in the main bronchus that is less than 2 cm from (but doesn't involve) the carina; or tumor that's accompanied by atelectasis or obstructive pneumonitis of the entire lung

T4 — tumor of any size that invades the mediastinum, heart, great vessels, trachea, esophagus, vertebral body, or carina; or tumor with malignant pleural effusion

N for nodal involvement
N refers to involvement of regional lymph nodes.

NX — regional lymph nodes can't be assessed

N0 — no detectable metastasis to regional lymph nodes

N1 — metastasis to the ipsilateral peribronchial or hilar lymph nodes or to both

N2 — metastasis to the ipsilateral mediastinal or subcarinal lymph nodes or to both

N3 — metastasis to the contralateral mediastinal or hilar lymph nodes, ipsilateral or contralateral scalene lymph nodes, or supraclavicular lymph nodes

M for metastasis
M refers to distant metastasis.

MX — distant metastasis can't be assessed

M0 — no evidence of distant metastasis

M1 — evidence of distant metastasis to scalene, cervical, or contralateral hilar lymph nodes or to the brain, bones, lungs, or liver

Staging categories
The T, N, and M factors may be combined into the following groups or stages:

Occult carcinoma — TX, N0, M0

Stage 0 — Tis, N0, M0

Stage I (potentially operable) — T1 or T2, N0, M0

Stage II (potentially operable) — T1 or T2, N1, M0

Stage IIIA (inoperable) — T1 or T2, N2, M0; or T3, N0, M0; T3, N1, M0; or T3, N2, M0

Stage IIIB (inoperable) — any T, N3, M0; or T4, any N, M0

Stage IV (inoperable) — any T, any N, M1

Based on the nursing diagnosis *impaired gas exchange,* develop appropriate patient outcomes. For example, your patient will:
• maintain partial pressure of arterial oxygen (PaO$_2$) above 60 mm Hg and partial pressure of arterial carbon dioxide (PaCO$_2$) below 45 mm Hg
• report that he feels comfortable breathing and is experiencing less dyspnea.

Based on the nursing diagnosis *ineffective airway clearance,* develop appropriate patient outcomes. For example, your patient will:
• maintain a patent airway
• report that he feels comfortable breathing
• expectorate sputum effectively
• report that he feels comfortable breathing.

Based on the nursing diagnosis *activity intolerance,* develop appropriate patient outcomes. For example, your patient will:
• develop a plan for daily living that includes periods of rest and routine activities
• participate in the activities he values
• perform activities of daily living (ADLs) to tolerance level
• identify people willing to assist him with ADLs and accept their help.

Based on the nursing diagnosis *anxiety,* develop appropriate patient outcomes. For example, your patient will:
• express his feelings of anxiety and grief
• identify and demonstrate three or more effective coping mechanisms
• participate in decisions about his care
• discuss his feelings about dying and death with members of his family (if appropriate).

Based on the nursing diagnosis *knowledge deficit,* develop appropriate patient outcomes. For example, your patient (or his caregiver) will:

• express understanding of methods for relieving pain and dyspnea
• demonstrate procedures (such as wound care) and the use of equipment (home health care)
• describe warning signs that must be reported to the doctor
• describe possible adverse effects of radiation therapy or chemotherapy and precautionary measures to avoid or lessen these effects.

Based on the nursing diagnosis *altered nutrition: less than body requirements,* develop appropriate patient outcomes. For example, your patient will:
• maintain body weight within 2% of ideal weight
• maintain caloric intake above recommended daily allowance for all food groups
• report symptoms that may prevent eating, including altered taste sensation, abdominal pain, or inflamed buccal cavities
• exhibit normal bowel movements and sounds
• maintain adequate muscle tone and strength.

IMPLEMENTATION

Treatment usually includes a combination of surgery, radiation therapy, and chemotherapy to address the spread of disease, and measures to alleviate pain and dyspnea. (See *Medical care of the patient with lung cancer,* page 285.)

Nursing interventions
• Encourage the patient to participate in decisions about his care.
• Administer prescribed analgesics for pain and assess the patient's response.
  Timesaving tip: You'll find it easier to prevent pain than to control it. So, instead of providing analgesics after pain occurs, determine the patient's pain pattern and administer analgesics on a 24-hour schedule to maintain effective blood levels. Use

Understanding bronchoscopy

Bronchoscopic examination of the tracheobronchial tree can help detect central lesions. The bronchoscope's open channel can accommodate biopsy forceps, a cytology brush, an anesthetic, or oxygen, as well as a suctioning catheter or lavage agents.

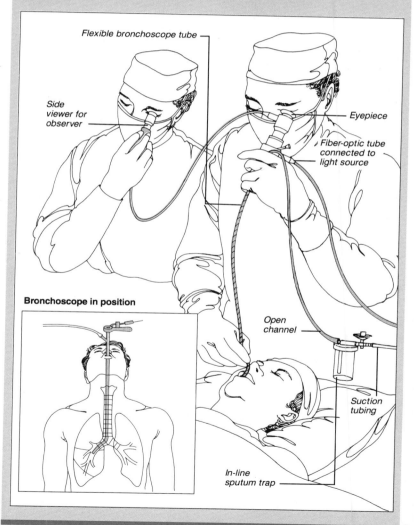

Flexible bronchoscope tube

Side viewer for observer

Eyepiece

Fiber-optic tube connected to light source

Bronchoscope in position

Open channel

Suction tubing

In-line sputum trap

oral analgesics whenever possible and titrate dosages individually to ensure the smallest *effective* dose. Keep in mind, however, that undermedication is a common problem in treating cancer pain.

• If narcotic analgesics are prescribed, anticipate adverse effects and implement preventive measures. Also remember that the patient's tolerance to the analgesic may increase. If you suspect increasing tolerance, collaborate with the doctor about adjusting the dosage or frequency.

• If the patient's pain can't be controlled, suggest that the doctor order patient-controlled analgesia.

• Use other measures, such as guided imagery, distraction, or relaxation exercises, to help alleviate pain.

• Administer oxygen, as prescribed, to help relieve dyspnea and reduce the patient's anxiety. Monitor arterial blood gas levels and assess the patient's respiratory status frequently.

• Help the patient into a position such as semi-Fowler's position that facilitates comfortable breathing. If the patient has severe dyspnea, sitting on a lounge chair or recliner or leaning forward often makes breathing easier.

• Encourage the patient to perform those activities that are within his ability, but to perform them slowly. Provide assistance with ADLs as needed.

• Provide adequate humidification and hydration to loosen secretions. Encourage the patient to cough effectively. If the patient is too weak to do so, maintain a patent airway using nasotracheal suctioning.

• Perform postural drainage and percussion, as tolerated by the patient or as needed.

• Administer bronchodilators and steroids, if prescribed, to help maintain a patent airway.

• Provide meticulous skin care to minimize the breakdown of skin over sites subjected to radiation therapy.

• Assess for fever and other signs of pulmonary infection. Administer prescribed antibiotics if infection occurs.

• Encourage the patient and family members to express their fears and concerns. Help the patient maintain a sense of control during treatment by describing all procedures and including him in decisions about care whenever possible.

• Help the patient identify effective methods for coping with his anxiety. Remember that controlling the patient's dyspnea and pain will help reduce anxiety.

• Encourage the patient to express his feelings of grief and loss and help him deal with these emotions. If necessary, consult with a mental health specialist.

• Provide the patient with a balanced diet that contains adequate calories for maintaining a desirable weight. Monitor caloric intake and weight. Consult with the dietician to plan appealing meals and snacks.

Timesaving tip: To quickly determine the minimum number of calories your patient needs each day to maintain his present weight, use the DeWys formula: Multiply your patient's body weight (in kilograms) by 20; then add 1,100 to get his daily minimum caloric requirement.

Thoracic surgery
Perform the following interventions if your patient has undergone thoracic surgery for lung cancer.

• Monitor the patient's vital signs and respirations. Report any signs or symptoms of complications, such as fever, tachypnea, difficulty breathing, cyanosis, frank bleeding, redness or swelling at the suture line, tachycardia, irregular heart rate, diaphoresis, hypotension, and abdominal distention.

• Position the patient on the surgical side to promote lung expansion.

• Maintain a patent airway. Monitor the patency of the chest tube and be

Treatments

Medical care of the patient with lung cancer

Treatment depends on the staging of the patient's cancer. Typically, it involves a combination of surgery, radiation therapy, and chemotherapy. However, because lung cancer usually is advanced at diagnosis, most treatment is palliative.

Surgery

Surgery is the preferred treatment for squamous cell carcinoma, adenocarcinoma, and large-cell carcinoma, unless the tumor can't be resected or the patient has a condition (for example, cardiovascular disease) that precludes surgery. Approximately two-thirds of all lung cancer patients aren't candidates for surgery because of metastasis, the location of the lesion, poor respiratory status, or poor general health.

Radiation therapy

Recommended for stage I and stage II tumors when surgery is contraindicated, radiation therapy also treats stage III tumors if the disease is localized. Using radiation to destroy malignant cells or curtail their growth helps relieve pain caused by chest wall metastasis, tumor compression, or bronchial obstruction.

Radiation therapy may be used after surgery to eradicate neoplastic cells undetected during surgery. It typically begins 4 to 6 weeks after surgery (after the wound heals) and focuses on the area most likely to incur metastasis. Occasionally, radiation therapy is administered before surgery to reduce tumor bulk; however, this practice has questionable value.

Although radiation therapy often reduces the risk of recurrence, it rarely improves the patient's chances for survival.

Chemotherapy

Useful for controlling residual disease or as an adjunct to surgery or radiation therapy, chemotherapy can induce tumor regression and prevent or delay metastasis. As a palliative treatment, chemotherapy aims to improve the patient's quality of life by relieving pain and other symptoms.

Commonly used chemotherapeutic drugs include:
- alkylating agents and nitrosoureas
- antimetabolites
- antitumor antibiotics
- plant alkaloids
- steroidal hormones.

Investigational therapies

Investigations of immunotherapy and laser therapy to treat lung cancer are currently underway.

Immunotherapy

Also called biotherapy, immunotherapy seeks to stimulate the patient's immune system to produce natural substances that kill abnormal cells or delay their growth. Nonspecific regimens using bacille Calmette-Guérin (BCG) vaccine or *Corynebacterium parvum* offer the most promise.

Laser therapy

This therapy directs a laser beam through a bronchoscope to destroy the tumor, thereby relieving hemoptysis, distal pneumonitis, and atelectasis. It can also help prevent death by strangulation. However, the patient may require further treatment.

sure it drains effectively. (Fluctuations in the water seal chamber during respirations will indicate that the chest tube is patent.) Monitor the system for air leaks and immediately report any that occur.

• Suction the patient to maintain a patent airway. Monitor and document the color and amount of chest drainage. Report any foul-smelling discharge or excessive drainage on surgical dressings. (Dressings are usually removed after 24 hours unless the wound appears infected.)

• Encourage the patient to begin using techniques for deep breathing and productive coughing as soon as possible after surgery. Frequently monitor the quality of secretions. (At first the patient's sputum will appear thick and dark with blood. After 24 hours, it should become thinner and grayish yellow.)

• Maintain adequate hydration. Monitor intake and output.

• Monitor for complications such as infection, shock, hemorrhage, atelectasis, dyspnea, mediastinal shift, or pulmonary embolism. Be prepared to intervene if complications arise.

• Help prevent pulmonary embolus by applying antiembolism stockings and encouraging the patient to perform range-of-motion exercises.

Chemotherapy

Add the following nursing interventions for patients undergoing chemotherapy.

• Provide soft, protein-rich meals (soft foods minimize irritation) and encourage high-calorie snacks between meals.

• Administer antiemetics and antidiarrheals as needed.

• Help the patient conserve energy by scheduling periods of rest in the plan of care.

Patient teaching

• Teach the patient and family members about lung cancer. Discuss progression of the disease, possible complications, and risk factors — especially cigarette smoking.

• Consult with the patient, family members, and the social services department about home health care arrangements. Help identify services that may be needed, such as nursing care, housekeeping, or a support service such as Meals on Wheels.

• Teach the patient techniques for managing pain. If pain control becomes inadequate, instruct him to notify the doctor.

• Teach him about measures that relieve dyspnea.

• Demonstrate the proper use of all equipment needed for home care. Teach the patient or caregiver how to perform essential procedures, such as incision care.

• Teach the patient techniques for deep breathing and productive coughing.

• Help him identify activities in his life that he values most. Provide guidelines for choosing activities that are interesting, but not physically demanding.

• Teach stress management techniques and methods for conserving energy during periods of activity. Explain the importance of rest periods.

• Assist the patient in identifying support services to help him perform ADLs and to provide additional care as needed.

• Explain all treatments to the patient, including their benefits and risks. Encourage the patient to ask questions during these discussions and answer them completely.

• If the patient is scheduled for surgery, supplement and reinforce the doctor's description of the disease and the surgical procedure. (See *Surgical options in lung cancer*.)

Teaching TimeSaver

Surgical options in lung cancer

Be prepared to teach the patient about surgical options in lung cancer and about his specific, scheduled procedure.

Lobectomy
If the tumor is confined to a lobe, with no evidence of lymph node involvement, the surgeon may remove a cancerous lobe from the lung.

Segmentectomy
The surgeon may remove one or more lung segments in an attempt to preserve functional tissue.

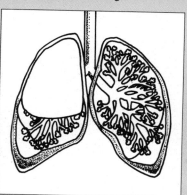

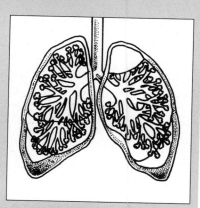

Pneumonectomy
If a lobectomy is insufficient or if the cancer has metastasized to lobar or hilar lymph nodes, the surgeon may remove an entire cancerous lung.

Wedge resection
If the patient has very small peripheral tumors, without lymph node involvement, the surgeon may remove lung tissue without regard for segmental planes.

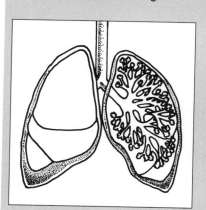

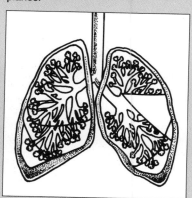

• If the patient will receive chemotherapy or radiation therapy, explain possible adverse effects of each, including reportable ones. Stress that each patient responds differently to these treatments. Explain measures for avoiding complications such as infection. If further treatment is scheduled, explain the importance of attending all follow-up appointments.
• Explain how to control nausea and diarrhea (two common adverse effects of treatment).
• Instruct the patient to wear loose-fitting clothing and to avoid sunburn. Demonstrate exercises that will prevent shoulder stiffness.
• Educate the patient about nutrition and his specific dietary requirements. Explain that a diet high in calories and protein will promote healing. If necessary, recommend nutritional supplements. Also recommend that he eat small, frequent meals.
• Tell the patient to weigh himself at least once each week. He should notify the doctor if he notes a weight loss of more than 2% of his discharge weight in any week.
• Provide the patient and family members with information about appropriate hospital and community sources of support, such as the local branch of the American Cancer Society.
• Provide referrals to a psychologist or religious or spiritual counselor, if appropriate, and help the patient arrange an appointment. Take the time to respond to the patient's questions about his illness; however, don't burden him with more information than he needs or wants. (See *Ensuring continued care for the patient with lung cancer.*)

EVALUATION

When evaluating the patient's response to your nursing care, gather reassessment data and compare this information to the patient outcomes specified

in your plan of care. During evaluation, review data relating to pain control, gas exchange, airway clearance, activity level, degree of anxiety, and nutrition.

Teaching and counseling
Begin by evaluating the effectiveness of your teaching and counseling. Consider the following questions:
• If pain control measures are inadequate, does the patient know who to call for assistance?
• Can he demonstrate techniques for effective coughing?
• Has he openly expressed his feelings of anxiety or grief?
• Has he started participating in daily activities that he considers important? Does he engage in all ADLs that he is capable of performing?
• Is he participating in decisions relating to his care?
• Can the patient or caregiver make appropriate food substitutions to maintain caloric intake?

Physical condition
Physical examination and diagnostic tests will also help evaluate the effectiveness of care. Consider the following questions:
• Is the patient free of pain? If not, has the pain decreased?
• Does he exhibit signs of improved comfort, such as absent or reduced tachycardia, restlessness, facial grimacing, and muscular tension?
• Does he have a patent airway and report feeling comfortable when breathing?
• Does he report fewer episodes of dyspnea?
• Has he been able to maintain a PaO_2 above 60 mm Hg and a $PaCO_2$ below 45 mm Hg?
• Has he experienced adverse reactions to surgery, radiation therapy, or chemotherapy?

Discharge TimeSaver

Ensuring continued care for the patient with lung cancer

Review the following teaching topics, referrals, and follow-up appointments to make sure that your patient is adequately prepared for discharge.

Teaching topics
Make sure that the following topics have been covered and that the patient's learning has been evaluated:
☐ nature of lung cancer, including its causes, symptoms, and complications
☐ applicable treatments, which may include surgery, chemotherapy, radiation therapy and, possibly, immunotherapy or laser therapy
☐ techniques for managing or minimizing adverse effects of treatments
☐ warning signs that must be reported to the doctor
☐ guidelines for activity and rest
☐ pain management techniques
☐ methods of relieving dyspnea
☐ techniques for productive coughing and deep breathing
☐ information about nutritional requirements
☐ infection control measures
☐ postural drainage and percussion (if needed)
☐ follow-up care and tests
☐ sources of information and support.

Referrals
Make sure that the patient has been provided with necessary referrals to:
☐ social services (for financial concerns)
☐ home health care agency or hospice program
☐ dietician
☐ support group
☐ mental health specialist.

Follow-up appointments
Make sure that the necessary follow-up appointments have been scheduled and that the patient has been notified:
☐ doctor
☐ surgeon
☐ additional diagnostic tests, if applicable
☐ radiation therapy or chemotherapy, if applicable.

● Has he maintained his weight within 2% of baseline?

Malignant mesothelioma

This cancer is linked to exposure to asbestos fibers. Even brief exposure or exposure that occurred years ago increases the risk for the disease. Incidence is highest among workers who manufactured or installed materials containing asbestos. Others at risk include members of the worker's family and residents of communities near asbestos processing sites or shipping routes.

Most patients with malignant mesothelioma are over age 50 at the time of diagnosis. In most cases, there is a 20- to 45-year gap between asbestos exposure and the onset of symptoms. The prognosis is poor; malignant mesothelioma is invariably fatal. Typically, less than 2 years pass between the onset of symptoms and death.

Complications of the disorder and its metastasis include severe dyspnea, infection, and problems associated with immobility, such as skin breakdown.

Causes

Malignant mesothelioma originates in the serosal lining of the pleural cavity, although the exact site and pathogenic mechanism are not known. Animal studies suggest that asbestos fibers migrate to mesothelial cells, penetrating the pleura. From there, pleural lymphatics carry them to the pleural surface. Signs and symptoms result from pleural effusion, restricted lung function, tumor mass, infection, and advanced disease.

In most cases, the patient's occupational history or area of residence will indicate where and when he was exposed to asbestos.

Health history

Chest pain and dyspnea are common chief complaints in malignant mesothelioma. The patient may also report a cough, hoarseness, anorexia, weight loss, weakness, or fatigue.

Physical examination

Inspection may reveal fever, shortness of breath and, in some cases, finger clubbing. You may discover dullness over affected lung fields during chest percussion and diminished breath sounds during auscultation.

Diagnostic test results

• Open pleural biopsy is performed to obtain a tissue specimen for histologic study to confirm the diagnosis.
• Chest X-ray typically reveals nodular, irregular, unilateral pleural thickening and varying degrees of unilateral pleural effusion.
• Computed tomography scan of the chest defines the tumor's size.

Common nursing diagnoses for a patient with malignant mesothelioma include:
• Knowledge deficit related to the disease process, treatments, and sources of support
• Pain related to lung surgery or pressure from the tumor
• Impaired gas exchange related to restricted lung expansion secondary to pleural effusion or tumor mass
• Anxiety related to dyspnea and poor prognosis.

Based on the nursing diagnosis *knowledge deficit,* develop appropriate patient outcomes. For example, your patient will:
• describe appropriate measures for relieving pain and dyspnea
• demonstrate proper use of equipment and procedures necessary for home health care
• identify three or more sources of support, such as a home health care agency, to help with activities of daily living
• describe warning signs that must be reported to the doctor
• identify the adverse effects of radiation therapy or chemotherapy and the precautions necessary to prevent them.

Based on the nursing diagnosis *pain,* develop appropriate patient outcomes. For example, your patient will:
• state that he is free of pain (or that any remaining pain is tolerable)
• exhibit improved comfort, as evidenced by reductions in tachycardia, restlessness, grimacing, and muscular tension.

Based on the nursing diagnosis *impaired gas exchange,* develop appropriate patient outcomes. For example, your patient will:
• maintain partial pressure of arterial oxygen above 60 mm Hg and partial

pressure of arterial carbon dioxide below 45 mm Hg
• experience fewer episodes of dyspnea.
  Based on the nursing diagnosis *anxiety,* develop appropriate patient outcomes. For example, your patient will:
• express his feelings of anxiety and grief
• identify and demonstrate three or more effective coping mechanisms
• participate in decisions about his care
• discuss his preferences about dying and death with members of the family at an appropriate time.

IMPLEMENTATION

No standard therapy exists for malignant mesothelioma. Your nursing care should focus on supportive measures, including teaching the patient and family members about malignant mesothelioma, controlling the patient's pain, and easing his anxiety. (See *Medical care of malignant mesothelioma,* page 292.)

Nursing interventions
• Listen to the patient's fears and concerns. Be sure to provide clear, concise explanations of all procedures. Remain with him during periods of severe anxiety.
• Encourage the patient to identify mechanisms that help him cope with anxiety. Involve members of the patient's family in the process of providing care.
• Include the patient and members of his family in decisions about care whenever possible.
• Help the patient and family members express and cope with their feelings of grief, loss, and anger. For example, the patient and family may have feelings of anger toward a job or situation that caused asbestos exposure.

• Administer prescribed pain medications. Monitor and document their effectiveness.
• Monitor the patient's respiratory status, including arterial blood gas levels, breath sounds, skin color, and mental status. Administer oxygen if prescribed. Help the patient find comfortable positions that facilitate chest expansion (Fowler's position, for example).
• If the patient's mobility decreases, turn him frequently and provide meticulous skin care, particularly over bony prominences. Encourage him to be as active as possible.
• Prevent infection by using strict aseptic technique during suctioning, during dressing changes, when establishing an I.V. line, and when performing any invasive procedure. Closely monitor the patient's temperature and white blood cell count.
• Monitor I.V. fluids to prevent circulatory overload and pulmonary congestion.
• Monitor for complications related to disease progression or treatments by observing and listening to the patient. Check vital signs frequently and review current laboratory findings.

Patient teaching
• Teach the patient about malignant mesothelioma, including its link to asbestos exposure, progression, and possible complications.
• Explain all procedures and treatments. Allow time to answer all of the patient's questions. (Include family members or the principle caregiver in these sessions.)
• Show the patient how to manage pain and dyspnea associated with progressive disease.
• Teach the patient how to minimize adverse effects of treatments; for example, by increasing his fluid intake after chemotherapy.

Treatments

Medical care of malignant mesothelioma

No standard treatment currently exists for malignant mesothelioma. Combinations of surgery, radiation therapy, and chemotherapy may be attempted; however, they seldom control the disease. Instead, therapy focuses on supportive measures, such as nutrition, energy conservation, and pain relief.

If surgery is selected, pleuropneumonectomy is the most common procedure. Chemotherapy may include combinations of cisplatin and mitomycin, which have proved more successful than other drug combinations in treating malignant mesothelioma.

• Explain the signs and symptoms that must be reported to the doctor, such as fever or hemoptysis.
• Teach the patient techniques to maximize breathing comfort and effectiveness and to prevent complications of immobility. (Include family members or the principal caregiver in these sessions.)
• Demonstrate infection prevention methods, such as meticulous hand washing, and describe aseptic techniques.
• Discuss the availability of counseling services and hospice or home health care agencies with the patient and members of his family. Provide the family with all necessary referrals. (See *Ensuring continued care for malignant mesothelioma*.)

EVALUATION

When evaluating the patient's response to your nursing care, gather reassessment data and compare this informa-

tion to patient outcomes specified in your plan of care.

Teaching and counseling

Begin by determining the effectiveness of your teaching and counseling. Because patients with malignant mesothelioma have such a poor prognosis, effective teaching and counseling is particularly important to help the patient and his family cope with the disease process and the changes it brings about in their lives.

Gather information by consulting with the patient, family members, and other members of the health care team. During your evaluation, consider the following questions:
• Does the patient understand the disease process, including its link to asbestos exposure?
• Does he understand the methods of treatment?
• Has he learned how to minimize adverse effects of treatment?
• Are the patient and family members aware of the warning signs and symptoms that must be reported to the doctor?
• Does he implement techniques for managing pain?
• Does he implement techniques for managing dyspnea?
• Does he appear to be more comfortable, as evidenced by reductions in tachycardia, restlessness, grimacing, and muscular tension?
• Does he state that he is experiencing less anxiety? Does his appearance suggest an increase or decrease in anxiety? Is he using effective coping mechanisms?
• Does he participate in decisions about his care?
• Can he identify sources of support within his community, such as a hospice (if appropriate) or a home health care agency? Does he appear willing to contact them?

Discharge TimeSaver
Ensuring continued care for the patient with malignant mesothelioma

Review the following teaching topics, referrals, and follow-up appointments to make sure that your patient is adequately prepared for discharge.

Teaching topics
Make sure that the following topics have been covered and that the patient's learning has been evaluated:
☐ disease process in malignant mesothelioma, including its link to asbestos exposure and potential complications
☐ follow-up treatments (including importance of attending appointments)
☐ managing or minimizing adverse effects of treatments
☐ warning signs that must be reported to the doctor
☐ pain management techniques
☐ methods of relieving dyspnea
☐ infection control measures
☐ sources of information and support.

Referrals
Make sure that the patient has been provided with necessary referrals to:
☐ social services (for financial concerns)
☐ dietician
☐ home health care agency or hospice program
☐ agencies that provide information and support.

Follow-up appointments
Make sure that the necessary follow-up appointments have been scheduled and that the patient has been notified:
☐ doctor
☐ surgeon
☐ additional diagnostic tests, if applicable
☐ radiation therapy or chemotherapy, if applicable.

Physical condition
Physical examination and diagnostic tests will provide additional information for your evaluation. Consider the following questions:
• Is the patient free of pain? If not, has he noted a reduction in pain?
• Has his dyspnea subsided? Does he report easier breathing?
• Has he experienced serious complications related to his illness or therapy?

Laryngeal cancer

In this type of cancer, a malignant growth occurs on the vocal cords or another part of the larynx. Squamous cell carcinoma accounts for 95% of all cases of laryngeal cancer. Rare forms include adenocarcinoma and sarcoma. Accurate identification of the site of the tumor in laryngeal cancer is important; spread of malignancy is directly related to tumor location. Tumors on the true vocal cord do not spread because the underlying connective tissue lacks lymph nodes. However, tumors on other parts of the larynx tend to spread early. (See *Key points about laryngeal cancer,* page 294.)

Causes
The exact cause of laryngeal cancer isn't known. Major risk factors include cigarette smoking and alcoholism. Minor risk factors include chronic inhalation of noxious fumes, genetic predis-

FactFinder

Key points about laryngeal cancer

- *Incidence:* Laryngeal cancer accounts for less than 2% of all cancers in North America. Men are five times more likely to be affected than women. Incidence is highest in patients ages 60 to 80.
- *Prognosis:* Early radiation therapy or surgery results in a 5-year survival rate of 85% to 95%.
- *Chief diagnostic method:* biopsy of specimen obtained by direct laryngoscopy.
- *Treatment:* typically, a combination of radiation therapy, laser surgery, and chemotherapy.
- *Leading complication:* metastasis.

position, and a history of laryngitis and vocal straining.

ASSESSMENT

Assessment findings will vary according to the tumor's location and stage. (See *Classifying laryngeal tumors,* opposite, and *Staging laryngeal cancer,* page 296.)

Health history
Usually, the patient's chief complaint is persistent hoarseness or throat irritation lasting longer than 2 weeks. If the disease has progressed, he may report a sore throat and trouble speaking louder than a stage whisper. Symptoms of advanced disease include a lump in the throat, pain radiating to the ear, dysphagia, dyspnea, and stridor. Anorexia and weight loss may also accompany advanced disease.

During the health history, investigate the patient's risk factors. Ask about cigarette smoking, use of alcohol, and any episodes of laryngitis.

Physical examination
In early-stage disease, physical examination may not reveal any signs. In advanced disease, palpation may detect a neck mass or enlarged cervical lymph nodes.

Diagnostic test results
- Indirect laryngoscopy with a laryngeal mirror may be performed initially to assess the condition of the larynx. Direct laryngoscopy may be used to obtain a biopsy specimen to confirm the diagnosis, and to determine the type, location, and extent of the tumor.
- Studies of the larynx and neck using computed tomography scans or magnetic resonance imaging help evaluate and stage the tumor. Scans of other sites, such as the brain, bone, and liver, and chest X-ray may be used to detect metastasis.
- Laboratory studies of hematologic, hepatic, and renal function provide further assessment data.

NURSING DIAGNOSIS

Common nursing diagnoses for a patient with laryngeal cancer include:
- Impaired verbal communication related to tumor on vocal cords or to surgery
- Impaired gas exchange related to tumorous mass causing airway obstruction
- Anxiety related to diagnosis, treatment, or threat of death
- Body image disturbance related to change in appearance and function due to tumor growth or treatment
- Altered nutrition: Less than body requirements, related to difficult or painful swallowing, surgery, or metastasis
- Knowledge deficit related to disease process, methods of treatment, and sources of support.

Classifying laryngeal tumors

Laryngeal cancer is classified according to tumor location.

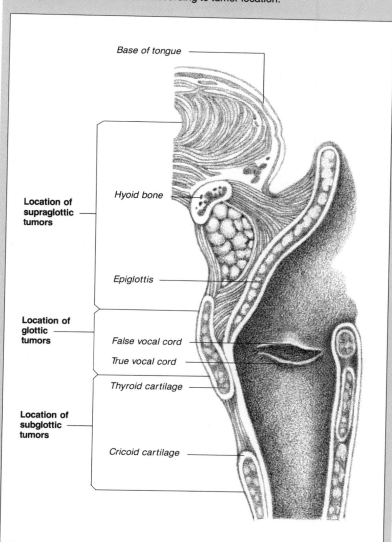

Base of tongue

Location of
supraglottic
tumors

Hyoid bone

Epiglottis

Location of
glottic
tumors

False vocal cord

True vocal cord

Thyroid cartilage

Location of
subglottic
tumors

Cricoid cartilage

Staging laryngeal cancer

The TNM (tumor, node, metastasis) system developed by the American Joint Committee on Cancer stages laryngeal cancer as follows.

T for primary tumor
TX — primary tumor can't be assessed
T0 — no evidence of primary tumor
Tis — carcinoma in situ

Supraglottic tumors
T1 — tumor confined to one subsite in supraglottis; vocal cords retain normal motion
T2 — tumor extends to other sites in supraglottis or to glottis; vocal cords retain motion
T3 — tumor confined to larynx, but vocal cords lose motion; or tumor extends to the postcricoid area, the pyriform sinus, or the preepiglottic space, and vocal cords lose motion; or both
T4 — tumor extends through thyroid cartilage; or to tissues beyond the larynx (such as the oropharynx or soft tissues of the neck); or both

Glottic tumors
T1 — tumor confined to vocal cords, which retain motion; may involve anterior or posterior commissures
T2 — tumor extends to supraglottis or subglottis; or both; vocal cords may lose motion
T3 — tumor confined to larynx, but vocal cords lose motion
T4 — tumor extends through thyroid cartilage; or to tissue beyond the larynx (such as the oropharynx or soft tissues of the neck); or both

Subglottic tumors
T1 — tumor is confined to the subglottis
T2 — tumor extends to vocal cords, which may lose motion

T3 — tumor is confined to larynx with vocal cord fixation
T4 — tumor extends through cricoid or thyroid cartilage; or to tissues beyond the larynx (such as the oropharynx or soft tissues of the neck); or both

N for nodal involvement (regional lymph nodes)
NX — regional lymph nodes can't be assessed
N0 — no evidence of regional lymph node metastasis
N1 — metastasis in a single ipsilateral lymph node, 3 cm or less in greatest dimension
N2 — metastasis in one or more ipsilateral lymph nodes, or in bilateral or contralateral nodes, larger than 3 cm but smaller than 6 cm in greatest dimension
N3 — metastasis in a node larger than 6 cm in greatest dimension

M for metastasis (distant)
MX — distant metastasis can't be assessed
M0 — no evidence of distant metastasis
M1 — distant metastasis

Staging categories
Laryngeal cancer progresses from mild to severe as follows:
Stage 0 — Tis, N0, M0
Stage I — T1, N0, M0
Stage II — T2, N0, M0
Stage III — T1 or T2, N1, M0; T3, N0 or N1, M0
Stage IV — T4, N0 or N1, M0; any T, N2 or N3, M0; any T, any N, M1

PLANNING

Based on the nursing diagnosis *impaired verbal communication,* develop appropriate patient outcomes. For example, your patient will:
• develop proficiency in alternative methods of communication
• communicate his needs without experiencing undue frustration.

Based on the nursing diagnosis *impaired gas exchange,* develop appropriate patient outcomes. For example, your patient will:
• maintain a patent airway
• maintain partial pressure of arterial oxygen (PaO_2) above 60 mm Hg and partial pressure of arterial carbon dioxide ($PaCO_2$) less than 45 mm Hg
• experience no episodes of severe dyspnea.

Based on the nursing diagnosis *anxiety,* develop appropriate patient outcomes. For example, your patient will:
• express his feelings of anxiety and grief
• identify three or more effective coping mechanisms
• participate in decisions about his care
• acknowledge a reduction in anxiety
• discuss his preferences about dying and death with members of the family at an appropriate time.

Based on the nursing diagnosis *body image disturbance,* develop appropriate patient outcomes. For example, your patient will:
• acknowledge changes in his body image
• perform self-care procedures
• resume his normal lifestyle within the limitations imposed by the illness and treatment
• participate in a support group
• communicate his acceptance of changes in his appearance or the way his body functions.

Based on the nursing diagnosis *altered nutrition: less than body requirements,* develop appropriate patient outcomes. For example, your patient will:
• maintain weight within 2% of his baseline
• adopt a nutritional diet that includes a specified number of calories and nutrients
• demonstrate proper technique during tube feedings (if warranted)
• tolerate tube feedings without adverse reactions.

Based on the nursing diagnosis *knowledge deficit,* develop appropriate patient outcomes. For example, your patient (or his caregiver) will:
• demonstrate stoma care and describe related measures and precautions
• demonstrate incision care
• identify three or more sources of support
• describe the warning signs that must be reported to the doctor
• describe the adverse effects of radiation therapy and chemotherapy
• describe plans for obtaining speech rehabilitation.

IMPLEMENTATION

Treatment may include surgery, radiation therapy and, possibly, chemotherapy. The exact regimen will depend on many factors, including the stage of the disease and the patient's age and general health. (See *Medical care of the patient with laryngeal cancer,* page 298.)

Nursing interventions
• Participate with the health care team (which may include an oncologist, surgeon, radiologist, mental health specialist, speech therapist, physical therapist, or dietician) in meeting the unique care needs of the patient, based on his treatment plan.
• Anticipate that the patient will be anxious. Explore specific causes of his anxiety and help the patient identify effective methods for coping with his anxiety.

Treatments

Medical care of the patient with laryngeal cancer

Treatment seeks to remove the tumor, preserve organ function, and minimize complications. Treatment options include surgery, radiation therapy, or both. Factors that affect the choice of therapy include the stage of the disease, general health and age of the patient, functions affected by the tumor, preferences of the doctor and patient, and ability of the patient to manage postoperative care.

Early-stage disease
Endoscopic laser surgery may be used to destroy precancerous lesions. Small lesions may be treated by radiation therapy.

Advanced disease
Recent evidence indicates that chemotherapy followed by radiation therapy is successful in returning function to about two-thirds of all patients with more advanced disease.

Laryngectomy is used when a patient fails to respond to less invasive measures, or if cancer recurs after initially responding to therapy. The type of procedure used will depend on the size and location of the tumor. Cordectomy, laryngofissure, vertical hemilaryngectomy, supraglottic partial laryngectomy, or total laryngectomy are all options. If cervical nodes are involved, a radical neck dissection may be performed.

• Encourage the patient and family members to express their fears and concerns. If the patient's condition warrants, help the patient and his family deal with feelings of loss and grief. The patient may be depressed or angry about possible disfigurement or loss of his voice. Encourage him to express his feelings. Consult with a mental health specialist as needed.
• Explain all procedures clearly to help the patient maintain a sense of control over his treatment and care.

Preoperative measures
• Listen to the patient's fears and concerns relating to scheduled surgery. Help him choose a temporary means of communicating after surgery, such as writing or using a communication board. If the patient is having a total laryngectomy, reassure him that speech rehabilitation will restore his ability to communicate. (See *Alternative methods of speech*.)

• In collaboration with the doctor and speech therapist, help the patient decide which communication method he will use after surgery, such as esophageal speech or an artificial larynx. If the patient is agreeable, arrange for a laryngectomee to visit him.

Postoperative measures in partial laryngectomy
• Administer I.V. fluids and tube feedings for 2 days after surgery; then resume oral fluids. Keep the tracheostomy tube in place until tissue edema subsides.
• Caution the patient against trying to speak until the doctor has given him permission (usually 2 to 3 days after surgery). Then tell the patient to whisper until healing is complete.

Postoperative care in laryngectomy
• When the patient returns from surgery, position him on his side and elevate his head 30 to 45 degrees. Re-

Alternative methods of speech

During convalescence, your patient should work with a speech pathologist who will teach him new ways to speak using esophageal speech, an artificial larynx, or a surgically implanted prosthesis.

Esophageal speech
By drawing air in through the mouth, trapping it in the upper esophagus, and releasing it slowly while forming words, the patient can communicate vocally. With training and practice, a highly motivated patient can master esophageal speech in about 1 month. The speech will sound choppy at first but become smooth and understandable with practice.

Because esophageal speech requires strength, older patients or patients with asthma or emphysema may find it too demanding to learn. Also, because it requires frequent sessions with a speech pathologist, a chronically ill patient may find learning esophageal speech overwhelming.

Artificial larynges
The throat vibrator and the Cooper-Rand device are basic artificial larynges. Both devices produce speech that's easy to understand but monotonous and mechanical.

To operate the throat vibrator, the patient holds the device against his neck. A pulsating disk in the device vibrates the throat tissue as he forms words with his mouth. The throat vibrator may be difficult to use immediately after surgery when the patient's neck wounds are still sore.

The Cooper-Rand device vibrates sounds piped into the patient's mouth through a thin tube, which the patient positions in the corner of his mouth. Easy to use, this device may be preferred soon after surgery.

Surgically implanted prostheses
Most surgical implants generate speech by vibrating when the patient manually closes the tracheostomy, forcing air upward. One such device is the Blom-Singer voice prosthesis. Within hours after it's inserted through an incision in the stoma, the patient can speak in a normal voice. The device may be implanted at the end of radiation therapy or within a few days, or even years, after laryngectomy.

To speak, the patient covers his stoma while exhaling. Exhaled air from the lungs travels through the trachea, through an airflow port on the bottom of the prosthesis, and exits through a slit at the esophageal end of the prosthesis, creating the vibrations needed to produce sound.

Tracheoesophageal puncture
Tracheoesophageal puncture is the surgical procedure used to insert a voice prosthesis. Not all patients are candidates for this procedure. Considerations include the extent of the laryngectomy, status of the pharyngoesophageal muscle, size and location of the stoma, as well as the patient's mental and emotional status, visual and auditory acuity, hand-eye coordination, bimanual dexterity, and self-care skills.

member to support the back of his neck as you move him to prevent tension on the sutures or the possibility of wound dehiscence.

• If the patient has a laryngectomy tube in place, care for it as you would a tracheostomy tube. It's shorter and thicker than a tracheostomy tube and stays in place until the stoma heals (about 7 to 10 days).

• Monitor the stoma for crusting and secretions that can cause skin breakdown. To prevent crusting, make sure the room is adequately humidified. Remove crusts with sterile moist gauze.

• Monitor vital signs. Be especially alert for fever, which indicates infection. Record fluid intake and output and watch for dehydration. Be alert for other postoperative complications and report all occurrences.

• Provide oral care frequently. Use a soft toothbrush or washcloth to clean the patient's tongue and sides of his mouth. Rinse his mouth with a mouthwash.

• Provide gentle suctioning through both the tube and the patient's nose because the patient can no longer blow air through his nose. Unless ordered, do not attempt deep suctioning, which could penetrate the suture line. Also, suction the patient's mouth gently.

• If a wound drainage tube is inserted (usually connected to a blood drainage system or a GI drainage system), do not stop the suctioning without the doctor's consent. After removing the tube, check the dressings for drainage.

• Administer prescribed analgesics. Keep in mind that opioid analgesics depress respiration and inhibit coughing.

• If the doctor orders nasogastric tube feeding, check tube placement, and elevate the patient's head to prevent aspiration. Because the patient may have difficulty swallowing, be prepared to perform nasotracheal suctioning when the nasogastric tube is removed and during the oral intake of fluids.

• Anticipate a period of grieving and provide the patient with emotional support. If his depression becomes severe, consider referring him for appropriate counseling.

Ongoing postoperative care

• Expect the patient to experience an identity disturbance related to loss of voice or to permanent hoarseness. In radical neck dissection, the patient may also react to the presence of a stoma and the change in his appearance. Help the patient express his fears and concerns, and identify realistic coping strategies.

• Encourage the patient to participate in his care, ask questions and, later, join a support group.

• Advise him to return to as normal a lifestyle as possible as soon as he can. (Many patients return to full-time employment within weeks of surgery.)

• Suggest that the patient wear loose-fitting clothing that covers the neck. If permitted, a female patient can apply cosmetics to cover any disfigurement.

• Refer the patient to a mental health specialist if his body image disturbance interferes with his ability to function normally.

• In advanced disease, administer prescribed oxygen therapy to ease respiratory distress, maintain a patent airway, and position the patient to help relieve dyspnea.

Patient teaching

• Teach the patient and family members about laryngeal cancer including its causes and possible complications.

• Explain all diagnostic procedures and their results.

• If surgery is planned, reinforce the doctor's explanation of the procedure. Make sure that the patient understands the nature of possible alterations in body function. Discuss plans for speech rehabilitation, if applicable. (See *Surgical options in laryngeal cancer.*)

• Prepare the patient for other functional losses. Explain that he will not be able to smell, blow his nose, whistle, gargle, sip, or suck on a straw.

(Text continues on page 304.)

Surgical options in laryngeal cancer

For many laryngeal cancer patients, treatment involves surgery. The information below will help you explain the purpose, extent, and effects of the planned surgery.

Endoscopy with laser surgery
This procedure, performed during laryngoscopy, uses a laser beam to remove or reduce the size of a glottic tumor that's confined to a small area, usually a single true vocal cord.
• Tell the patient that he'll retain his voice and that he can resume his usual activities shortly after the procedure.

Transoral cordectomy
This procedure, performed during laryngoscopy, resects an early, small tumor limited to the true vocal cords.
• Tell the patient that the cure rate is high and that he'll retain his normal voice.

Laryngofissure
This procedure removes larger glottic tumors confined to a single vocal cord. The surgeon makes an incision in the thyroid cartilage and removes the diseased vocal cord.
• Tell the patient that this procedure has a high cure rate.
• Explain that after surgery he'll have a temporary tracheostomy and his voice may be hoarse, but that hoarseness will abate as scar tissue replaces the vocal cord.

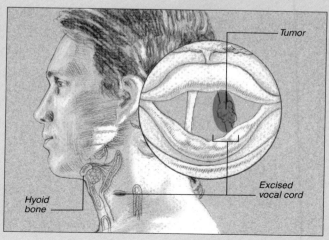

(continued)

Teaching TimeSaver

Surgical options in laryngeal cancer *(continued)*

Vertical hemilaryngectomy
This procedure removes a widespread tumor. The surgeon excises about one-half of the thyroid cartilage and the subglottic cartilage, one false vocal cord, and one true vocal cord and then rebuilds the area with strap muscles.
• Tell the patient that he'll have a temporary tracheostomy and that postoperative hoarseness will subside.

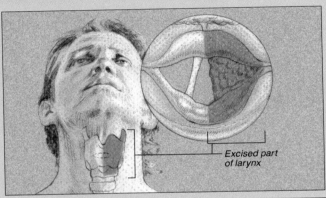

Excised part
of larynx

Horizontal supraglottic laryngectomy
This operation removes a large supraglottic tumor. The surgeon removes the epiglottis, the hyoid bone, and the false vocal cords, but leaves the true vocal cords.
• Tell the patient that he'll have a temporary tracheostomy and that he won't lose his voice but may have swallowing difficulties.

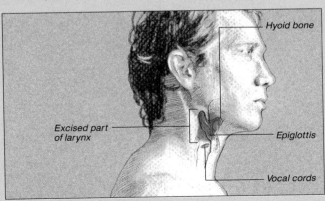

Hyoid bone

Excised part
of larynx

Epiglottis

Vocal cords

Surgical options in laryngeal cancer *(continued)*

Total laryngectomy
This procedure removes the true vocal cords, false vocal cords, epiglottis, hyoid bone, cricoid cartilage, and two or three tracheal rings. Nearby tissue may also be removed, depending on the tumor's extent. The procedure may be performed to remove a large glottic or supraglottic tumor attached to the vocal cord.
• Tell the patient that he'll have a permanent tracheostomy and a laryngeal stoma and that he'll lose his voice. Explain that a speech pathologist will help him learn alternative methods of speech.

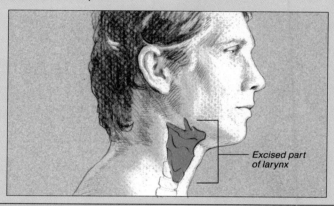

Excised part of larynx

Radical neck dissection
When cancer spreads to surrounding tissues and glands, the surgeon extends the supraglottic or total laryngectomy to remove the cervical chain of lymph nodes, the sternomastoid muscle, the fascia, and the internal jugular vein on the side of the lesion.
• Tell the patient he may experience shoulder discomfort for months after surgery. Instruct him to use heat and massage to relieve discomfort.
• Explain to the patient that during surgery some of the nerves in one of his shoulder muscles were severed and that some muscle tissue was lost. Caution him not to lie on the affected side and not to lift more than 2 lb (1 kg) with the affected arm. Tell him that he'll need to perform rehabilitation exercises to strengthen accessory support muscles. However, caution him to wait to perform exercises until his neck incision has healed and he has received permission from his doctor.
• If the patient had a laryngectomy, teach him stoma and tracheostomy care and arrange for follow-up visits with a speech pathologist.
• Because this surgery disfigures the patient's face and neck, be prepared to provide strong emotional support during your teaching sessions before surgery as well as throughout the recovery period.

• If a horizontal supraglottic laryngectomy is planned, refer the patient to a health professional, such as a speech or occupational therapist, who specializes in teaching swallowing techniques. Swallowing techniques help to prevent food and fluids from entering the trachea.
• Before partial or total laryngectomy, teach the patient about proper oral hygiene.
• Explain all preoperative procedures and care measures.
• Teach the patient about postoperative procedures, such as suctioning, nasogastric tube feeding, tracheostomy care, humidified oxygen, I.V. therapy, neck drains and dressings (with radical neck dissection), deep breathing and positioning, and monitoring equipment.

Timesaving tip: Teaching sessions are easier and quicker when you use an anatomic diagram or a model of the larynx. For example, you can use an inexpensive styrofoam head (used to store wigs) to illustrate tracheostomy care. Cut a 1½" (4-cm) hole at the normal tracheostomy site, and apply a thin layer of clear nail polish to the edges to prevent crumbling. Then use this simulator to teach care of a tracheostomy, laryngectomy tube, and stoma. (Antiseptic agents will not harm the styrofoam.)

• Teach the patient how to care for the incision and stoma. Include members of his family in these teaching sessions. Make sure that they perform the procedures correctly.
• If the patient has undergone a total laryngectomy, explain that laughing, coughing, or sneezing may cause a sudden expectoration of mucus from the stoma and that he can avoid embarrassment by gently covering the stoma with a handkerchief.
• Explain the importance of a high-protein, high-calorie diet of soft foods (when tube feedings are discontinued).

Tell the patient to weigh himself weekly for the first few months and to notify the doctor if he loses weight.
• If warranted, teach the patient rehabilitation exercises that strengthen neck, shoulder, and arm muscles. Collaborate with the physical therapist as necessary.
• Recommend that the patient wear a medical identification bracelet and carry an identification card that explains emergency resuscitation (mouth to stoma) measures necessary for a laryngectomee.
• Describe potential complications of surgery, radiation therapy, and chemotherapy, if applicable. Teach the patient precautions that will prevent or minimize complications. For example, if the patient has a stoma or tube, explain that he should not go swimming and that he should use a stoma guard when showering.
• Explain the necessity of follow-up appointments.
• Encourage the patient to contact support groups, such as the American Speech-Learning-Hearing Association, the International Association of Laryngectomees, the American Cancer Society, or a local chapter of the Lost Chord Club or Speak Easy. Provide referrals as necessary. (See *Ensuring continued care for the patient with laryngeal cancer.*)

EVALUATION

When evaluating the patient's response to your nursing care, gather reassessment data and compare this information to the patient outcomes specified in your plan of care.

Teaching and counseling
Begin by evaluating the effectiveness of your teaching and counseling. Consider the following questions:

Ensuring continued care for the patient with laryngeal cancer

Review the following teaching topics, referrals, and follow-up appointments to make sure that your patient is adequately prepared for discharge.

Teaching topics
Make sure that the following topics have been covered and that the patient's learning has been evaluated:
☐ nature of laryngeal cancer, including risk factors and potential complications
☐ care associated with radiation therapy or chemotherapy (if scheduled)
☐ techniques for managing or minimizing adverse effects of treatments
☐ personal care measures, such as incision care, stoma care, tracheal suctioning, and rehabilitation exercises
☐ alternative speech methods
☐ speech rehabilitation
☐ warning signs that must be reported to the doctor
☐ diet and nutrition guidelines
☐ rationale for follow-up care and testing
☐ sources of information and support
☐ rationale for obtaining a medical identification bracelet and card.

Referrals
Make sure that the patient has been provided with necessary referrals to:
☐ social services (for financial concerns or psychosocial support)
☐ dietician
☐ home health care agency or hospice program
☐ mental health specialist
☐ speech therapist
☐ physical therapist
☐ support group.

Follow-up appointments
Make sure that the necessary follow-up appointments have been scheduled and that the patient has been notified:
☐ doctor
☐ surgeon
☐ additional diagnostic testing, if applicable
☐ radiation therapy or chemotherapy, if applicable.

• Do the patient and members of his family understand the disease process and methods of treatment?

• Can they demonstrate proper stoma or incision care?

• Do they know the warning signs and symptoms of infection that must be reported to the doctor?

• Do they understand the adverse effects of radiation therapy and chemotherapy (if applicable)?

• Does the patient use an alternative speech method effectively? Can he communicate without experiencing frustration?

• Has he been able to come to terms with changes in his ability to speak?

• Has his level of anxiety about treatment or the possibility of death diminished?

• Does he understand and use effective coping mechanisms?

• Does he initiate self-care?

• Has he implemented dietary changes to maintain the recommended number of calories and nutrients in his diet?

• Does he demonstrate proper tube feeding without adverse effects (if applicable)?

• Is his body image improving? Does he express acceptance of the alteration in his appearance?

• Has he resumed a normal lifestyle within the limitations imposed by his illness or treatment?

• Has the patient, if terminally ill, talked with his family about making arrangements in the event of his death?
• Can he identify three or more sources of support, such as family, friends, or support groups?
• Is he willing to participate in a support group?

Physical condition
Physical examination and diagnostic tests will provide additional information for your evaluation. Note whether or not the patient:
• maintains a patent airway
• maintains a PaO_2 above 60 mm Hg and a $PaCO_2$ below 45 mm Hg
• maintains a weight within 2% of his baseline
• experiences continued episodes of dyspnea (if yes, how frequently?)
• experiences serious complications related to his illness or therapy.

Appendices and index

Quick reference to respiratory treatments

Breathing techniques: Deep diaphragmatic

In deep diaphragmatic breathing, the diaphragm is used for maximal inspiration, improving both basilar inflation and inferior segmental expansion.

To perform this technique, have the patient lie on his back with his knees bent; place a pillow under his head, elevating it 15 to 20 degrees. Tell the patient to place his hands or a book lightly on his abdomen. Then have him inhale using the diaphragm. If effective, deep diaphragmatic breathing should cause the patient's hands or the book to rise and then fall during expiration. Instruct the patient to perform this technique for about 30 minutes several times a day.

Indications
• To manage dyspneic episodes (used with pursed-lip breathing) in patients with chronic obstructive pulmonary disease (COPD)
• To increase cough effectiveness (performed for 4 to 5 minutes before a coughing technique)
• To prevent and treat atelectasis

Complications
• Hyperventilation (if deep breathing is performed at an increased respiratory rate)

Breathing techniques: Pursed-lip

For this technique, place the patient in a sitting position or a semi-Fowler position with his hips and knees flexed. Instruct him to take a deep breath through his nose and then to exhale slowly through pursed lips (lips shaped for a whistle). This helps rid the lungs of air that has been trapped in the alveoli, whereas rapid, forceful expiration will only trap more air by causing bronchial collapse. The patient should strive for a relaxed (not forced) expiration that's twice as long as inspiration.

Indications
• To help relieve dyspneic episodes in patients with COPD

Complications
• Collapse of damaged airways and increased air trapping (may be caused by poor technique)

Continuous positive-airway pressure (CPAP)

CPAP maintains positive pressure in the airways throughout the respiratory cycle. It increases oxygenation by enhancing functional residual capacity (FRC) and lung compliance. Used for a patient who is breathing spontaneously, CPAP allows him to exhale against the positive pressure. The pressure is applied — using a continuous flow or demand flow system — with an endotracheal, nasotracheal, or tracheostomy tube or through a continuous flow, tight-fitting face mask.

Indications
• To treat patients who can ventilate adequately but who have inadequate oxygenation because of decreased FRC
• To help wean a patient from mechanical ventilation
• To treat sleep apnea

Complications
• Gastric distention, vomiting, and aspiration (when CPAP is delivered through a mask)
• Respiratory muscle fatigue

Cough technique: Assisted

This technique involves manual compression of the patient's abdomen to compensate for paralyzed abdominal muscles. To perform controlled coughing, place the patient in a supine position and slightly elevate his head. Place your hands on his abdomen, midway between the umbilicus and the xiphoid process. Instruct him to take a deep breath and attempt to cough. When he reaches end inspiration and begins to cough, perform one or two abdominal thrusts, rapidly pressing inward and upward on the abdomen.

Indications
• To increase cough effectiveness in paralyzed patients who can't contract their abdominal muscles

Complications
• Injury to abdominal organs or fractured ribs (may be caused by incorrect hand placement)
• Vomiting. (Avoid performing after eating.)

Coughing technique: Controlled

In controlled coughing, the patient should sit upright, leaning slightly forward, with his feet supported. A postoperative patient will need to splint his incision. To perform controlled coughing, he should:
• begin with maximal inhalation
• hold his breath for 2 seconds
• cough twice with his mouth slightly open. (The first cough loosens mucus; the second helps remove it.)
• pause briefly, then inhale through his nose by sniffing gently
• rest.

Indications
• To treat excessive mucus
• To prevent respiratory complications, such as atelectasis, after thoracic or abdominal surgery

Complications
• Fatigue, throat irritation, new or worsened bronchospasm (may be caused by excessive coughing)

Cough technique: Huff

In this technique, the patient coughs while the glottis remains open. Have the patient sit upright, leaning slightly forward, with his feet supported. Instruct the patient to take a deep breath and to exhale forcefully through an open mouth while saying the word *huff.*

Indications
• To treat patients with retained secretions who have difficulty producing a cough because of pain
• To treat COPD patients who experience significant airway collapse on forced expiration

Complications
• Fatigue and throat irritation (may be caused by excessive coughing)

Endotracheal intubation

This procedure involves the oral or nasal insertion of a flexible tube through the larynx into the trachea to mechanically ventilate the patient. Recently, endotracheal tubes have been used to deliver emergency medications. Associated care involves frequent assessment of airway status, suctioning to maintain a patent airway, maintenance of proper cuff pressure to prevent tissue ischemia and necrosis, careful repositioning of the tube to avoid traumatic manipulation, and constant monitoring for complications.

Indications
• To provide an open airway during cardiopulmonary resuscitation (CPR) and airway obstruction when other efforts have failed
• To provide a controlled airway for mechanical ventilation (may be used in nonemergency situations, such as before surgery)

Complications
• Apnea (caused by reflex breath-holding or interruption of oxygen delivery)
• Bronchospasm

- Aspiration of blood, secretions, or gastric contents
- Tooth damage or loss
- Injury to the lips, mouth, pharynx, or vocal cords
- Laryngeal edema and erosion
- Tracheal stenosis, erosion, and necrosis
- Nasal bleeding, laceration, sinusitis, and otitis media (may be caused by nasotracheal intubation)

Incentive spirometry

This procedure uses a breathing device called an incentive spirometer, which is designed to provide a visual incentive to encourage the patient to achieve maximal ventilation. Some incentive spirometers contain plastic floats that are raised according to the amount of air the patient pulls through the device when he inhales. The device measures respiratory flow or volume and encourages the patient to take a deep breath (while his lips are closed tightly around the device's mouthpiece) and hold it for several seconds. The deep breath produces increased lung volume and inflation of alveoli and facilitates venous return. In addition, deep breathing establishes alveolar hyperventilation, thus preventing or reversing alveolar collapse that produces atelectasis and pneumonitis.

Indications
- To treat patients on prolonged bed rest
- To treat patients after thoracic or abdominal surgery
- To prevent and treat atelectasis

Complications
- Nausea (if used at mealtimes)
- Hyperventilation (if performed at an increased respiratory rate)

Mechanical ventilation

A ventilator can totally control the patient's respirations or can assist respirations. Major types include positive pressure, negative pressure, and high-frequency ventilation (HFV).

Positive-pressure systems push air into the chest — the opposite of normal physiologic function. Expiration occurs passively at the end of inspiration. These systems include volume-cycled or pressure-cycled ventilators and may deliver positive end-expiratory pressure or CPAP. Volume-cycled ventilators deliver a preset volume of gas that provides consistent tidal volume despite changes in airway resistance or lung compliance. Pressure-cycled ventilators terminate inspiration at a preset pressure of gas; however, they deliver varying amounts of tidal volume over varying time intervals.

Negative pressure systems provide ventilation for patients who can't generate adequate inspiratory pressures, such as those with neuromuscular disorders.

HFV systems provide high ventilation rates with low peak airway pressures.

Indications
- To treat apnea, acute ventilatory failure, and impending acute ventilatory failure, resulting from interruption of the normal regulatory mechanism of respiration
- To treat fatigue or paralysis of respiratory muscles, restriction of chest wall movement, or impaired gas exchange

Complications
- Respiratory distress from ventilator malfunction
- Airway malfunction
- Barotrauma
- Pneumothorax
- Oxygen toxicity
- Respiratory infection
- Atelectasis
- Decreased venous return and resulting reduced cardiac output
- GI complications, such as stress ulcer
- Asynchronous breathing
- Ventilator dependence
- Adverse psychological effects

Oronasopharyngeal suction

Used to maintain a patent airway, oronasopharyngeal suction removes secretions from the pharynx by means of a suction catheter inserted through the mouth or nostril.

Indications
• To treat patients who can't clear the upper airway effectively with coughing (for example, unconscious or debilitated patients)
• To treat intubated patients with secretions pooled above the cuff of the artificial airway

Complications
• Hypoxia (secondary to removal of oxygen with secretions)
• Mucosal trauma, possibly with bleeding
• Nosocomial infection

Oxygen therapy

This treatment provides tissues with sufficient oxygen to carry on metabolic processes. Oxygen delivery devices include nasal cannula, face mask, partial rebreather mask, nonrebreather mask, Venturi mask, transtracheal oxygen, and CPAP mask. Additionally, aerosolized oxygen from a nebulizer may be delivered by face mask, hood, tent, tracheostomy collar, or T tube.

Indications
• To treat patients with decreased partial pressure of oxygen in arterial blood, decreased cardiac output, reduced blood oxygen-carrying capacity, or increased oxygen demand

Complications
• Skin breakdown from oxygen delivery device
• Dry mucous membranes
• Oxygen toxicity
• Absorption atelectasis
• Retrolental fibroplasia
• Death (possible because high-frequency oxygen in a patient with COPD may cause depression of the hypoxic drive and may thereby inhibit breathing)

Percussion

Percussion is usually performed sequentially, with the patient placed in the appropriate postural drainage position for the involved pulmonary segment. In percussion, you first cup your hands to create maximum air pockets. Then clap over the involved pulmonary segments to cause rhythmic waves that help mechanically dislodge thick, tenacious secretions from the bronchial walls.

Indications
• To treat patients with large amounts of retained thick, tenacious sputum — for example, patients with cystic fibrosis and bronchiectasis

Complications
• Fractured ribs, especially in a patient with osteoporosis (may be caused by vigorous percussion)
• Kidney pain or damage (may be caused by percussing too low posteriorly)
• Increased bronchospasm (especially when combined with postural drainage)

Positive end-expiratory pressure (PEEP)

PEEP applies positive pressure at the end of each expiration to keep open collapsed alveoli. It's used for a patient who isn't breathing spontaneously. It may be administered with positive-pressure mechanical ventilation. Alternatively, it may be performed during manual ventilation by attaching a PEEP valve to the manual resuscitation bag.

Indications
• To treat patients with diffuse restrictive lung disease or hypoxemic respiratory failure that's unresponsive to mechanically delivered oxygen alone

Complications
• Decreased cardiac output (may be related to high intrathoracic pressures)
• Pneumothorax or subcutaneous emphysema (may be caused by pulmonary

barotrauma from increased intrapulmonary pressure)

Postural drainage

Also known as bronchial drainage, postural drainage uses specific body positions to facilitate gravity drainage of secretions from affected lung segments into major airways. Optimal drainage occurs when the involved segmental bronchus lies perpendicular to the floor. Secretions then move from the involved peripheral airways toward the segmental bronchus and up the bronchial tree to the trachea for expectoration. During postural drainage, the patient should maintain each position no longer than 20 minutes. Monitor how well the patient tolerates the procedure.

Indications
• To drain excessive amounts of retained secretions

Complications
• Impaired respiratory excursion, possibly leading to hypoxia or postural hypotension (caused by pressure on the diaphragm by abdominal contents)

Thoracentesis

During thoracentesis, the doctor inserts a needle or catheter into the pleural space to aspirate fluid or air (to relieve pulmonary compression or respiratory distress) or to instill chemotherapeutic or other drugs.

Indications
• To treat pleural effusion in patients with cancer, tuberculosis, empyema, or pleurisy

Complications
• Pneumothorax or hemothorax
• Abdominal injury
• Infection
• Injury to diaphragm
• Hemorrhage
• Hypovolemic shock
• Protein depletion

Thoracic drainage

In a patient with chest trauma, one or more chest tubes may be surgically inserted and connected to a thoracic drainage system. Normally, negative pressure in the pleural cavity exerts a suction force that keeps the lungs expanded. Chest trauma that upsets this pressure may cause lung collapse. Thoracic drainage uses gravity and possibly suction to restore negative pressure and remove any material that collects in the pleural cavity. An underwater seal in the drainage system allows air and fluid to escape from the pleural cavity but doesn't allow air to reenter.

Indications
• To help treat pneumothorax, hemothorax, empyema, pleural effusion, or chylothorax
• To restore negative pressure in the pleural cavity after a thoracotomy

Complications
• Tension pneumothorax
• Atelectasis (from decreased chest expansion and infection)

Thoracotomy

This surgical opening of the thoracic cavity is usually performed to remove all or part of the lung. Lung excision may involve pneumonectomy (excision of an entire lung), lobectomy (removal of one of the five lobes), segmental resection (removal of one or more lung segments), or wedge resection (removal of a small portion of the lung without regard to segments).

Indications
• To locate tumors or sources of bleeding
• To remove diseased lung tissue, which may result from lung cancer, tuberculosis, lung abscess, bronchiectasis, benign tumors, or fungal infections
• To obtain a biopsy specimen to identify the cause of lung dysfunction

Complications
- Hemorrhage
- Infection
- Tension pneumothorax
- Bronchopleural fistula
- Empyema
- Persistent air space that the remaining lung tissue doesn't expand to fill

Tracheal suction

This procedure removes secretions from the trachea or bronchi by means of a catheter inserted through the mouth, nose, tracheal stoma, tracheostomy tube, or endotracheal tube. Besides removing secretions to help maintain a patent airway, tracheal suctioning also stimulates the cough reflex.

Indications
- To treat patients with retained tracheobronchial secretions who can't produce an effective cough (for example, patients with neuromuscular weakness caused by Guillain-Barré syndrome, paralysis, respiratory muscle fatigue, or decreased level of consciousness)

Complications
- Hypoxemia
- Arrhythmias
- Hypotension
- Hypertension
- Respiratory tract infection
- Mucosal trauma with bleeding
- Increased intracranial pressure, especially in high-risk patients
- Laryngospasm or bronchospasm

Tracheotomy

A tracheotomy involves the surgical creation of an external opening — called a tracheostomy — into the trachea and insertion of an indwelling tube to maintain the airway's patency. The procedure may be performed during an emergency or during a more controlled situation; it may be a permanent or temporary measure. Associated care involves assessing airway status, suctioning secretions, cleaning the cannula, caring for the stoma, and maintaining proper cuff pressure.

Indications
- To maintain a patent airway in patients with complete upper airway obstruction (for example, from laryngeal edema, foreign body obstruction, or tumor) when endotracheal intubation is impossible; usually preferred for long-term intubation

Complications
- Airway obstruction from improper tube placement or buildup of secretions
- Hemorrhage
- Edema
- Infection
- Perforated esophagus
- Subcutaneous or mediastinal emphysema
- Aspiration of secretions
- Tracheal necrosis (from cuff pressure)
- Laceration of arteries, veins, or nerves

Vibration

Vibration helps mobilize secretions from the bronchial tree to the trachea. It causes less complications than percussion and may be used with or as an alternative to percussion in a patient who is frail, in pain, or recovering from thoracic surgery or trauma.

To perform this procedure, hold your hands flat against the patient's chest wall and then, as the patient exhales, vibrate your hands by tensing your arm and shoulder muscles.

Indications
- To help mobilize retained secretions in such conditions as cystic fibrosis, COPD, bronchiectasis, and pneumonia

Complications
- Fractured ribs (may be caused by vigorous therapy)

Quick reference to respiratory drugs

acetylcysteine

General
Brand names: Airbron, Mucomyst, Mucosil
Pharmacologic classification: amino acid (L-cysteine) derivative
Therapeutic classification: mucolytic agent

Indications and dosage
• Pneumonia, bronchitis, tuberculosis, cystic fibrosis, emphysema, atelectasis (adjunct). *Adults:* by direct instillation into trachea — 1 to 2 ml 10% to 20% solution as often as every hour. By mouthpiece instillation — 3 to 5 ml 20% solution or 6 to 10 ml 10% solution, t.i.d. or q.i.d. The 20% solution may be diluted with 0.9% sodium chloride solution.

Adverse reactions
EENT: *rhinorrhea,* hemoptysis
GI: *stomatitis, nausea, vomiting*
Other: ***bronchospasm*** (especially in asthmatics), allergic reactions

acyclovir sodium (acycloguanosine)

General
Brand name: Zovirax
Pharmacologic classification: synthetic purine nucleoside
Therapeutic classification: antiviral

Indications and dosage
• Pneumonia caused by herpes simplex types 1 and 2 and varicella zoster. *Adults:* 5 to 10 mg/kg q 8 hours as a 1-hour infusion.

Adverse reactions
Blood: neutropenia, thrombocytopenia
CNS: lethargy, obtundation, ***seizures,*** tremor, hallucinations
GI: *nausea, vomiting,* anorexia, abdominal pain

GU: *increased blood urea nitrogen (BUN) and creatinine levels,* ***anuria,*** painful urination
Other: *pain on injection,* hypotension, altered liver function studies, rash

albuterol
albuterol sulfate (salbutamol, salbutamol sulphate)

General
Brand names: Proventil, Proventil Repetabs, Ventolin, Ventolin Rotacaps
Pharmacologic classification: adrenergic
Therapeutic classification: bronchodilator

Indications and dosage
• Prevention and treatment of bronchospasm in patients with reversible obstructive airway disease. *Adults and children over age 12:* 1 to 2 inhalations q 4 to 6 hours. More frequent administration or a greater number of inhalations is not recommended.
  Oral tablets or syrup — 2 to 4 mg t.i.d. or q.i.d. Maximum dosage is 8 mg q.i.d.
  Extended-release tablets — 4 to 8 mg q 12 hours. Maximum dosage is 16 mg b.i.d.
• Prevention of exercise-induced asthma. *Adults:* 2 inhalations 15 minutes before exercise.

Adverse reactions
CNS: *tremor, nervousness,* dizziness, insomnia, headache
CV: tachycardia, palpitations, hypertension
EENT: drying and irritation of nose and throat (with inhaled form)
GI: heartburn, nausea, vomiting
Other: muscle cramps, hypokalemia (with high doses)

Common reactions are in *italics;* life-threatening reactions are in ***bold italics.***

aminophylline (theophylline ethylenediamine)

General
Brand names: Aminophyllin, Phyllocontin, Somophyllin-DF
Pharmacologic classification: xanthine derivative
Therapeutic classification: bronchodilator

Indications and dosage
• Symptomatic relief of bronchospasm. *Patients not currently receiving theophylline who require rapid relief of symptoms:* Loading dose is 6 mg/kg (equivalent to 4.7 mg/kg anhydrous theophylline) I.V. slowly (less than or equal to 25 mg/minute), then maintenance infusion.
Adults (nonsmokers): 0.5 mg/kg/hour. *Otherwise healthy adult smokers:* 0.9 mg/kg/hour.
Older patients and adults with cor pulmonale: 0.3 mg/kg/hour.
Adults with congestive heart failure (CHF) or liver disease: 0.1 to 0.2 mg/kg/hour.
Patients currently receiving theophylline: aminophylline bolus doses of 0.63 mg/kg (0.5 mg/kg anhydrous theophylline) over 20 to 40 minutes will increase plasma levels of theophylline by 1 mcg/ml. Some clinicians recommend a dose of 3.1 mg/kg (2.5 mg/kg anhydrous theophylline) if no obvious signs of theophylline toxicity are present and theophylline levels are unknown.
• Chronic bronchial asthma. *Adults:* 600 to 1,600 mg P.O. daily divided t.i.d. or q.i.d.
Note: All doses are adjusted for a desired serum theophylline level of 8 to 20 mcg/ml.

Adverse reactions
CNS: *nervousness, restlessness, dizziness,* headache, *insomnia,* light-headedness, **seizures**, muscle twitching
CV: *palpitations, sinus tachycardia,* extrasystoles, flushing, marked hypotension, increase in respiratory rate

GI: *nausea, vomiting, anorexia,* bitter aftertaste, dyspepsia, heavy feeling in stomach, diarrhea
Local: rectal suppositories may cause irritation
Skin: urticaria

aminosalicylate sodium

General
Brand names: Nemasol Sodium, PAS Sodium, Tubasal
Pharmacologic classification: aminobenzoic acid analogue
Therapeutic classification: antitubercular

Indications and dosage
• Adjunctive treatment of tuberculosis. *Adults:* 10 to 12 g P.O. daily, divided in three or four doses, given with meals.

Adverse reactions
Blood: leukopenia, **agranulocytosis**, eosinophilia, thrombocytopenia, **hemolytic anemia**
CNS: encephalopathy
CV: vasculitis
GI: *nausea, vomiting, diarrhea,* abdominal pain, peptic ulcer, gastric ulcer, malabsorption (folic acid, vitamin B_{12}, iron, lipids)
GU: albuminuria, **hematuria, crystalluria**
Hepatic: *jaundice,* **hepatitis**
Metabolic: *acidosis, hypokalemia, goiter*
Skin: *rash, pruritus*
Other: *infectious mononucleosis–like syndrome, fever, lymphadenopathy*
Note: Drug should be discontinued if patient shows signs of hypersensitivity reaction, bone marrow toxicity, or hepatic failure.

amoxicillin/clavulanate potassium

General
Brand names: Augmentin, Clavulin
Pharmacologic classification: aminopenicillin and beta-lactamase inhibitor

---

Common reactions are in *italics;* life-threatening reactions are in ***bold italics***.

Therapeutic classification: antibacterial

Indications and dosage
• Lower respiratory infections, otitis media, and sinusitis caused by susceptible strains of gram-positive and gram-negative organisms. *Adults:* 250 mg (based on the amoxicillin component) P.O. q 8 hours. For more severe infections, 500 mg q 8 hours.

Adverse reactions
Blood: anemia, ***thrombocytopenia***, thrombocytopenic purpura, eosinophilia, ***leukopenia***
GI: *nausea,* vomiting, *diarrhea,* pseudomembranous colitis
Other: hypersensitivity (erythematous maculopapular rash, urticaria, ***anaphylaxis***, overgrowth of nonsusceptible organisms

amoxicillin trihydrate

General
Brand names: Amoxil, Axicillin, Novamoxin, Polymox, Trimox, Wymox
Pharmacologic classification: aminopenicillin
Therapeutic classification: antibacterial

Indications and dosage
• Systemic infections caused by susceptible strains of gram-positive and gram-negative organisms. *Adults:* 750 mg to 1.5 g P.O. daily in divided doses given q 8 hours.

Adverse reactions
Blood: anemia, ***thrombocytopenia,***
thrombocytopenic purpura, eosinophilia, ***leukopenia***
GI: *nausea,* vomiting, *diarrhea*
Other: hypersensitivity (erythematous maculopapular rash, urticaria, ***anaphylaxis***), overgrowth of nonsusceptible organisms

amphotericin B

General
Brand name: Fungizone
Pharmacologic classification: polyene macrolide
Therapeutic classification: antifungal

Indications and dosage
• Systemic fungal infections (histoplasmosis, coccidioidomycosis, blastomycosis, cryptococcosis, disseminated moniliasis, aspergillosis, phycomycosis). *Adults:* initially, 1 mg in 250 ml of dextrose 5% in water (D_5W) infused over 2 to 4 hours; or 0.25 mg/kg daily by slow infusion over 6 hours. Increase daily dosage gradually as patient tolerance develops to maximum 1 mg/kg daily or 1.5 mg/kg every other day. If drug is discontinued for 1 week or more, administration must resume with initial dose and again increase gradually.

Adverse reactions
Blood: normochromic, normocytic anemia
CNS: headache, peripheral neuropathy
CV: hypotension, ***cardiac arrhythmias, asystole***
GI: *anorexia, weight loss, nausea,* vomiting, dyspepsia, diarrhea, epigastric cramps
GU: abnormal renal function with hypokalemia, azotemia, hyposthenuria, hypomagnesemia, renal tubular acidosis, nephrocalcinosis; with large doses — permanent renal impairment, anuria, oliguria
Local: burning, stinging, irritation, tissue damage with extravasation, *thrombophlebitis,* pain at site of injection
Other: arthralgia, myalgia, muscle weakness secondary to hypokalemia, *fever, chills,* malaise, generalized pain

---

Common reactions are in *italics;* life-threatening reactions are in ***bold italics.***

ampicillin
ampicillin sodium
ampicillin trihydrate

General
Brand names: Apo-Ampi, Novo Ampicillin, Omnipen, Penbritin, Principen, Polycillin, Totacillin
Pharmacologic classification: aminopenicillin
Therapeutic classification: antibacterial

Indications and dosage
• Systemic infections caused by susceptible strains of gram-positive and gram-negative organisms. *Adults:* 1 to 4 g P.O. daily, divided into doses given q 6 hours; 2 to 12 g I.M. or I.V. daily, divided into doses given q 4 to 6 hours.

Adverse reactions
Blood: anemia, **thrombocytopenia,** thrombocytopenic purpura, eosinophilia, **leukopenia**
GI: *nausea,* vomiting, *diarrhea,* glossitis, stomatitis
Local: pain at injection site, vein irritation, thrombophlebitis
Other: hypersensitivity (erythematous maculopapular rash, urticaria, **anaphylaxis**), overgrowth of nonsusceptible organisms

azithromycin

General
Brand name: Zithromax
Pharmacologic classification: azalide macrolide
Therapeutic classification: antibacterial

Indications and dosage
• Acute bacterial exacerbations of chronic obstructive pulmonary disease (COPD) caused by *Haemophilus influenzae, Moraxella (Branhamella) catarrhalis,* or *Streptococcus pneumoniae;* pneumonias caused by *H. influenzae* or *S. pneumoniae* or *Mycobacterium avium-intracellulare. Adults and adolescents ages 16 and over:* initially,

500 mg P.O. as a single dose on day 1, followed by 250 mg daily on days 2 through 5. Total dose is 1.5 g. Dose is doubled if used to treat pneumonia caused by *M. avium-intracellulare.*

Adverse reactions
CNS: dizziness, vertigo, headache, fatigue, somnolence
CV: palpitations, chest pain
GI: *nausea, vomiting, diarrhea, abdominal pain,* dyspepsia, flatulence, melena, cholestatic jaundice, pseudomembranous colitis
GU: monilia, vaginitis, nephritis
Skin: rash, photosensitivity
Other: angioedema

beclomethasone dipropionate

General
Brand names: Beconase Nasal Inhaler, Beclovent, Vancenase AQ Nasal Spray, Vanceril
Pharmacologic classification: glucocorticoid
Therapeutic classification: antiasthmatic, anti-inflammatory

Indications and dosage
• Steroid-dependent asthma. *Adults:* 2 to 4 oral inhalations t.i.d. or q.i.d.; maximum of 20 inhalations daily. Alternatively, 12 to 16 nasal sprays daily, reduced to 2 sprays t.i.d. or q.i.d. as tolerated.
• Relief of symptoms of seasonal or perennial rhinitis. *Adults and children over age 12:* usual dosage is 1 spray (42 mcg) in each nostril b.i.d. to q.i.d. (total dosage 168 to 336 mcg daily). Most patients require 1 spray in each nostril t.i.d. (252 mcg daily).

Adverse reactions (oral form)
CNS: headache
EENT: hoarseness, fungal infections of mouth and throat, throat irritation
GI: dry mouth

Adverse reactions (nasal form)
CNS: headache
EENT: *mild transient nasal burning and stinging,* nasal congestion, sneezing, epistaxis, watery eyes

Common reactions are in *italics;* life-threatening reactions are in ***bold italics.***

GI: nausea, vomiting
Other: development of nasopharyngeal fungal infections

cefaclor

General
Brand name: Ceclor
Pharmacologic classification: second-generation cephalosporin
Therapeutic classification: antibacterial

Indications and dosage
• Infections of respiratory tract; otitis media caused by *Haemophilus influenzae, Streptococcus pneumoniae, S. pyogenes, Escherichia coli, Proteus mirabis, Klebsiella* species, and staphylococci. *Adults:* 250 to 500 mg P.O. q 8 hours. Total daily dosage should not exceed 4 g.

Adverse reactions
Blood: transient leukopenia, lymphocytosis, anemia, eosinophilia
CNS: dizziness, headache, somnolence
GI: *nausea,* vomiting, *diarrhea,* anorexia, pseudomembranous colitis
GU: red and white cells in urine, vaginal moniliasis, vaginitis
Skin: *maculopapular rash,* dermatitis
Other: *hypersensitivity,* fever, cholestatic jaundice

cefazolin sodium

General
Brand names: Ancef, Kefzol
Pharmacologic classification: first-generation cephalosporin
Therapeutic classification: antibacterial

Indications and dosage
• Serious infections of respiratory tract caused by *Escherichia coli,* gonococci, *Klebsiella, Proteus mirabilis, Staphylococcus aureus, Streptococcus pneumoniae,* and group A beta-hemolytic streptococci. *Adults:* 500 mg I.M. or I.V. q 8 hours to 1 g q 6 hours. Maximum 12 g/day in life-threatening situations.

Total daily dosage is same for I.M. or I.V. administration and depends on susceptibility of organism and severity of infection. In patients with impaired renal function, doses or frequency of administration must be modified according to degree of renal impairment, severity of infection, and susceptibility of organism. Should be injected deep I.M. into a large muscle mass, such as gluteus or lateral aspect of thigh.

Adverse reactions
Blood: transient neutropenia, leukopenia, eosinophilia, anemia
CNS: dizziness, headache, malaise, paresthesia
GI: pseudomembranous colitis, nausea, anorexia, vomiting, *diarrhea,* glossitis, dyspepsia, abdominal cramps, anal pruritus, tenesmus, oral candidiasis (thrush)
GU: genital pruritus and moniliasis, vaginitis
Local: *at injection site — pain, induration, sterile abscesses, tissue sloughing; phlebitis and thrombophlebitis with I.V. injection*
Skin: *maculopapular and erythematous rashes, urticaria*
Other: *hypersensitivity,* dyspnea

cefixime

General
Brand name: Suprax
Pharmacologic classification: third-generation cephalosporin
Therapeutic classification: antibacterial

Indications and dosage
• Acute bronchitis and acute exacerbations of chronic bronchitis caused by *Streptococcus pneumoniae* and *Haemophilus influenzae* (beta-lactamase positive and negative strains). *Adults:* 400 mg P.O. daily as a single 400-mg tablet or 200 mg q 12 hours.

Adverse reactions
Blood: thrombocytopenia, leukopenia, eosinophilia
CNS: headache, dizziness

Common reactions are in *italics;* life-threatening reactions are in ***bold italics***.

GI: *diarrhea,* loose stools, abdominal pain, nausea, vomiting, dyspepsia, flatulence, pseudomembranous colitis
GU: genital pruritus, vaginitis, genital candidiasis
Skin: pruritus, rash, urticaria
Other: drug fever, ***hypersensitivity reactions***

---

cefotaxime sodium

General
Brand name: Claforan
Pharmacologic classification: third-generation cephalosporin
Therapeutic classification: antibacterial

Indications and dosage
• Serious infections of the lower respiratory tract. Among susceptible microorganisms are streptococci, including *Streptococcus pneumoniae* and *S. pyogenes; Escherichia coli; Klebsiella; Haemophilus influenzae; Enterobacter; Proteus;* and *Peptostreptococcus.* Adults: usual dose is 1 g I.V. or I.M. q 4 to 12 hours. Up to 12 g daily can be administered in life-threatening infections. Total daily dosage is same for I.M. or I.V. administration and depends on susceptibility of organism and severity of infection. In adults with impaired renal function, doses or frequency of administration must be modified according to degree of renal impairment, severity of infection, and susceptibility of organism. Should be injected deep I.M. into a large muscle mass, such as gluteus or lateral aspect of thigh.

Adverse reactions
Blood: transient neutropenia, eosinophilia, hemolytic anemia
CNS: headache, malaise, paresthesia, dizziness
GI: pseudomembranous colitis, nausea, anorexia, vomiting, *diarrhea,* glossitis, dyspepsia, abdominal cramps, tenesmus, anal pruritus, oral candidiasis (thrush)
GU: genital pruritus and moniliasis
Local: *at injection site — pain, induration, sterile abscesses, fever, tissue*

sloughing; *phlebitis and thrombophlebitis with I.V. injection*
Skin: *maculopapular and erythematous rashes, urticaria*
Other: ***hypersensitivity,*** dyspnea, elevated temperature

---

cefotetan disodium

General
Brand name: Cefotan
Pharmacologic classification: second-generation cephalosporin
Therapeutic classification: antibacterial

Indications and dosage
• Serious infections of the lower respiratory tract. Among susceptible microorganisms are streptococci, *Staphylococcus epidermidis, Escherichia coli, Klebsiella, Enterobacter, Proteus, Haemophilus influenzae, Neisseria gonorrhoeae,* and *Bacteroides,* including *B. fragilis.* Adults: 1 to 2 g I.V. or I.M. q 12 hours. Up to 6 g daily in life-threatening infections.
Total daily dosage is same for I.M. or I.V. administration and depends on susceptibility of organism and severity of infection. In patients with impaired renal function, doses or frequency of administration must be modified according to degree of renal impairment, severity of infection, and susceptibility of organism. Should be injected deep I.M. into a large muscle mass, such as gluteus or lateral aspect of thigh.

Adverse reactions
Blood: transient neutropenia, eosinophilia, hemolytic anemia, hypoprothrombinemia, bleeding
CNS: headache, malaise, paresthesia, dizziness
GI: pseudomembranous colitis, nausea, anorexia, vomiting, *diarrhea,* glossitis, dyspepsia, abdominal cramps, tenesmus, anal pruritus
GU: genital pruritus and moniliasis
Local: *at injection site — pain, induration, sterile abscesses, tissue sloughing; phlebitis and thrombophlebitis with I.V. injection*

Common reactions are in *italics;* life-threatening reactions are in ***bold italics.***

Skin: *maculopapular and erythematous rashes, urticaria*
Other: *hypersensitivity,* dyspnea, elevated temperature

cefoxitin sodium

General
Brand name: Mefoxin
Pharmacologic classification: second-generation cephalosporin
Therapeutic classification: antibacterial

Indications and dosage
• Serious infections of respiratory tract. Susceptible organisms include *Escherichia coli* and other coliform bacteria, streptococci, *Klebsiella,* and *Bacteroides,* including *B. fragilis. Adults:* 1 to 2 g q 6 to 8 hours for uncomplicated forms of infection. Up to 12 g daily in life-threatening infections.
Total daily dosage is same for I.M. or I.V. administration and depends on susceptibility of organism and severity of infection. In patients with impaired renal function, doses or frequency of administration must be modified according to degree of renal impairment, severity of infection, and susceptibility of organism. Should be injected deep I.M. into a large muscle mass, such as gluteus or lateral aspect of thigh.

Adverse reactions
Blood: transient neutropenia, eosinophilia, hypothrombinemia, **hemolytic anemia**
CNS: headache, malaise, paresthesia, dizziness
GI: pseudomembranous colitis, nausea, anorexia, vomiting, *diarrhea,* glossitis, dyspepsia, abdominal cramps, tenesmus, anal pruritus, oral candidiasis (thrush)
GU: genital pruritus and moniliasis
Local: *at injection site — pain, induration, sterile abscesses, tissue sloughing; phlebitis and thrombophlebitis with I.V. injection*
Skin: *maculopapular and erythematous rashes, urticaria*
Other: *hypersensitivity,* dyspnea, fever

cefpodoxime proxetil

General
Brand name: Vantin
Pharmacologic classification: second-generation cephalosporin
Therapeutic classification: antibacterial

Indications and dosage
• Community-acquired pneumonia, pharyngitis, and tonsillitis caused by susceptible species of *Streptococcus pneumoniae, Haemophilus influenzae,* and *Moraxella (Branhamella) catarrhalis. Adults:* 100 to 200 mg b.i.d. with food.

Adverse reactions
Blood: transient leukopenia, lymphocytosis, anemia, eosinophilia
CNS: dizziness, headache, somnolence
GI: *nausea,* vomiting, *diarrhea,* anorexia, pseudomembranous colitis
GU: red and white cells in urine, vaginal moniliasis, vaginitis
Skin: *maculopapular rash,* dermatitis
Other: *hypersensitivity,* fever, cholestatic jaundice

cefprozil

General
Brand name: Cefzil
Pharmacologic classification: second-generation cephalosporin
Therapeutic classification: antibacterial

Indications and dosage
• Exacerbations of chronic bronchitis, pharyngitis, and tonsillitis caused by *Streptococcus pyogenes, Haemophilus influenzae,* and *Moraxella (Branhamella) catarrhalis. Adults:* 500 mg daily or b.i.d.

Adverse reactions
Blood: transient leukopenia, lymphocytosis, anemia, eosinophilia
CNS: dizziness, headache, somnolence
GI: *nausea,* vomiting, *diarrhea,* anorexia, pseudomembranous colitis
GU: red and white cells in urine, vaginal moniliasis, vaginitis

---

Common reactions are in *italics;* life-threatening reactions are in ***bold italics***.

Skin: *maculopapular rash*, dermatitis
Other: ***hypersensitivity***, fever, cholestatic jaundice

ceftazidime

General
Brand names: Fortaz, Tazicef, Tazidime
Pharmacologic classification: third-generation cephalosporin
Therapeutic classification: antibacterial

Indications and dosage
• Serious infections of the lower respiratory tract. Among susceptible microorganisms are streptococci, including *Streptococcus pneumoniae* and *S. pyogenes; Escherichia coli; Klebsiella; Proteus; Enterobacter; Haemophilus influenzae;* and *Pseudomonas. Adults:* 1 g I.V. or I.M. q 8 to 12 hours; up to 6 g daily in life-threatening infections.

Adverse reactions
Blood: eosinophilia, thrombocytosis, leukopenia
CNS: headache, dizziness
GI: pseudomembranous colitis, nausea, vomiting, diarrhea, dysgeusia, abdominal cramps
GU: genital pruritus and moniliasis
Hepatic: transient elevation in liver enzymes
Local: *at injection site — pain, induration, sterile abscesses, tissue sloughing; phlebitis and thrombophlebitis with I.V. injection*
Skin: *maculopapular and erythematous rashes, urticaria*
Other: ***hypersensitivity***, dyspnea, elevated temperature

ceftriaxone sodium

General
Brand name: Rocephin
Pharmacologic classification: third-generation cephalosporin
Therapeutic classification: antibacterial

Indications and dosage
• Serious infections of the lower respiratory tract. Susceptible microorganisms are streptococci, including *Streptococcus pneumoniae* and *S. pyogenes; Escherichia coli; Klebsiella; Haemophilus influenzae; Neisseria meningitidis; N. gonorrhoeae; Enterobacter; Proteus; Pseudomonas; Peptostreptococcus,* and *Serratia marcescens. Adults:* 1 to 2 g I.M. or I.V. daily or in equally divided doses b.i.d. Total daily dosage should not exceed 4 g. No dosage adjustment is needed for patients with renal dysfunction.

Adverse reactions
Blood: eosinophilia, thrombocytosis, leukopenia
CNS: headache, dizziness
GI: pseudomembranous enterocolitis, nausea, vomiting, diarrhea, dysgeusia, abdominal cramps
GU: genital pruritus and moniliasis
Hepatic: transient elevation in liver enzymes, biliary sludge
Local: *at injection site — pain, induration, sterile abscesses, tissue sloughing; phlebitis and thrombophlebitis with I.V. injection*
Skin: *maculopapular and erythematous rashes, urticaria*
Other: ***hypersensitivity***, dyspnea, elevated temperature

cefuroxime axetil
cefuroxime sodium

General
Brand names: Ceftin, Kefurox, Zinacef
Pharmacologic classification: second-generation cephalosporin
Therapeutic classification: antibacterial

Indications and dosage
• Oral and injectable forms are used for treatment of serious infections of the lower respiratory tract. Among susceptible organisms are *Streptococcus pneumoniae* and *S. pyogenes, Haemophilus influenzae, Klebsiella, Staphylococcus aureus, Escherichia coli, Enterobacter,* and *Neisseria gonorrhoeae. Adults:* usu-

al dosage of cefuroxime sodium is 750 mg to 1.5 g I.M. or I.V. q 8 hours, usually for 5 to 10 days. For life-threatening infections and infections caused by less susceptible organisms, 1.5 g I.M. or I.V. q 6 hours.

Alternatively, administer cefuroxime axetil 250 mg P.O. q 12 hours. For severe infections or for less susceptible organisms, dosage may be increased to 500 mg P.O. q 12 hours.

Adverse reactions
Blood: transient neutropenia, eosinophilia, *hemolytic anemia,* decrease in hemoglobin and hematocrit
CNS: headache, malaise, paresthesia, dizziness
GI: pseudomembranous colitis, nausea, anorexia, vomiting, *diarrhea,* glossitis, dyspepsia, abdominal cramps, tenesmus, anal pruritus
GU: genital pruritus and moniliasis
Local: *at injection site — pain, induration, sterile abscesses, temperature elevation, tissue sloughing; phlebitis and thrombophlebitis with I.V. injection*
Skin: *maculopapular and erythematous rashes, urticaria*
Other: *hypersensitivity,* dyspnea

cephalexin monohydrate

General
Brand names: Keflex, Keftab, Novolexin
Pharmacologic classification: first-generation cephalosporin
Therapeutic classification: antibacterial

Indications and dosage
• Infections of respiratory tract caused by *Escherichia coli* and other coliform bacteria, group A beta-hemolytic streptococci, *Haemophilus influenzae, Klebsiella, Proteus mirabilis, Streptococcus pneumoniae,* and staphylococci. *Adults:* 250 mg to 1 g P.O. q 6 hours.

Adverse reactions
Blood: transient neutropenia, eosinophilia, anemia
CNS: dizziness, headache, malaise, paresthesia

GI: pseudomembranous colitis, *nausea, anorexia,* vomiting, *diarrhea,* glossitis, dyspepsia, abdominal cramps, anal pruritus, tenesmus, oral candidiasis (thrush)
GU: genital pruritus and moniliasis, vaginitis
Skin: *maculopapular and erythematous rashes, urticaria*
Other: *hypersensitivity,* dyspnea

cephalothin sodium

General
Brand names: Ceporacin, Keflin
Pharmacologic classification: first-generation cephalosporin
Therapeutic classification: antibacterial

Indications and dosage
• Serious infections of respiratory tract. Susceptible organisms include *Escherichia coli* and other coliform bacteria, Enterobacteriaceae, enterococci, gonococci, group A beta-hemolytic streptococci, *Haemophilus influenzae, Klebsiella, Proteus mirabilis, Salmonella, Staphylococcus aureus, Shigella, Streptococcus pneumoniae* and *S. viridans,* and staphylococci. *Adults:* 500 mg to 1 g I.M. or I.V. (or intraperitoneally) q 4 to 6 hours; in life-threatening infections, up to 2 g q 4 hours.

Adverse reactions
Blood: transient neutropenia, eosinophilia, *hemolytic anemia*
CNS: headache, malaise, paresthesia, dizziness
GI: pseudomembranous colitis, nausea, anorexia, vomiting, *diarrhea,* glossitis, dyspepsia, abdominal cramps, tenesmus, anal pruritus, oral candidiasis (thrush)
GU: nephrotoxicity, genital pruritus and moniliasis
Local: *at injection site — pain, induration, sterile abscesses, tissue sloughing; phlebitis and thrombophlebitis with I.V. injection*
Skin: *maculopapular and erythematous rashes, urticaria*
Other: *hypersensitivity,* dyspnea, fever

Common reactions are in *italics;* life-threatening reactions are in *__bold italics.__*

cephradine

General
Brand names: Anspor, Velosef
Pharmacologic classification: first-generation cephalosporin
Therapeutic classification: antibacterial

Indications and dosage
• Serious infections of respiratory tract. Among susceptible organisms are *Escherichia coli* and other coliform bacteria, group A beta-hemolytic streptococci, *Haemophilus influenzae, Klebsiella, Proteus mirabilis, Staphylococcus aureus, Streptococcus pneumoniae* and *S. viridans,* and staphylococci. *Adults:* 500 mg to 1 g I.M. or I.V. b.i.d. to q.i.d.; do not exceed 12 g daily. Or 250 to 500 mg P.O. q 6 hours. Severe or chronic infections may require larger or more frequent doses, or both (up to 1 g P.O. q 6 hours). Parenteral therapy may be followed by oral treatment. Injections should be given deep I.M. into a large muscle mass, such as gluteus or lateral aspect of thigh.

Adverse reactions
Blood: transient neutropenia, eosinophilia
CNS: dizziness, headache, malaise, paresthesia
GI: pseudomembranous colitis, *nausea, anorexia,* vomiting, heartburn, glossitis, dyspepsia, abdominal cramping, *diarrhea,* tenesmus, anal pruritus, oral candidiasis (thrush)
GU: genital pruritus and moniliasis, vaginitis
Local: *at injection site — pain, induration, sterile abscesses, tissue sloughing; phlebitis and thrombophlebitis with I.V. injection*
Skin: *maculopapular and erythematous rashes, urticaria*
Other: *hypersensitivity,* dyspnea

ciprofloxacin

General
Brand names: Cipro, Cipro I.V.

Pharmacologic classification: quinolone antibiotic
Therapeutic classification: antibacterial

Indications and dosage
• Mild to moderate respiratory tract infections. *Adults:* 250 to 500 mg P.O. or 200 to 400 mg I.V. q 12 hours.
• Severe respiratory tract infections. *Adults:* 750 mg P.O. q 12 hours.

Adverse reactions
CNS: *headache,* restlessness, tremor, *light-headedness,* confusion, hallucinations, **seizures**
GI: *nausea, diarrhea,* vomiting, abdominal pain or discomfort, oral candidiasis
GU: crystalluria
Local: (with I.V. administration) thrombophlebitis, burning, pruritus, paresthesia, erythema, swelling
Other: *rash,* eosinophilia, photosensitivity

clarithromycin

General
Brand name: Biaxin
Pharmacologic classification: macrolide
Therapeutic classification: antibacterial

Indications and dosage
• Pneumonia caused by *Streptococcus pneumoniae* or *Mycoplasma pneumoniae. Adults:* 250 mg P.O. q 12 hours for 7 to 14 days.
• Acute exacerbations of chronic bronchitis caused by *Haemophilus influenzae. Adults:* 500 mg P.O. q 12 hours for 7 to 14 days.
• Pneumonia caused by *Mycobacterium avium-intracellulare. Adults:* 1,000 mg q 12 hours (in combination with other antimycobacterials) for weeks to months.

Adverse reactions
CNS: headache
GI: *diarrhea, nausea, abnormal taste,* dyspepsia, abdominal pain or discomfort

---

Common reactions are in *italics;* life-threatening reactions are in ***bold italics***.

clindamycin hydrochloride
clindamycin palmitate
clindamycin phosphate hydrochloride

General
Brand names: Cleocin, Dalacin C
Pharmacologic classification: lincomycin derivative
Therapeutic classification: antibacterial

Indications and dosage
• Infections caused by sensitive staphylococci, streptococci, pneumococci, *Bacteroides, Fusobacterium, Clostridium perfringens,* and other sensitive aerobic and anaerobic organisms. *Adults:* 150 to 450 mg P.O. q 6 hours; or 300 mg I.M. or I.V. q 6, 8, or 12 hours. Up to 2,700 mg I.M. or I.V. daily, divided q 6, 8, or 12 hours. May be used for severe infections.

Adverse reactions
Blood: transient leukopenia, eosinophilia, thrombocytopenia
GI: *nausea,* vomiting, abdominal pain, *diarrhea,* pseudomembranous colitis, esophagitis, flatulence, anorexia, *bloody or tarry stools, dysphagia*
Hepatic: elevated levels of aspartate aminotransferase (AST), formerly SGOT; alkaline phosphatase; and bilirubin
Local: *pain,* induration, *sterile abscess with I.M. injection;* thrombophlebitis, erythema, and pain after I.V. administration
Skin: maculopapular rash, urticaria
Other: unpleasant or bitter taste, *anaphylaxis*

codeine phosphate
codeine sulfate

General
Brand name: Paveral
Pharmacologic classification: opioid
Therapeutic classification: antitussive
Controlled Substance Schedule: II

Indications and dosage
• Nonproductive cough. *Adults:* 10 to 20 mg P.O. q 4 to 6 hours. Maximum dosage is 120 mg/24 hours.

Adverse reactions
CNS: *sedation, clouded sensorium, euphoria,* dizziness, seizures with large doses
CV: *hypotension,* bradycardia
GI: *nausea, vomiting, constipation, dry mouth,* ileus
GU: *urine retention*
Skin: pruritus, flushing
Other: *respiratory depression,* physical dependence

co-trimoxazole
(sulfamethoxazole-trimethoprim)

General
Brand names: Apo-Sulfatrim, Bactrim, Bactrim DS, Bactrim I.V. Infusion, Cotrim, Cotrim D.S., Septra, Septra DS, Septra I.V. Infusion, SMZ-TMP
Pharmacologic classification: sulfonamide and folate antagonist
Therapeutic classification: antibacterial

Indications and dosage
• *Pneumocystis carinii* pneumonitis. *Adults:* 20 mg/kg trimethoprim/100 mg/kg sulfamethoxazole P.O. per 24 hours, in equally divided doses q 6 hours for 14 days. If indicated, give by I.V. infusion 15 to 20 mg/kg/day (based on trimethoprim component) in three or four divided doses q 6 to 8 hours for up to 14 days. Reduce dosage for patients with renal impairment.
• Chronic bronchitis. *Adults:* 160 mg trimethoprim/800 mg sulfamethoxazole P.O. q 12 hours for 10 to 14 days.

Adverse reactions
Blood: *agranulocytosis, aplastic anemia,* megaloblastic anemia, thrombocytopenia, leukopenia, *hemolytic anemia*
CNS: headache, mental depression, seizures, hallucinations

GI: *nausea, vomiting,* diarrhea, abdominal pain, anorexia, stomatitis
GU: *toxic nephrosis with oliguria and anuria,* crystalluria, hematuria
Hepatic: jaundice
Skin: *erythema multiforme (Stevens-Johnson syndrome),* generalized skin eruption, *epidermal necrolysis, exfoliative dermatitis,* photosensitivity, urticaria, pruritus
Other: *hypersensitivity, serum sickness, drug fever, anaphylaxis*

---

cromolyn sodium (sodium cromoglycate)

General
Brand names: Gastrocrom, Intal, Intal Inhaler, Intal Spincaps, Nalcrom, Nasalcrom, Opticrom
Pharmacologic classification: chromone derivative
Therapeutic classification: mast cell stabilizer, antiasthmatic

Indications and dosage
• Adjunct in treatment of severe perennial bronchial asthma. *Adults:* contents of 20-mg capsule inhaled orally q.i.d. at regular intervals. Or administer 2 metered sprays using inhaler q.i.d. at regular intervals. Also available as an aqueous solution administered through a nebulizer.
• Prevention and treatment of allergic rhinitis. *Adults:* spray in each nostril t.i.d or q.i.d. May give up to six times daily.
• Prevention of exercise-induced bronchospasm. *Adults:* contents of 20-mg capsule or 2 metered sprays inhaled no more than 1 hour before anticipated exercise.

Adverse reactions
CNS: dizziness, headache
EENT: *irritation of the throat and trachea, cough, bronchospasm after inhalation of dry powder;* esophagitis; nasal congestion; pharyngeal irritation; wheezing
GI: nausea
GU: dysuria, urinary frequency
Skin: rash, urticaria

Other: joint swelling and pain, lacrimation, swollen parotid gland, *angioedema, eosinophilic pneumonia*

---

dexamethasone dexamethasone sodium phosphate

General
Brand names: Decadrol, Decadron, Decadron Phosphate Turbinaire (nasal), Dexasone, Dexone, Hexadrol, (systemic)
Pharmacologic classification: glucocorticoid
Therapeutic classification: antiasthmatic, anti-inflammatory

Indications and dosage
• Inflammatory conditions, allergic reactions. *Adults:* 0.25 to 4 mg P.O. b.i.d., t.i.d., or q.i.d.; or 2 sprays (phosphate) in each nostril b.i.d. or t.i.d. Maximum 12 sprays daily. Each spray delivers 0.1 mg dexamethasone sodium phosphate equal to 0.084 mg dexamethasone. May be preceded by 4 to 8 mg I.M.
• Asthma. *Adults:* 300 mcg by oral inhalation t.i.d. or q.i.d. to a maximum of 1,200 mcg daily; or 2 to 4 mg I.V. or P.O. b.i.d. to q.i.d.

Adverse reactions (systemic use)
Most adverse reactions of corticosteroids are dose- or duration-dependent.
CNS: *euphoria, insomnia,* psychotic behavior, pseudotumor cerebri
CV: *CHF,* hypertension, edema
EENT: cataracts, glaucoma
GI: *peptic ulcer,* GI irritation, increased appetite
Local: atrophy at I.M. injection sites
Metabolic: hypokalemia, hyperglycemia, growth suppression in children
Skin: delayed wound healing, acne, various skin eruptions
Other: muscle weakness, pancreatitis, hirsutism, susceptibility to infections
Acute adrenal insufficiency may follow increased stress (infection, surgery, or trauma) or abrupt withdrawal after long-term therapy. *Withdrawal symptoms:* rebound inflammation, fatigue, weakness, arthralgia, fever, dizziness, lethargy, de-

---

Common reactions are in *italics;* life-threatening reactions are in ***bold italics***.

pression, fainting, orthostatic hypotension, dyspnea, anorexia, hypoglycemia. *Sudden withdrawal may be fatal.*

Adverse reactions (nasal use)
EENT: nasal irritation, dryness, rebound nasal congestion
Other: hypersensitivity, systemic effects with prolonged use (pituitary-adrenal suppression, sodium retention, headaches, masking of infection)

dextromethorphan hydrobromide

General
Brand names: Benylin DM, Hold, Pertussin 8 Hour Cough Formula. More commonly available in combination products such as Contac Cough and Sore Throat Formula, Novahistine DMX Liquid, Robitussin-DM
Pharmacologic classification: levorphanol derivative (dextrorotatory methyl ether)
Therapeutic classification: antitussive (nonnarcotic)

Indications and dosage
• Nonproductive cough. *Adults:* 10 to 20 mg P.O. q 4 hours, or 30 mg q 6 to 8 hours. Or the controlled-release liquid 60 mg b.i.d.; maximum 120 mg daily.

Adverse reactions
CNS: drowsiness, dizziness
GI: nausea, vomiting, stomach pain

dicloxacillin sodium

General
Brand names: Dycill, Dynapen, Pathocil
Pharmacologic classification: penicillinase-resistant penicillin
Therapeutic classification: antibiotic

Indications and dosage
• Upper and lower respiratory tract infections caused by penicillinase-producing staphylococci. *Adults:* 1 to 2 g daily P.O., divided into doses given q 6 hours.

Adverse reactions
Blood: eosinophilia
CNS: neuromuscular irritability, seizures
GI: *nausea,* vomiting, *epigastric distress,* flatulence, *diarrhea*
Other: hypersensitivity (pruritus, urticaria, rash, **anaphylaxis**), overgrowth of nonsusceptible organisms

diphenhydramine hydrochloride

General
Brand names: Allerdryl, Benadryl, Benylin Cough
Pharmacologic classification: ethanolamine-derivative antihistamine
Therapeutic classification: antihistamine (H_1-receptor antagonist), antitussive

Indications and dosage
• Rhinitis, allergy symptoms. *Adults:* 25 to 50 mg P.O. t.i.d. or q.i.d.; or 10 to 50 mg deep I.M. or I.V. Maximum dosage is 400 mg daily.
• Nonproductive cough. *Adults:* 25 mg P.O. q 4 hours (not to exceed 100 mg daily).

Adverse reactions
CNS: (especially in elderly patients) *drowsiness,* confusion, insomnia, headache, vertigo
CV: palpitations
EENT: diplopia, nasal stuffiness
GI: *nausea,* vomiting, diarrhea, *dry mouth,* constipation
GU: dysuria, urine retention
Skin: urticaria, photosensitivity

doxycycline
doxycycline hyclate
doxycycline monohydrate

General
Brand names: Monodox, Vibramycin, Vibra-Tabs
Pharmacologic classification: tetracycline antibiotic
Therapeutic classification: antibacterial

Indications and dosage
• Infections caused by sensitive gram-negative and gram-positive organisms and *Mycoplasma. Adults:* 100 mg P.O. q 12 hours on first day, then 100 mg P.O. daily; or 200 mg I.V. on first day in one or two infusions, then 100 to 200 mg I.V. daily.

Give I.V. infusion slowly (minimum 1 hour). Infusion must be completed within 12 hours (within 6 hours in lactated Ringer's solution or dextrose 5% in lactated Ringer's solution).

Adverse reactions
Blood: neutropenia, eosinophilia
CNS: *intracranial hypertension*
CV: pericarditis
EENT: sore throat, glossitis, dysphagia
GI: anorexia, *epigastric distress, nausea,* vomiting, *diarrhea,* enterocolitis, anogenital inflammation
Local: thrombophlebitis
Skin: *maculopapular and erythematous rashes, photosensitivity, increased pigmentation, urticaria*
Other: *hypersensitivity, fungal overgrowth*

---

epinephrine
epinephrine bitartrate
epinephrine hydrochloride

General
Brand names: Adrenalin, Bronkaid Mist, Primatene Mist Solution, Sus-Phrine
Pharmacologic classification: adrenergic
Therapeutic classification: bronchodilator, cardiac stimulant

Indications and dosage
• Bronchospasm, hypersensitivity reactions, anaphylaxis. *Adults:* 0.1 to 0.5 mg S.C. or I.M; repeat q 10 to 15 minutes, p.r.n. Or 0.1 to 0.25 mg I.V. or 0.5 mg S.C. q 6 hours (suspension).
• Acute asthmatic attacks (inhalation). *Adults:* 1 or 2 inhalations q 1 to 5 minutes until relief is obtained; 0.2 mg/dose of usual content.

Adverse reactions
CNS: *nervousness,* tremor, euphoria, anxiety, coldness of extremities, vertigo, *headache,* sweating, disorientation, agitation; in patients with Parkinson's disease, drug increases rigidity and tremor
CV: *palpitations;* widened pulse pressure; *hypertension; tachycardia; ventricular fibrillation; CVA;* anginal pain; electrocardiogram changes, including a decrease in the T-wave amplitude
Metabolic: *hyperglycemia, glycosuria*
Other: *pulmonary edema, dyspnea, pallor*

---

erythromycin base
erythromycin estolate
erythromycin ethylsuccinate
erythromycin gluceptate
erythromycin lactobionate
erythromycin stearate

General
Brand names: E-Mycin, Erythrocin, Ilosone, Ilotycin
Pharmacologic classification: erythromycin
Therapeutic classification: antibacterial

Indications and dosage
• Mild to moderately severe respiratory tract infections caused by sensitive group A beta-hemolytic streptococci, *Diplococcus pneumoniae, Mycoplasma pneumoniae, Corynebacterium diphtheriae, Bordetella pertussis, Listeria monocytogenes. Adults:* 250 to 500 mg (erythromycin base, estolate, stearate) P.O. q 6 hours or 333 mg q 8 hours; or 400 to 800 mg (erythromycin ethylsuccinate) P.O. q 6 hours; or 15 to 20 mg/kg I.V. daily, divided q 6 hours.
• Legionnaire's disease. *Adults:* 500 mg to 1 g I.V. or P.O. (base, estolate, stearate) or 800 to 1,600 mg (ethylsuccinate) q 6 hours for 21 days.

Adverse reactions
EENT: hearing loss with high I.V. doses
GI: *abdominal pain and cramping, nausea, vomiting, diarrhea*
Hepatic: cholestatic jaundice

Common reactions are in *italics;* life-threatening reactions are in ***bold italics.***

Local: *venous irritation, thrombophlebitis after I.V. injection*
Skin: urticaria, rashes
Other: overgrowth of nonsusceptible bacteria or fungi; *anaphylaxis;* fever
  Note: Concomitant use with terfenadine or astemizole may cause cardiac toxicity.

ethambutol hydrochloride

General
Brand names: Etibi, Myambutol
Pharmacologic classification: semisynthetic antitubercular
Therapeutic classification: antitubercular

Indications and dosage
• Adjunctive treatment in pulmonary tuberculosis. *Adults:* initial treatment for patients who have not received previous antitubercular therapy is 15 mg/kg P.O. daily single dose.
  Retreatment: 25 mg/kg P.O. daily as a single dose for 60 days with at least one other antitubercular drug; then decrease to 15 mg/kg daily as a single dose.

Adverse reactions
CNS: headache, dizziness, mental confusion, possible hallucinations, peripheral neuritis (numbness and tingling of extremities)
EENT: optic neuritis (vision loss and loss of color discrimination, especially red and green)
GI: anorexia, nausea, vomiting, abdominal pain
Metabolic: *elevated uric acid levels*
Other: *anaphylactoid reactions,* fever, malaise, bloody sputum

fluconazole

General
Brand name: Diflucan
Pharmacologic classification: imidazole derivative
Therapeutic classification: antifungal

Indications and dosage
• Pneumonia caused by susceptible species of *Candida. Adults:* 200 mg b.i.d. on day 1, followed by 200 mg once daily I.V. or P.O.

Adverse reactions
CNS: headache
GI: *nausea,* diarrhea
Hepatic: altered liver function tests, *hepatitis*
Skin: rash, *Stevens-Johnson syndrome*

gentamicin sulfate

General
Brand names: Cidomycin, Garamycin
Pharmacologic classification: aminoglycoside
Therapeutic classification: antibacterial

Indications and dosage
• Serious infections caused by sensitive *Pseudomonas aeruginosa, Escherichia coli, Proteus, Klebsiella, Serratia, Enterobacter, Citrobacter,* and *Staphylococcus.* Adults: 3 mg/kg daily in divided doses q 8 hours I.M. or I.V. infusion (in 50 to 200 ml of 0.9% sodium chloride solution or D_5W infused over 30 minutes to 2 hours). For life-threatening infections, patient may receive up to 5 mg/kg daily in three or four divided doses. Adjust dose based on serum levels.

Adverse reactions
CNS: headache, lethargy, *neuromuscular blockade*
EENT: *ototoxicity (tinnitus, vertigo, hearing loss)*
GU: *nephrotoxicity (cells or casts in the urine; oliguria; proteinuria; decreased creatinine clearance; increased BUN, nonprotein nitrogen, and serum creatinine levels)*
Other: *hypersensitivity reactions, hepatic necrosis*, hypomagnesemia

guaifenesin (glyceryl guaiacolate)

General
Brand names: Resyl, Robitussin

Pharmacologic classification: propanediol derivative
Therapeutic classification : expectorant

Indications and dosage
• Expectorant. *Adults:* 100 to 400 mg P.O. q 4 hours. Maximum is 2,400 mg daily.

Adverse reactions
CNS: drowsiness
GI: stomach pain, diarrhea, vomiting and nausea occur with large doses

ipratropium bromide

General
Brand name: Atrovent
Pharmacologic classification: anticholinergic
Therapeutic classification: bronchodilator

Indications and dosage
• Maintenance treatment of bronchospasm in COPD; 2 inhalations (26 mcg) q.i.d. Additional inhalations may be needed. However, total inhalations should not exceed 12 in 24 hours.

Adverse reactions
CNS: nervousness, dizziness, headache
CV: palpitations
EENT: cough, blurred vision
GI: nausea, GI distress, dry mouth
Skin: rash

isoetharine hydrochloride
isoetharine mesylate

General
Brand names: Bronkometer, Bronkosol
Pharmacologic classification: adrenergic
Therapeutic classification: bronchodilator

Indications and dosage
• Bronchial asthma and reversible bronchospasm occurring with bronchitis and emphysema in adults. Isoetharine hydrochloride may be administered by hand nebulizer, oxygen aerosolization, or intermittent positive-pressure breathing (IPPB).
Oxygen aerosolization: 0.5 to 1 ml of a 0.5% solution or 0.25 to 0.5 ml of a 1% solution diluted 1:3 with sterile water or 0.9% sodium chloride solution.
Undiluted aerosolization: 2 to 4 ml of a 0.125% solution, 2.5 ml of a 0.2% solution, or 2 ml of a 0.25% solution.
IPPB solution: 0.5 to 1 ml of a 0.5% solution or 0.25 to 1 ml of a 1% solution diluted 1:3 with sterile water or 0.9% sodium chloride solution.
Undiluted IPPB: 2 to 4 ml of a 0.125% solution, 2.5 ml of a 0.2% solution, or 2 ml of a 0.25% solution.
Hand nebulizer: 3 to 7 inhalations of undiluted 0.5% or 1% solution.
Isoetharine mesylate may be administered by aerosol.
Metered aerosol: 1 to 2 inhalations. Occasionally, more may be required.

Adverse reactions
CNS: *tremor, headache,* dizziness, excitement
CV: *palpitations,* increased heart rate
GI: nausea, vomiting

isoniazid (INH)

General
Brand names: Isotamine, Nydrazid
Pharmacologic classification: isonicotinic acid hydrazine
Therapeutic classification: antitubercular

Indications and dosage
• Primary treatment against actively growing tubercle bacilli. *Adults:* 5 mg/kg P.O. or I.M. daily as a single dose, up to 300 mg/day, continued for 6 months to 2 years.
• Preventive therapy against tubercle bacilli of those closely exposed or those with a positive skin test whose chest X-rays and bacteriologic studies are consistent with nonprogressive tuberculous disease. *Adults:* 300 mg P.O. daily as a single dose, continued for 1 year.

Adverse reactions
Blood: *agranulocytosis, hemolytic anemia, aplastic anemia,* eosinophilia, leukopenia, neutropenia, thrombocytopenia, methemoglobinemia, pyridoxine-responsive hypochromic anemia
CNS: *peripheral neuropathy* (especially in malnourished, alcoholic, and diabetic patients and in slow acetylators), usually preceded by paresthesia of hands and feet; psychosis
GI: nausea, vomiting, epigastric distress, constipation, dryness of the mouth
Hepatic: *hepatitis, occasionally severe and sometimes fatal, especially in elderly patients*
Local: irritation at I.M. injection site
Metabolic: hyperglycemia, metabolic acidosis
Other: rheumatic syndrome and systemic lupus erythematosus–like syndrome; hypersensitivity (fever, rash, lymphadenopathy, vasculitis).

itraconazole

General
Brand name: Sporanox
Pharmacologic classification: imidazole derivative
Therapeutic classification: antifungal

Indications and dosage
• Pulmonary histoplasmosis and blastomycosis. *Adults:* 200 mg P.O. daily or b.i.d. May give 200 mg t.i.d. for the first 3 days in life-threatening infections.

Adverse reactions
CNS: headache, dizziness
GI: *nausea,* vomiting, diarrhea, abdominal pain
Hepatic: *hepatitis,* liver function test abnormalities
Skin: *rash,* pruritus
Other: edema, fatigue, fever, hypertension, hypokalemia
Note: Concomitant use with terfenadine or astemizole may result in cardiac arrhythmias and death.

loracarbef

General
Brand name: Lorabid
Pharmacologic classification: second-generation cephalosporin
Therapeutic classification: antibacterial

Indications and dosage
• Pneumonia, exacerbations of chronic bronchitis, pharyngitis, and tonsillitis caused by susceptible species of *Streptococcus pneumoniae, S. pyogenes, Haemophilus influenzae,* and *Moraxella (Branhamella) catarrhalis. Adults:* 200 to 400 mg b.i.d.

Adverse reactions
Blood: transient leukopenia, lymphocytosis, anemia, eosinophilia
CNS: dizziness, headache, somnolence
GI: *nausea,* vomiting, *diarrhea,* anorexia, pseudomembranous colitis
GU: red and white cells in urine, vaginal moniliasis, vaginitis
Skin: *maculopapular rash,* dermatitis
Other: *hypersensitivity,* fever, cholestatic jaundice

metaproterenol sulfate

General
Brand names: Alupent, Metaprel
Pharmacologic classification: adrenergic
Therapeutic classification: bronchodilator

Indications and dosage
• Acute episodes of bronchial asthma. *Adults:* 2 to 3 inhalations. Should not repeat inhalations more often than q 3 to 4 hours. Should not exceed 12 inhalations daily.
• Bronchial asthma and reversible bronchospasm. *Adults:* 20 mg P.O. q 6 to 8 hours.

Adverse reactions
CNS: nervousness, weakness, drowsiness, tremor

Common reactions are in *italics;* life-threatening reactions are in ***bold italics***.

CV: tachycardia, hypertension, palpitations; *with excessive use,* **cardiac arrest**
GI: vomiting, nausea, bad taste in mouth
Other: paradoxical bronchiolar constriction with excessive use

nafcillin sodium

General
Brand names: Nafcil, Nallpen, Unipen
Pharmacologic classification: penicillinase-resistant penicillin
Therapeutic classification: antibacterial

Indications and dosage
• Systemic infections caused by penicillinase-producing staphylococci.
Adults: 2 to 4 g P.O. daily, divided into doses given q 6 hours; or 2 to 12 g I.M. or I.V. daily, divided into doses given q 4 to 6 hours.
Note: Drug is not well absorbed orally; alternative penicillins are recommended.

Adverse reactions
Blood: transient leukopenia; neutropenia; granulocytopenia; ***thrombocytopenia*** with high doses
GI: *nausea,* vomiting, diarrhea
Local: vein irritation, thrombophlebitis
Other: hypersensitivity (chills, fever, rash, pruritus, urticaria, ***anaphylaxis***)

ofloxacin

General
Brand name: Floxin
Pharmacologic classification: fluoroquinolone
Therapeutic classification: antibacterial

Indications and dosage
• Lower respiratory tract infections caused by susceptible strains of *Haemophilus influenzae* or *Staphylococcus* species and other gram-negative organisms, including *Pseudomonas aeruginosa. Adults:* 200 to 400 mg P.O. or I.V. q 12 hours.
If creatinine clearance is 10 to 50 ml/minute, decrease dosage interval to once q 24 hours. If creatinine clearance is below 10 ml/minute, give half the recommended dose q 24 hours.

Adverse reactions
CNS: *headache,* restlessness, tremor, *light-headedness,* confusion, hallucinations, *seizures*
GI: *nausea, diarrhea,* vomiting, abdominal pain or discomfort, oral candidiasis
GU: crystalluria
Local: (with I.V. administration) thrombophlebitis, burning, pruritus, paresthesia, erythema, swelling
Other: *rash,* eosinophilia, photosensitivity

penicillin G potassium
penicillin G sodium

General
Brand names: Crystapen, Megacillin, Pfizerpen
Pharmacologic classification: natural penicillin
Therapeutic classification: antibacterial

Indications and dosage
• Moderate to severe systemic infections caused by streptococci. *Adults:*
Potassium: 1.6 to 3.2 million units P.O. daily in divided doses given q 6 hours (1 mg = 1,600 units); or 1.2 to 24 million units I.M. or I.V. daily in divided doses given q 4 hours.
Sodium: 1.2 to 24 million units daily I.M. or I.V., divided into doses given q 4 hours.

Adverse reactions
Blood: hemolytic anemia, leukopenia, thrombocytopenia
CNS: arthropathy (sodium); neuropathy, *seizures* with high doses (potassium and sodium)
Local: vein irritation (sodium); *thrombophlebitis, pain at injection site* (potassium and sodium)
Metabolic: *potassium poisoning with high doses* (hyperreflexia, seizures, coma, cardiac arrest); hypokalemia, salt and water retention (sodium)

Other: hypersensitivity (rash, urticaria, maculopapular eruptions, *exfoliative dermatitis,* chills, fever, edema, *anaphylaxis*), overgrowth of nonsusceptible organisms

penicillin V potassium (phenoxymethylpenicillin potassium)

General
Brand names: Beepen-VK, Betapen-VK, Ledercillin VK, NovoPen-VK, Pen Vee K, PVF K, Robicillin VK, V-Cillin K, VC-K, Veetids
Pharmacologic classification: natural penicillin
Therapeutic classification: antibacterial

Indications and dosage
• Mild to moderate systemic infections caused by streptococci. *Adults:* 250 to 500 mg (400,000 to 800,000 units) P.O. q 6 hours.

Adverse reactions
Blood: eosinophilia, hemolytic anemia, leukopenia, thrombocytopenia
CNS: neuropathy
GI: *epigastric distress,* vomiting, diarrhea, *nausea*
Other: hypersensitivity (rash, urticaria, chills, fever, edema, *anaphylaxis*), overgrowth of nonsusceptible organisms

pentamidine isethionate

General
Brand names: NebuPent, Pentam 300
Pharmacologic classification: diamidine derivative
Therapeutic classification: antiprotozoal

Indications and dosage
• Prophylaxis and treatment of pneumonia caused by *Pneumocystis carinii. Adults:* 4 mg/kg I.V. or I.M. once a day for 14 days.
• Prevention of *Pneumocystis carinii* pneumonia in high-risk individuals.

Adults: 300 mg by inhalation (using a Respirgard II nebulizer) once q 4 weeks.

Adverse reactions
Blood: *leukopenia,* thrombocytopenia, anemia
CNS: confusion, hallucinations
CV: *hypotension,* tachycardia
Endocrine: *hypoglycemia,* hyperglycemia, hypocalcemia
GI: nausea, anorexia, metallic taste
GU: *elevated serum creatinine,* renal toxicity, *acute renal failure*
Hepatic: elevated liver enzymes
Local: *sterile abscess, pain or induration at injection site,* phlebitis
Skin: rash, facial flushing, pruritus; *cough, bronchospasm* (inhalation)
Other: fever

piperacillin sodium

General
Brand name: Pipracil
Pharmacologic classification: extended-spectrum penicillin, acylaminopenicillin
Therapeutic classification: antibacterial

Indications and dosage
• Systemic infections caused by susceptible strains of gram-positive and especially gram-negative organisms (including *Proteus, Pseudomonas aeruginosa, Serratia, Enterobacter*). *Adults:* 100 to 300 mg/kg daily divided q 4 to 6 hours I.V. or I.M.

Adverse reactions
Blood: *bleeding with high doses,* neutropenia, eosinophilia, leukopenia, *thrombocytopenia*
CNS: neuromuscular irritability, *seizures,* headache, dizziness
GI: nausea, diarrhea
Local: pain at injection site, vein irritation, phlebitis
Metabolic: *hypokalemia*
Other: hypersensitivity (edema, fever, chills, rash, pruritus, urticaria, *anaphylaxis*), overgrowth of nonsusceptible organisms

---

Common reactions are in *italics;* life-threatening reactions are in ***bold italics***.

prednisone

General
Brand names: Apo-Prednisone, Liquid Pred, Meticorten, Orasone
Pharmacologic classification: adrenocorticoid
Therapeutic classification: antiasthmatic, anti-inflammatory

Indications and dosage
• Asthma, exacerbations of COPD. *Adults:* 2.5 to 15 mg P.O. b.i.d., t.i.d., or q.i.d. Maintenance dosage given once daily or every other day. Dosage must be individualized.
• Adjunctive therapy of *Pneumocystis carinii* pneumonia. *Adults:* 40 mg b.i.d. P.O. for 5 days, tapering to 20 mg/day over 2 weeks.
• Sarcoidosis. *Adults:* 40 to 80 mg P.O. daily.

Adverse reactions
Most adverse reactions of corticosteroids are dose- or duration-dependent.
CNS: *euphoria, insomnia,* psychotic behavior, pseudotumor cerebri
CV: ***CHF,*** hypertension, edema
EENT: cataracts, glaucoma
GI: *peptic ulcer,* GI irritation, increased appetite
Metabolic: hypokalemia, hyperglycemia, growth suppression in children
Skin: delayed wound healing, acne, various skin eruptions
Other: muscle weakness, pancreatitis, hirsutism, susceptibility to infections
Acute adrenal insufficiency may occur with increased stress (infection, surgery, or trauma) or abrupt withdrawal after long-term therapy. *Withdrawal symptoms:* rebound inflammation, fatigue, weakness, arthralgia, fever, dizziness, lethargy, depression, fainting, orthostatic hypotension, dyspnea, anorexia, hypoglycemia. ***Sudden withdrawal may be fatal.***

pseudoephedrine hydrochloride
pseudoephedrine sulfate

General
Brand names: Afrinol Repetabs, Eltor, Sudafed
Pharmacologic classification: adrenergic
Therapeutic classification: decongestant

Indications and dosage
• Nasal and eustachian tube decongestant. *Adults:* 30 to 60 mg P.O. q 4 hours. Maximum dosage is 240 mg daily.
Extended-release form: *Adults and children over age 12:* 120 mg P.O. q 12 hours.

Adverse reactions
CNS: *anxiety,* transient stimulation, tremor, dizziness, headache, insomnia, *nervousness*
CV: arrhythmias, *palpitations,* tachycardia.
EENT: dry mouth
GI: anorexia, nausea, vomiting
GU: difficulty in urinating
Skin: pallor

pyrazinamide

General
Brand name: PMS Pyrazinamide
Pharmacologic classification: synthetic pyrazine analogue of nicotinamide
Therapeutic classification: antitubercular

Indications and dosage
• Adjunctive treatment of tuberculosis (when primary and secondary antitubercular drugs can't be used or have failed). *Adults:* 20 to 35 mg/kg P.O. daily, divided in three to four doses. Maximum dosage is 3 g daily.

Adverse reactions
Blood: sideroblastic anemia, possible bleeding tendency due to thrombocytopenia
GI: anorexia, nausea, vomiting, diarrhea

Common reactions are in *italics;* life-threatening reactions are in ***bold italics.***

GU: dysuria
Hepatic: *hepatitis*
Metabolic: interference with control in diabetes mellitus, *hyperuricemia*
Other: malaise, fever, arthralgia

---

rifabutin

General
Brand name: Mycobutin
Pharmacologic classification: ansamycin derivative
Therapeutic classification: antimycobacterial

Indications and dosage
• Prevention of disseminated infections caused by *Mycobacterium avium intracellulare* in patients with human immunodeficiency virus infection. *Adults:* 300 mg daily in one or two doses.

Adverse reactions
Blood: *leukopenia,* thrombocytopenia, anemia
GI: *nausea,* anorexia, diarrhea, abdominal pain
GU: *discolored urine*
Hepatic: *altered liver function tests*
Skin: *rash*
Other: altered taste, headache

---

rifampin (rifampicin)

General
Brand names: Rifadin, Rimactane, Rofact
Pharmacologic classification: semisynthetic rifamycin B derivative (macrocyclic antibiotic)
Therapeutic classification: antitubercular

Indications and dosage
• Primary treatment in pulmonary tuberculosis. *Adults:* 600 mg P.O. daily as a single dose 1 hour before or 2 hours after meals. May also be given I.V., 600 mg once daily. Rifampin is usually given in combination with other antituberculars to prevent or delay resistance.

Adverse reactions
Blood: eosinophilia, thrombocytopenia, transient leukopenia, hemolytic anemia
CNS: headache, fatigue, *drowsiness,* ataxia, dizziness, mental confusion, generalized numbness
GI: epigastric distress, anorexia, nausea, vomiting, abdominal pain, diarrhea, flatulence, sore mouth and tongue
Hepatic: *serious hepatotoxicity as well as transient abnormalities in liver function tests*
Metabolic: hyperuricemia
Skin: pruritus, urticaria, rash
Other: flulike syndrome, red-orange discoloration of body fluids

---

streptomycin sulfate

General
Pharmacologic classification: aminoglycoside
Therapeutic classification: antibacterial

Indications and dosage
• Primary and adjunctive treatment in tuberculosis. *Adults with normal renal function:* 1 g I.M. daily for 2 to 3 months, then 1 g two or three times weekly. Inject deeply into upper outer quadrant of buttocks.
Adults with impaired renal function: initial dose is same as for those with normal renal function. Subsequent doses and frequency determined by renal function study results.

Adverse reactions
CNS: *neuromuscular blockade*
EENT: *ototoxicity (tinnitus, vertigo, hearing loss)*
Local: *pain, irritation, and sterile abscesses at injection site*
Skin: *exfoliative dermatitis*
Other: *hypersensitivity* (rash, fever, urticaria, and angioneurotic edema), headache, *transient agranulocytosis*

Common reactions are in *italics;* life-threatening reactions are in ***bold italics***.

terbutaline sulfate

General
Brand names: Brethaire, Brethine, Bricanyl
Pharmacologic classification: adrenergic (beta$_2$-adrenergic agonist)
Therapeutic classification: bronchodilator

Indications and dosage
• Relief of bronchospasm in patients with reversible obstructive airway disease. *Adults:* 2 inhalations separated by a 60-second interval, repeated q 4 to 6 hours. May also administer 2.5 to 5 mg P.O. q 8 hours or 0.25 mg S.C.

Adverse reactions
CNS: *nervousness, tremor, headache,* drowsiness, sweating
CV: palpitations, increased heart rate
EENT: drying and irritation of nose and throat (with inhaled form)
GI: vomiting, nausea
Other: hypokalemia (with high doses)

terfenadine

General
Brand name: Seldane
Pharmacologic classification: butyrophenone derivative
Therapeutic classification: antihistamine (H$_1$-receptor antagonist)

Indications and dosage
• Rhinitis, allergy symptoms. *Adults:* 60 mg P.O. b.i.d.

Adverse reactions
CNS: fatigue, dizziness, headache, sedation
CV: *arrhythmias* (with overdose)
GI: abdominal distress, nausea
EENT: dry throat and mouth, nasal stuffiness
Other: alopecia, cholestatic jaundice.
Note: Concomitant use with erythromycin or ketoconazole may cause cardiac arrhythmias.

tetracycline hydrochloride

General
Brand names: Achromycin V, Apo-Tetra, Panmycin, Robitet, Sumycin
Pharmacologic classification: tetracycline
Therapeutic classification: antibacterial

Indications and dosage
• Infections caused by sensitive gram-negative and gram-positive organisms; *Mycoplasma* pneumonia. *Adults:* 250 to 500 mg P.O. q 6 hours.

Adverse reactions
Blood: neutropenia, eosinophilia
CNS: *intracranial hypertension*
CV: pericarditis
EENT: sore throat, glossitis, dysphagia
GI: anorexia, *epigastric distress, nausea,* vomiting, *diarrhea,* enterocolitis, anogenital inflammation
Skin: *maculopapular and erythematous rashes, photosensitivity, increased pigmentation, urticaria*
Other: *hypersensitivity, fungal overgrowth*

theophylline

General
Brand names: Elixophyllin, Slo-Phyllin, Theo-Dur, Theo-24
Pharmacologic classification: xanthine derivative
Therapeutic classification: bronchodilator

Indications and dosage
• Prophylaxis and symptomatic relief of bronchial asthma, bronchospasm of chronic bronchitis and emphysema. *Adults:* 6 mg/kg P.O. followed by 2 to 3 mg/kg q 4 hours for two doses. Maintenance dosage is 1 to 3 mg/kg or 6 to 20 mg/kg/day divided q 6 hours (immediate-release).

Most oral timed-release forms are given q 8 to 12 hours. Several products, however, may be given q 24 hours.

Common reactions are in *italics;* life-threatening reactions are in ***bold italics.***

• Parenteral theophylline for patients not currently receiving theophylline. *Loading dose:* 4.7 mg/kg I.V. slowly; then maintenance infusion. *Adults (nonsmokers):* 0.4 mg/kg/hour. *Otherwise-healthy adult smokers:* 0.8 mg/kg/hour. *Older adults with cor pulmonale:* 0.25 mg/kg/hour. *Adults with CHF or liver disease:* 0.1 to 0.15 mg/kg/hour.

Switch to oral theophylline as soon as patient shows adequate improvement.

• Symptomatic relief of bronchospasm in patients currently receiving theophylline. *Adults:* each 0.5 mg/kg I.V. or P.O. (loading dose) will increase plasma levels by 1 mcg/ml. Ideally, dose is based on current theophylline level. In emergency situations, some clinicians recommend a 2.5 mg/kg I.V. or P.O. dose of rapidly absorbed form if no obvious signs of theophylline toxicity are present.

Note: All doses are adjusted for a decreased serum theophylline level of 8 to 20 mg/ml.

Adverse reactions
CNS: *nervousness, restlessness, dizziness,* headache, *insomnia,* light-headedness, **seizures,** muscle twitching
CV: *palpitations, sinus tachycardia,* extrasystoles, flushing, marked hypotension, increase in respiratory rate
GI: *nausea, vomiting, anorexia,* bitter aftertaste, dyspepsia, heavy feeling in stomach, diarrhea
Skin: urticaria

ticarcillin disodium

General
Brand name: Ticar
Pharmacologic classification: extended-spectrum penicillin, alpha-carboxypenicillin
Therapeutic classification: antibacterial

Indications and dosage
• Severe systemic infections caused by susceptible strains of gram-positive and especially gram-negative organisms (including *Pseudomonas, Proteus*). *Adults:* 12 to 18 g I.V. or I.M. daily, divided into doses given q 4 to 6 hours.

Adverse reactions
Blood: neutropenia, eosinophilia, leukopenia, *thrombocytopenia*
CNS: neuromuscular irritability, **seizures,** headache, dizziness
GI: nausea, diarrhea
Local: pain at injection site, vein irritation, phlebitis
Metabolic: *hypokalemia*
Other: hypersensitivity (edema, fever, chills, rash, pruritus, urticaria, **anaphylaxis**), overgrowth of nonsusceptible organisms

ticarcillin disodium/ clavulanate potassium

General
Brand name: Timentin
Pharmacologic classification: extended-spectrum penicillin, beta-lactamase inhibitor
Therapeutic classification: antibacterial

Indications and dosage
• Infections of the lower respiratory tract caused by beta-lactamase-producing strains of bacteria or by ticarcillin-susceptible organisms, including *Staphylococcus, Bacteroides, Pseudomonas, Proteus,* and *Serratia. Adults:* 1 vial (ticarcillin 3 g and clavulanate potassium 0.1 g) administered by I.V. infusion q 4 to 6 hours.

Adverse reactions
Blood: neutropenia, eosinophilia, leukopenia, *thrombocytopenia*
CNS: neuromuscular irritability, **seizures,** headache, dizziness
GI: nausea, diarrhea
Local: pain at injection site, vein irritation, phlebitis
Metabolic: hypokalemia
Other: hypersensitivity (edema, fever, chills, rash, pruritus, urticaria, **anaphylaxis**), overgrowth of nonsusceptible organisms

---

Common reactions are in *italics;* life-threatening reactions are in **bold italics**.

tobramycin sulfate

General
Brand name: Nebcin
Pharmacologic classification: aminoglycoside
Therapeutic classification: antibacterial

Indications and dosage
• Serious infections caused by sensitive strains of *Escherichia coli, Proteus, Klebsiella, Enterobacter, Serratia, Staphylococcus aureus, Pseudomonas, Citrobacter,* and *Providencia. Adults:* 3 mg/kg I.M. or I.V. daily divided q 8 hours. Up to 5 mg/kg I.M. or I.V. daily divided q 6 to 8 hours for life-threatening infections. Adjust dose based on serum levels of drug.

Adverse reactions
CNS: headache, lethargy, ***neuromuscular blockade***
EENT: *ototoxicity (tinnitus, vertigo, hearing loss)*
GU: *nephrotoxicity (cells or casts in the urine; oliguria; proteinuria; decreased creatinine clearance; increased BUN, nonprotein nitrogen, and serum creatinine levels)*
Other: ***hypersensitivity reactions, hepatic necrosis,*** hypomagnesemia

triamcinolone acetonide

General
Brand name: Azmacort
Pharmacologic classification: glucocorticoid
Therapeutic classification: antiasthmatic, anti-inflammatory

Indications and dosage
• Steroid-dependent asthma. *Adults:* 2 inhalations t.i.d. to q.i.d. Maximum dosage is 16 inhalations daily.

Adverse reactions
EENT: hoarseness, fungal infections of mouth and throat
GI: dry mouth

Common reactions are in *italics;* life-threatening reactions are in ***bold italics***.

Index

i refers to an illustration; t, to a table

i refers to an illustration; t, to a table

i refers to an illustration; t, to a table